DECISION MAKING IN INFERTILITY

CLINICAL DECISION MAKING℠ SERIES

Consulting Editor
Ben Eiseman, M.D.

DECISION MAKING IN INFERTILITY

Alan H. DeCherney, M.D.

The John Slade Ely Professor
Department of Obstetrics and Gynecology
Yale University School of Medicine
New Haven, Connecticut

Mary Lake Polan, M.D., Ph.D.

Associate Professor
Department of Obstetrics and Gynecology
Yale University School of Medicine
New Haven, Connecticut

Ronald D. Lee, M.D.

Assistant Professor
Department of Surgery, Section of Urology
Yale University School of Medicine
New Haven, Connecticut

Stephen P. Boyers, M.D.

Assistant Professor
Department of Obstetrics and Gynecology
Yale University School of Medicine
New Haven, Connecticut

1988

B.C. Decker Inc • Toronto • Philadelphia

Publisher

B.C. Decker Inc
3228 South Service Road
Burlington, Ontario   L7N 3H8

B.C. Decker Inc
320 Walnut Street
Suite 400
Philadelphia, Pennsylvania   19106

Sales and Distribution

United States and Possessions	**The C.V. Mosby Company** 11830 Westline Industrial Drive Saint Louis, Missouri 63146
Canada	**The C.V. Mosby Company, Ltd.** 5240 Finch Avenue East, Unit No. 1 Scarborough, Ontario M1S 4P2
United Kingdom, Europe and the Middle East	**Blackwell Scientific Publications, Ltd.** Osney Mead, Oxford OX2 OEL, England
Australia	**Harcourt Brace Jovanovich** 30–52 Smidmore Street Marrickville, N.S.W. 2204 Australia
Japan	**Igaku-Shoin Ltd.** Tokyo International P.O. Box 5063 1–28–36 Hongo, Bunkyo-ku, Tokyo 113, Japan
Asia	**Info-Med Ltd.** 802–3 Ruttonjee House 11 Duddell Street Central Hong Kong
South Africa	**Libriger Book Distributors** Warehouse Number 8 "Die Ou Looiery" Tannery Road Hamilton, Bloemfontein 9300
South America (non-stock list representative only)	**Inter-Book Marketing Services** Rua das Palmeiras, 32 Apto. 701 222–70 Rio de Janeiro RJ, Brazil

Decision Making in Infertility   ISBN 155664–015–3

Library of Congress catalog card number: 87–71768

10 9 8 7 6 5 4 3 2 1

CONTRIBUTORS

ROMAINE B. BAYLESS, M.D.

Postdoctoral Associate, Department of Obstetrics and Gynecology, Yale University School of Medicine, New Haven, Connecticut

STEPHEN P. BOYERS, M.D.

Assistant Professor, Department of Obstetrics and Gynecology, Yale University School of Medicine, New Haven, Connecticut

ROBERT G. BRZYSKI, M.D.

Chief Resident, Department of Obstetrics and Gynecology, Yale University School of Medicine, New Haven, Connecticut

MICHAEL P. DIAMOND, M.D.

Assistant Professor, Department of Obstetrics and Gynecology, Yale University School of Medicine, New Haven, Connecticut

ROBERT A. GRAEBE, M.D.

Director of Reproductive Endocrinology, Monmouth and Riverview Medical Centers, Monmouth, New Jersey

LAWRENCE GRUNFELD, M.D.

Postdoctoral Associate, Department of Obstetrics and Gynecology, Yale University School of Medicine, New Haven, Connecticut

ERVIN E. JONES, M.D., Ph.D.

Assistant Professor, Department of Obstetrics and Gynecology, Yale University School of Medicine, New Haven, Connecticut

GAD LAVY, M.D.

Assistant Professor, Department of Obstetrics and Gynecology, Yale University School of Medicine, New Haven, Connecticut

RONALD D. LEE, M.D.

Assistant Professor, Department of Surgery, Section of Urology, Yale University School of Medicine, New Haven, Connecticut

AVI LIGHTMAN, M.D., M.Sc.

Postdoctoral Fellow in Reproductive Endocrinology, On Leave from Department of Obstetrics and Gynecology, Rambam Medical Center, Haifa, Israel

MARY LAKE POLAN, M.D., Ph.D.

Associate Professor, Department of Obstetrics and Gynecology, Yale University School of Medicine, New Haven, Connecticut

JEFFREY B. RUSSELL, M.D.

Postdoctoral Associate, Department of Obstetrics and Gynecology, Yale University School of Medicine, New Haven, Connecticut

BRUCE S. SHAPIRO, M.D.

Postdoctoral Associate, Department of Obstetrics and Gynecology, Yale University School of Medicine, New Haven, Connecticut

JAMES M. WHEELER, M.D.

Robert Wood Johnson Clinical Scholar, Yale University School of Medicine, New Haven, Connecticut

Decision trees provide an intriguing and innovative way to learn. In fact, much of the information currently found in formal textbooks on the management of the infertile couple is predicated on this type of thinking. Thus *Decision Making in Infertility* is an attempt to formalize the concept of decision making and to approach it in an encyclopedic fashion. Descriptive detail is by necessity absent. However, an attempt has been made to cover the physiologic, pathologic, and surgical aspects of infertility and its ramifications. Special emphasis has been placed on the reproductive endocrine components of male and female infertility and on the latest information on laparoscopic surgery, in vitro fertilization, and embryo transfer; the offshoots of GIFT and embryo freezing have also been included.

A major effort has been expended to coordinate the overlapping areas. Our major goal was to define and conceptualize patterns for patient referral.

The text represents the "Yale Way" to approach the problems of infertility.

Alan H. DeCherney, M.D.
Mary Lake Polan, M.D., Ph.D.
Ronald D. Lee, M.D.
Stephen P. Boyers, M.D.

CONTENTS

ENDOMETRIOSIS

ENDOSCOPY AND LASERS IN REPRODUCTIVE SURGERY

INTRODUCTION

Decision making is crucial to the diagnostic and therapeutic work-up of the infertile couple. Although there are specific therapies for specific disease entities, most infertile couples require extensive diagnostic and therapeutic measures to solve their problem.

Some topics are presented in a single tree; several are presented in a series of trees arranged sequentially. However, the focus of every chapter is the decision tree. The text amplifies the information presented in the tree, but is usually not essential for following the decision-making process. The references have been selected to support and to elucidate each chapter.

EPIDEMIOLOGY OF INFERTILITY

James M. Wheeler, M.D.
Mary Lake Polan, M.D., Ph.D.

A. Most clinicians diagnose infertility when conception does not occur after a couple actively attempts pregnancy for 1 year; 80 to 90 percent of couples who achieve pregnancy do so within 1 year. In younger patients, or in those in whom regular sexual exposure is doubted, some clinicians delay the active investigation and treatment of infertility for up to 2 years. The couple's contraceptive history must be taken into account in the definition of infertility; after discontinuation of oral contraceptives, certain medications (e.g., Thorazine, danazol), or intrauterine devices, the first 2 to 3 months may be less than optimal for achieving pregnancy owing to temporary ovulatory dysfunction or an unfavorable endometrium. Infertility is becoming more prevalent; current textbooks estimate the overall incidence of infertility as 10 to 15 percent of married couples. Many of these couples can be helped; current techniques offer an overall pregnancy incidence of 50 percent in infertile couples. Reports of success must be compared to age-specific cohorts; no longer will tubal anastomoses be 80 percent successful, because even "fertile" people in their late 30s and 40s will conceive only 50 to 60 percent of the time. This realization will prompt technological advancement and stimulate research into methods to "preserve" gametes (in vivo and in vitro) until pregnancy is desired. Technological advancement of in vitro fertilization has initiated discussion as to the limits of who can conceive at what cost. Ethical considerations are being raised daily in infertility practices.

B. For over a century, observant clinicians have noted spontaneous "cures" for sterility, recognizing such "successes" as being a coincidence rather than a consequence of treatment. In a study published in 1969, 35 percent of 1,145 infertile patients conceived without treatment: 7 percent after interview and sperm count, 4 percent after vaginal examination and removal of tenacious cervical mucus, and another 17 percent after performance of a tubal patency test. A more recent article compared 597 couples treated for infertility with 548 untreated couples; pregnancy incidences did not significantly vary between the groups—41 percent vs. 35 percent respectively. Furthermore, many of the pregnancies in the "treated" group were sufficiently remote from therapy that the question of treatment-independent success was raised. The authors conclude the need for untreated control groups in fertility studies, because 23 percent of the 1,145 couples conceived without therapy.

C. The most common clinical classification of infertility is that distinguishing between primary and secondary infertility. "Primary infertility" means that the couple has never achieved pregnancy.

D. "Secondary infertility" implies a previous conception within the couple. Less clear in this distinction is the situation where one (or both) members of a couple seeking evaluation for infertility have had pregnancies with another partner. It is much preferred to detail the reproductive experience of each member of the couple. Similarly, use of the word "sterility" should be relegated to patients with permanent conditions irreversible by today's treatment options (e.g., congenital absence of the uterus or ovaries).

E. Pregnancy wastage is defined as the inability to carry a conceptus to live birth and includes both spontaneous abortion and stillbirth in the strict sense. However, infertility specialists typically refer to pregnancy wastage as first- and second-trimester spontaneous abortions. Demographic usage of "infertility" includes both infecundity and pregnancy wastage. Spontaneous abortion is the form of pregnancy wastage of greatest concern to the clinician treating infertility. Approximately 15 percent of clinically recognized pregnancies end in spontaneous abortion; according to sensitive assays of human chorionic gonadotropin (hCG), as many as 40 to 60 percent of fertilized ova fail to survive. The traditional definition of habitual abortion mandates 3 or more confirmed pregnancy losses prior to evaluation. In current practice, most specialists will evaluate a couple with two or more first or second trimester losses (see p 72).

References

Collins JA, Wrixon W, Janes LB, Wilson EH. Treatment-independent pregnancy among infertile couples. N Engl J Med 1983; 309:1201–1206.

Mosher WD. Infertility trends among U.S. couples: 1965–1976. Fam Plan Perspect 1982; 14:22–27.

United States Bureau of the Census: Fertility of American women: June, 1980. Curr Popul Rep (P-20) No. 375, 1982.

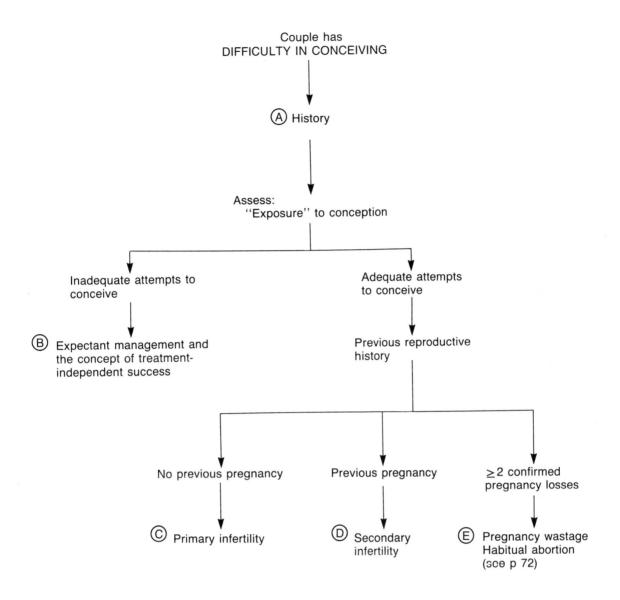

Couple has
DIFFICULTY IN CONCEIVING

Ⓐ History

Assess:
"Exposure" to conception

Inadequate attempts to
conceive

Adequate attempts
to conceive

Ⓑ Expectant management and
the concept of treatment-
independent success

Previous reproductive
history

No previous pregnancy

Previous pregnancy

≥2 confirmed
pregnancy losses

Ⓒ Primary infertility

Ⓓ Secondary
infertility

Ⓔ Pregnancy wastage
Habitual abortion
(see p 72)

EPIDEMIOLOGIC FACTORS: HISTORICAL CLUES

James M. Wheeler, M.D.
Mary Lake Polan, M.D., Ph.D.

A. The initial evaluation should include investigation of the couple as a unit. In particular, a careful sexual history should be elicited. Frequency of intercourse appears related to the age of both partners as well as the duration of the relationship. In fertile couples, a weekly frequency of four times produced the highest conception incidences; in infertile couples, instructions are usually given for intercourse to occur every other day during the week surrounding ovulation.

A general history and physical examination of both the male and female are included in the initial consultation regarding infertility; family history of genitourinary anomalies, endometriosis, leiomyoma uteri, and varicocele should be sought. Following couple interview, investigation of the woman and man proceeds.

B. Women stopping oral contraceptives have a longer interval to delivery than women using other methods; this difference disappears 30 to 42 months after discontinuing the pill. Although some intrauterine devices (IUDs) are associated with pelvic inflammatory disease, there is no direct effect on delaying fecundity. There is no evidence that spermicides or barrier methods adversely affect fertility.

C. Severe disturbances in nutrition (e.g., famine, anorexia nervosa), weight loss (e.g., medical or psychiatric disease), and strenuous activity (e.g., marathon runners, ballet dancers) are associated with ovulatory disturbances. Obesity may also be associated with anovulatory cycles because of tonic increase in estrogen levels.

D. Severe stress causes anovulation and amenorrhea. Emotional tension may be associated with sexual dysfunction, including vaginismus and dyspareunia. Substance abuse should be investigated, although the association of recreational drugs and infertility is speculative. There is no clear association between excessive coffee drinking or cigarette smoking and infertility.

E. Exposure to lead in the pottery or smelting industries, carbon disulfide in textiles, and benzene as a solvent in many industrial processes are examples known to increase the risk of infertility and pregnancy wastage.

F. Infertility may affect all ethnic groups and socioeconomic classes. Patterns of etiology may vary because of class differences in nutritional status, exercise, genetic factors, and exposure to sexually transmitted diseases. In population studies, the probability of conception decreases with age. The expected percentages of nonsterile women who will conceive in 12 months of unprotected intercourse drops from 86 percent in the 20- to 24-year-old group to 52 percent in the 35- to 39-year-old group. Women over 35 years of age have a two-fold increase in spontaneous abortion compared to those 20 years of age or younger.

G. In the male, gonorrhea can cause a blocked vas deferens; *Chlamydia* can cause urethritis and *Mycoplasma* may impair spermatogenesis. Mumps complicated by orchitis is the most common viral etiology, although fertility impairment from mumps orchitis is unusual. Hernia operations may compromise testicular blood supply. Scrotopexy of cryptorchid testes is associated with variable semen quality. Congenital anomalies and repair of the urinary tract or sacrum may affect ejaculation. Previously diagnosed varicocele is not an uncommon history.

H. Any severe febrile illness may depress semen quality. Diabetics may have retrograde ejaculation. Cancer chemotherapy often permanently destroys the male's germinal epithelium.

I. Impotence is often related to stress. There are case reports of azoospermia caused by severe anxiety, which is reversible upon alleviation of the stress. Marked abuse of alcohol and marijuana may induce a state of hypogonadism with abnormal spermatogenesis. Moderate quantities of alcohol and cigarettes seem to have no significant effect on semen quality. Certain medications such as cancer chemotherapeutic drugs, sulfasalazine, and tranquilizers may contribute to poor sperm quality. Males exposed to diethylstilbestrol in utero have an increased incidence of genital tract abnormalities, including epididymal cysts, maldescended and hypoplastic testes, and varicocele.

J. Exposure to excessive heat or chemicals, especially benzene and petroleum products, may depress semen quality. Military personnel may have toxic exposures during active duty.

K. Conception is more likely when the husband is less than 25 years of age compared with the husband 25 years or older, with a marked reduction in success when over 35 years of age. However, conceptions are known to occur at advanced age when men have minimal erectile function and semen quality.

References

Hendershot GE, Mosher WD, Pratt WF. Infertility and age: an unresolved issue. Fam Plan Perspect 1982; 14:287–289.

Schwartz D, Mayaux MJ. Female fecundity as a function of age: results of artificial insemination in 2193 nulliparous women with azoospermic husbands. N Engl J Med 1982; 306:404–406.

Virro MR, Shewchuk AB. Pregnancy outcome in 242 conceptions after artificial insemination with donor sperm and effects of maternal age on the prognosis for successful pregnancy. Am J Obstet Gynecol 1984; 148:518–524.

EPIDEMIOLOGIC FACTORS: HISTORICAL CLUES

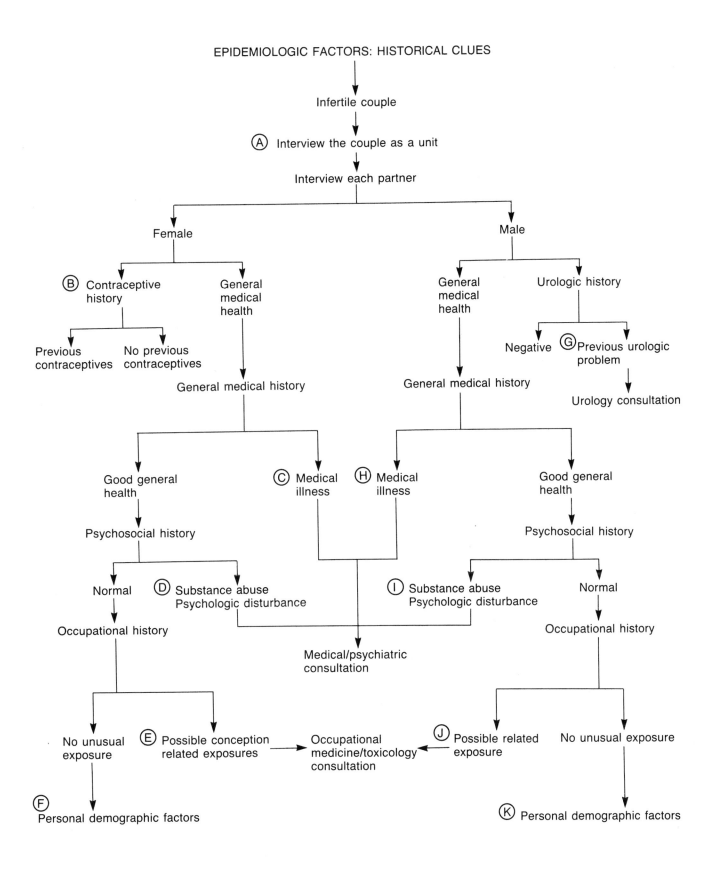

ETIOLOGY OF INFERTILITY: FEMALE FACTORS

James M. Wheeler, M.D.
Mary Lake Polan, M.D., Ph.D.

A. Infertility is diagnosed and treated within the context of a couple unit; the proportion of couples with female factors equals the proportion of couples with male factors, and many couples have multiple reasons for their infertility. Female factors are implicated in about 50 percent of couples conceiving; often, male factors are involved in addition to a suspected female factor.

B. Ovulation can be proven only by direct observation of oocyte release from the ovaries. Clinically, biphasic basal body temperature charts, midluteal progesterone greater than 12 ng per milliliter, and secretory endometrium on biopsy suggest normal ovulatory cycles. Late luteal biopsy may also detect qualitative ovulatory dysfunction in the form of luteal phase defects.

C. As usually cycling women may have an occasional anovulatory cycle, any diagnostic test suggesting anovulation should be repeated or confirmed with another type of test. About 15 percent of all infertile couples are diagnosed with anovulation. The hypothalamus may mediate anovulation in anorexia nervosa, states of extreme physical exertion (e.g., ballerinas, marathon runners), or stress. Disruption of the normal hypothalamic pituitary tracts by tumors or vascular events can perturb gonadotropin release; hyperprolactinemia also produces anovulation via the hypothalamic-pituitary axis. Excess androgen production can arise from adrenal (tumor or hyperplasia) or ovarian (polycystic ovarian syndrome) sources; high tonic levels of circulating estrogen may be associated with obesity, estrogen secreting tumors, or exogenous estrogens. Diseases such as diabetes, Cushing's disease and syndrome, Addison's disease, and hyper- and hypothyroidism may be associated with anovulation. Lately, much controversy centers upon women who develop follicles but fail to release ova despite luteinization (luteinized unruptured follicle syndrome [LUF]). An inadequate luteal phase may be associated with LUF.

D. In 5 percent of couples, the lower female genital tract hinders conception. Developmental abnormalities may inhibit conception in obvious ways as seen in transverse vaginal septa, or more subtle ways as in diethylstilbestrol-associated anatomic changes. Abnormalities of the cervix produced by surgery (conization, cautery) or infection (Chlamydia) decrease sperm penetration. Cervical mucus may possess antibodies that limit sperm motility and ascent into the uterus and tubes.

E. Hysterosalpingography (HSG) may produce the first suggestion of uterotubal disease.

F. Intrauterine adhesions are being diagnosed more frequently owing to the increased use of diagnostic hysteroscopy. However, the contribution to infertility of the various degrees and locations of intrauterine adhesions remains to be well defined. Hysteroscopy or HSG may also detect uterine developmental malformations and submucosal leiomyomas that distort the uterine cavity. Endometrial biopsy, in addition to its use in evaluating the luteal phase, may suggest chronic endometritis caused by infection (e.g., tuberculosis).

G. Intrinsic tubal mucosal damage and external tubal distortion may be suggested by an abnormal HSG that requires confirming ovulation and treatment. See chapters on evaluation of tubal disease (pp 86, 88) and chapters on treatment of tubal obstruction (pp 94, 96, 98).

H. Laparoscopy reveals tuboperitoneal disease in 20 percent of women with normal HSG; conversely, 5 percent of women with abnormal HSG have no disease identified at laparoscopy. Some form of tuboperitoneal factor is implicated in one-fourth of infertile couples. Previous salpingitis is perhaps the most common of these factors; the endosalpingitis typical of pelvic inflammatory disease is usually more devastating to tubal function than the exosalpingitis typical of postabortal salpingitis or periappendicitis. Endometriosis is diagnosed more frequently today because laparoscopy is usually included in the evaluation of the infertile couple; furthermore, as various forms of early endometriosis are identified, sometimes with the aid of light or electron microscopy, the prevalence of this diagnosis will probably increase.

I. After thorough investigation, 10 percent of couples will lack a distinct diagnosis of their cause(s) of infertility. A complete review of the couple's evaluation is warranted to assure no oversights; a repeat history may reveal sexual dysfunction, nonproductive timing of intercourse, or the use of spermicidal agents as lubricants. Borderline test results may need to be repeated. Assuming satisfaction with the couple's evaluation, a period of expectant management will result in pregnancy in some couples. Artificial insemination techniques may then be elected (see pp 148, 152). In vitro fertilization and gamete intrafallopian transfer are the final options for the couple with unexplained infertility (see p 194).

References

Kovacs GT, Newman GB, Henson GL. The postcoital test: what is normal? Br Med J 1978; 1:818.

Pauerstein CJ, Eddy CA. The role of the oviduct in reproduction: our knowledge and our ignorance. J Reprod Fertil 1979; 55:223–229.

Schwabe MG, Shapiro SS, Haning RV Jr. Hysterosalpingography with oil contrast medium enhances fertility in patients with infertility of unknown etiology. Fertil Steril 1983; 40:604–606.

ETIOLOGY OF INFERTILITY: FEMALE FACTORS

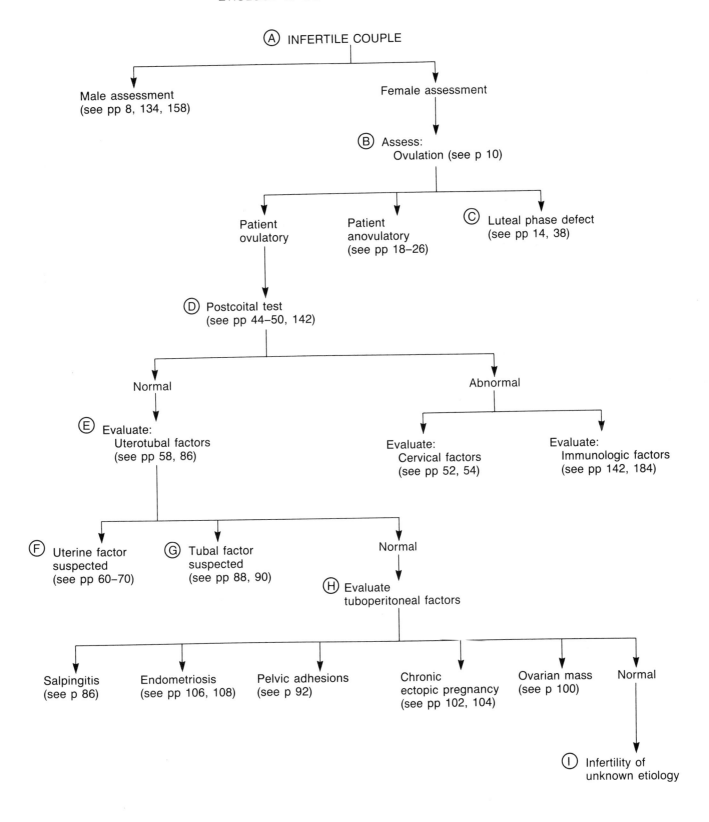

Ⓐ INFERTILE COUPLE

Male assessment
(see pp 8, 134, 158)

Female assessment

Ⓑ Assess:
Ovulation (see p 10)

Patient
ovulatory

Patient
anovulatory
(see pp 18–26)

Ⓒ Luteal phase defect
(see pp 14, 38)

Ⓓ Postcoital test
(see pp 44–50, 142)

Normal

Abnormal

Ⓔ Evaluate:
Uterotubal factors
(see pp 58, 86)

Evaluate:
Cervical factors
(see pp 52, 54)

Evaluate:
Immunologic factors
(see pp 142, 184)

Ⓕ Uterine factor
suspected
(see pp 60–70)

Ⓖ Tubal factor
suspected
(see pp 88, 90)

Normal

Ⓗ Evaluate
tuboperitoneal factors

Salpingitis
(see p 86)

Endometriosis
(see pp 106, 108)

Pelvic adhesions
(see p 92)

Chronic
ectopic pregnancy
(see pp 102, 104)

Ovarian mass
(see p 100)

Normal

Ⓘ Infertility of
unknown etiology

7

ETIOLOGY OF INFERTILITY: MALE FACTORS

James M. Wheeler, M.D.
Mary Lake Polan, M.D., Ph.D.

A. Male factors are suspected of contributing to infertility in almost half of infertile couples. Although the gynecologic infertility therapist must have a working knowledge of the differential diagnosis of male factor, the evaluation and treatment of the male partner are best accomplished in consultation with a urologist experienced in male infertility.

B. Semen analysis (SA) involves evaluation of semen volume and viscosity, sperm density, motility and morphology (see p 136). More advanced methods include migration testing (see p 138), penetration testing (see pp 50, 144), and immunologic testing (see pp 142, 184). Semen quality is variable over time in an individual, and there are rare absolute characteristics (e.g., azoospermia) preventing fertilization. SA should be repeated over time, certainly at decision-making points in the investigation of both male and female partners. Just as ovulation is periodically assessed in the infertile woman with a regular cycle, so should spermatogenesis be followed in an infertile man with one normal SA.

C. Klinefelter's syndrome (47,XXY) is the most frequent abnormality of sex chromatin in infertile males; not all patients with a 47,XXY karyotype have typical clinical findings of Klinefelter's syndrome. Other genetic abnormalities associated with male infertility are XXXY, XXXXY, XXYY, XX/XXY and XY/XXY patterns. Autosomal translocations may also be associated with subfertility.

D. Varicoceles, although found in many fertile men, are associated with abnormal semen analyses that may improve after spermatic vein ligation. Less frequently, spermatozoa are obstructed by congenital defects including partial/total absence of the vas deferens, and epispadias or hypospadias. Spermatocele caused by previous surgery can obstruct the vas. Retrograde ejaculation due to innervation problems (e.g., diabetes mellitus, spinal cord trauma) can be successfully treated in many men with medical therapy and special collection techniques.

E. Orchitis may result from mumps, tuberculosis, syphilis, or pancreatitis. Epididymitis may be caused by gonorrhea, *Chlamydia trachomatis*, or tuberculosis. Prostatitis is usually bacterial in origin and notoriously difficult to treat. The seminal vesicles may be infected with *Trichomonas vaginalis* or tuberculosis. Urethritis is usually caused by *Chlamydia*, gonorrhea, or *Ureaplasma* organisms. Temperature elevation from any cause can produce a transient suppression of spermatogenesis. Autoimmune damage to the testicles may occur, as that seen associated with leprosy. The lack of intrascrotal abnormalities does not rule out the possibility of infections or immunologic abnormality. Seminal plasma and blood may contain antibodies that immobilize spermatozoa in typically anatomically normal men. Other occult causes of male factor include toxic exposure. Many drugs, most notably several classes of antihypertensive and neuroleptics, may impair sexual function. Environmental toxins such as heavy metals or dyes may contribute to infertility. Drug abuse, including ethanol, may suppress spermatogenesis. Radiation may cause testicular fibrosis.

F. Hypogonadotropic states in the male may have a pituitary etiology, such as Cushing's disease, acromegaly, pituitary tumor or failure, or isolated gonadotropin deficiency. A hypothalamic process (e.g., tumor, stalk trauma) may produce a hypogonadotropic hypogonadal state. Hypo- or hyperthyroidism may contribute to hypothalamus-pituitary-mediated male infertility. Hypergonadotropic states are due to testicular insufficiency of an idiopathic nature or secondary to trauma or inflammation. Androgen synthesis or receptor abnormalities may be implicated more frequently in the future.

G. Certain histologic diagnoses such as hypospermatogenesis, maturational arrest, and Sertoli-cell-only syndrome have unknown etiologies. A careful history of trauma (torsion), groin surgery, toxin exposure, and infection is imperative in the male partner of the infertile couple.

References

Curie-Cohen M, Luttrell L, Shapiro S. Current practice of artificial insemination by donor in the United States. N Engl J Med 1979; 300:585–590.

Collins JA, Wrixon W, Janes LB, Wilson EH. Treatment-independent pregnancy among infertile couples. N Engl J Med 1983; 309:1201–1206.

Mosher WD. Infertility trends among U.S. couples: 1965–1976. Fam Plan Perspect 1982; 14:22–27.

United States Bureau of the Census. Fertility of American women: June 1980. Curr Popul Rep (P–20) No. 375, 1982.

White RM, Glass RH. Intrauterine insemination with husband's sperm. Obstet Gynecol 1976; 47:119–121.

ETIOLOGY OF INFERTILITY: MALE FACTORS

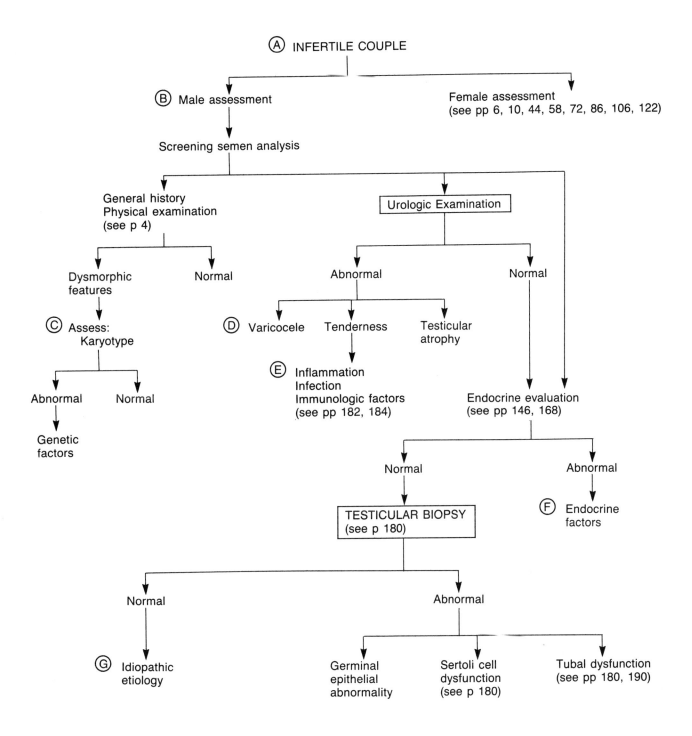

OVULATORY FUNCTION EVALUATION

Stephen P. Boyers, M.D.
Ervin E. Jones, M.D., Ph.D.

A. Ovulatory dysfunction accounts for 10 to 25 percent of the instances of female infertility. Fortunately most cases of anovulatory infertility can be treated successfully. The history and physical examination are the most important tools for evaluating ovulatory status. Since infertility and menstrual dysfunction are often indicative of potentially serious underlying diseases, these should be excluded or treated before focusing on infertility and ovulation induction per se. Testing is tailored according to the menstrual history and whether hirsutism, galactorrhea, or other evidence of underlying disease exists.

B. Hirsutism is usually a reflection of hyperandrogenism. Mild to moderate hirsutism is usually associated with functional hyperandrogenism, most often polycystic ovarian disease or adult onset adrenal hyperplasia. Severe hirsutism, especially with virilization, may be caused by androgen-producing ovarian or adrenal tumors. Serum testosterone and dehydroepiandrosterone sulfate (DHEA-S) levels are helpful in distinguishing functional from tumor-related hyperandrogenism. The work-up for hirsutism should be completed before focusing on infertility and the ovulatory status.

C. Galactorrhea frequently reflects hyperprolactinemia, which may be caused by a variety of drugs as well as by hypothyroidism and pituitary adenomas. Hyperprolactinemia interferes with ovulatory function and may cause a spectrum of disorders, from the inadequate luteal phase through oligo-ovulation to complete anovulation and amenorrhea. Galactorrhea should be thoroughly evaluated, including thyroid stimulating hormone (TSH) and prolactin levels, before focusing on infertility, especially since restoration of normal prolactin levels may also restore regular ovulatory cycles and fertility.

D. In patients without hirsutism, galactorrhea, or other evidence of serious underlying disease, evaluation of the ovulatory status is directed by the menstrual history. Eumenorrhea is defined as regular menstrual cycles every 21 to 36 days. Oligomenorrhea is defined as menstrual cycles more infrequent than every 36 days, and amenorrhea as absence of menses for more than 6 months in a previously eumenorrheic woman.

E. Eumenorrhea, implying menstrual cycle regularity, is not necessarily indicative of ovulation. Anovulatory bleeding can occur with relative regularity. Regular menstrual bleeding in cycles accompanied by dysmenorrhea, mid-cycle cervical mucorrhea or mittelschmerz, and premenstrual molimina is almost invariably ovulatory. The basal body temperature (BBT) pattern is helpful in confirming ovulation, and the duration of the luteal phase temperature rise provides a clue to luteal phase adequacy.

F. A patient with eumenorrhea and a normal biphasic BBT pattern may still have an inadequate luteal phase. Documentation of luteal phase adequacy requires a late luteal endometrial biopsy with histologic evidence of an in-phase secretory endometrium. A midluteal serum progesterone determination may also be helpful in assessing luteal phase adequacy.

G. Amenorrhea frequently reflects a serious underlying disease, and a thorough evaluation is necessary before embarking on a program of nonspecific ovulation induction. All patients of reproductive age with amenorrhea should be considered pregnant until proven otherwise. A negative serum β-hCG level reliably excludes pregnancy. Hyperprolactinemia is commonly found in amenorrheic patients, even in the absence of galactorrhea. When TSH and prolactin levels are normal, the diagnosis hinges on the response to a progestin challenge and an assessment of follicle stimulating hormone (FSH) and luteinizing hormone (LH) concentrations.

H. Oligomenorrhea implies, at best, infrequent ovulation and, at worst, anovulation. Because both are indications for ovulation induction, it is not necessary to distinguish between ovulatory and anovulatory bleeding in these infertile patients. It is important, however, to exclude thyroid dysfunction and hyperprolactinemia, since both are easily discovered and require specific therapies that may correct ovulatory function, making clomiphene or other ovulation inducing drugs unnecessary.

I. Hypergonadotropic hypogonadism implies ovarian failure, which may be primary or secondary. Gonadal dysgenesis is responsible for most cases of primary gonadal failure. Surgery or exposure to antineoplastic drugs or radiation may cause secondary premature ovarian failure. Autoimmune oophoritis has been implicated in other cases, and many cases have no discernible etiology. Ovulation induction is usually not successful, but hormonal substitution and the use of donor oocytes and in vitro fertilization may offer these patients a chance to carry a pregnancy.

J. Hypoestrogenism with low or normal levels of FSH and LH confirms the diagnosis of hypogonadotropic hypogonadism. Both hypothalamic and pituitary disorders are responsible for this common form of amenorrhea. In many series, weight loss and anorexia nervosa are the most common causes. Exercise induced amenorrhea also falls into this category. Central nervous system tumors are potentially life threatening, and a thorough neurologic assessment and imaging study are essential before beginning ovulation induction in these patients. When gonadotropin levels are normal and bleeding fails to occur after an estrogen and progestin challenge, end organ failure should be suspected and the endometrial cavity evaluated by hysterosalpingography, biopsy, and hysteroscopy.

References

Cox LW. Infertility: a comprehensive programme. Br J Obstet Gy-

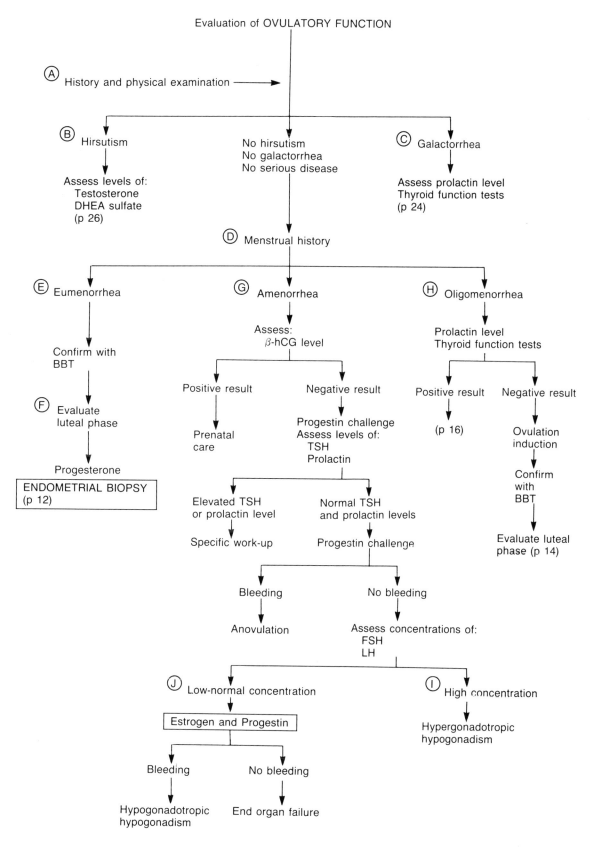

Evaluation of OVULATORY FUNCTION

Ⓐ History and physical examination →

Ⓑ Hirsutism

Assess levels of:
Testosterone
DHEA sulfate
(p 26)

No hirsutism
No galactorrhea
No serious disease

Ⓒ Galactorrhea

Assess prolactin level
Thyroid function tests
(p 24)

Ⓓ Menstrual history

Ⓔ Eumenorrhea

Confirm with
BBT

Ⓕ Evaluate
luteal phase

Progesterone

ENDOMETRIAL BIOPSY
(p 12)

Ⓖ Amenorrhea

Assess:
β-hCG level

Positive result

Prenatal
care

Negative result

Progestin challenge
Assess levels of:
TSH
Prolactin

Elevated TSH
or prolactin level

Specific work-up

Normal TSH
and prolactin levels

Progestin challenge

Bleeding

Anovulation

No bleeding

Assess concentrations of:
FSH
LH

Ⓙ Low-normal concentration

Estrogen and Progestin

Bleeding

Hypogonadotropic
hypogonadism

No bleeding

End organ failure

Ⓘ High concentration

Hypergonadotropic
hypogonadism

Ⓗ Oligomenorrhea

Prolactin level
Thyroid function tests

Positive result

(p 16)

Negative result

Ovulation
induction

Confirm
with
BBT

Evaluate luteal
phase (p 14)

necol 1975; 82:2–6.

Jacobs HS, Hull MGR, Murray MAF, Franks S. Therapy-oriented diagnosis of secondary amenorrhea. Horm Res 1975; 6:268–287.

Jewelewicz R. Management of infertility resulting from anovulation. Am J Obstet Gynecol 1975; 122:909–920.

Thorneycroft IH, Boyers SP. The human menstrual cycle: correlation of hormonal patterns and clinical signs and symptoms. Obstet Gynecol Annu 1983; 12:199–225.

Vollman RF. The menstrual cycle. Philadelphia: WB Saunders, 1977.

OVARIAN EVALUATION: EUMENORRHEA

Ervin E. Jones, M.D., Ph.D.
Stephen P. Boyers, M.D.

A. The history and physical examination are the most important tools for evaluating ovulatory status. Infertility and menstrual dysfunction often indicate potentially serious underlying diseases. These should be excluded, and hirsutism and galactorrhea should be thoroughly evaluated before focusing on infertility and the ovulatory status per se.

B. In patients without hirsutism, galactorrhea, or other evidence of serious underlying disease, the evaluation of ovulatory status is directed by the menstrual history. Eumenorrhea, defined as regular menstrual bleeding every 21 to 36 days, is not definitive evidence of ovulation, since anovulatory bleeding can occur with relative regularity. Ovulation should be confirmed by the menstrual history, basal body temperature (BBT) pattern, and serum progesterone concentration if necessary.

C. A thorough menstrual history is valuable in determining the ovulatory status. Each phase of the menstrual cycle has characteristic differences revealed when ovulatory cycles are compared to anovulatory cycles. The menstrual or early follicular phase in ovulatory cycles is characteristically accompanied by dysmenorrhea and often systemic prostaglandin-related symptoms. At midcycle, ovulating patients may experience mittelschmerz and cervical mucorrhea. Finally, the presence of regular premenstrual moliminal symptoms, such as breast tenderness, abdominal bloating, and mood changes, is good evidence of ovulation in eumenorrheic cycles.

D. Historical evidence of ovulation should be supported by recording the BBT (Fig. 1). A biphasic BBT pattern reflects ovulation, with the caveat that actual release of the ovum from the follicle cannot be confirmed by any measure of corpus luteum function as luteinization without ovulation is possible. It has been reported that a monophasic BBT pattern may exist despite a progesterone rise, but our experience and that of Vollman suggest an extremely low incidence of monophasic BBT patterns in ovulatory women.

E. It should almost never be necessary to measure the serum progesterone level merely to distinguish between ovulation and anovulation. That information is better obtained from the menstrual history and BBT pattern. In patients who are poor historians and simply cannot chart BBTs reliably, however, a single luteal phase serum progesterone level of 3.0 ng or higher per milliliter confirms ovulation. We rarely measure the serum progesterone level to distinguish ovulation from anovulation, but rather reserve that test for assessment of luteal phase adequacy.

F. In eumenorrheic patients the documentation of ovulation should be followed by an assessment of luteal phase adequacy. Although short cycles with an attenuated BBT rise make one suspect luteal dysfunction, a normal cycle length and a normal BBT rise are not adequate to insure an adequate luteal phase. That should be done by a late luteal endometrial biopsy (days 25 to 26 of a 28-day cycle), dated histologically. Endometrial biopsy is essential. A midluteal serum progesterone measurement may provide additional data.

References

Israel R, Mishell DR, Stone SC, Thorneycroft IH, Moyer DL. Single luteal phase serum progesterone assay as an indicator of ovulation. Am J Obstet Gynecol 1972; 112:1043–1046.

Lundstrom V, Green K. Endogenous levels of prostaglandin $F_{2\alpha}$ and its main metabolites in plasma and endometrium of normal and dysmenorrheic women. Am J Obstet Gynecol 1978; 130:640–646.

Magyar DM, Boyers SP, Marshall JR. Regular menstrual cycles and premenstrual molimina as indicators of ovulation. Obstet Gynecol 1979; 53:441.

Thorneycroft IH, Boyers SP. The human menstrual cycle: correlation of hormonal patterns and clinical signs and symptoms. Obstet Gynecol Annu 1983; 12:199–225.

Vollman RF. The menstrual cycle. Philadelphia: WB Saunders, 1977.

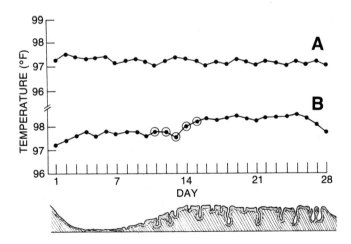

Figure 1 *A,* No ovulation: irregular BBT pattern. *B,* Normal ovulation: temperature rise on day 12.

OVARIAN EVALUATION: EUMENORRHEA

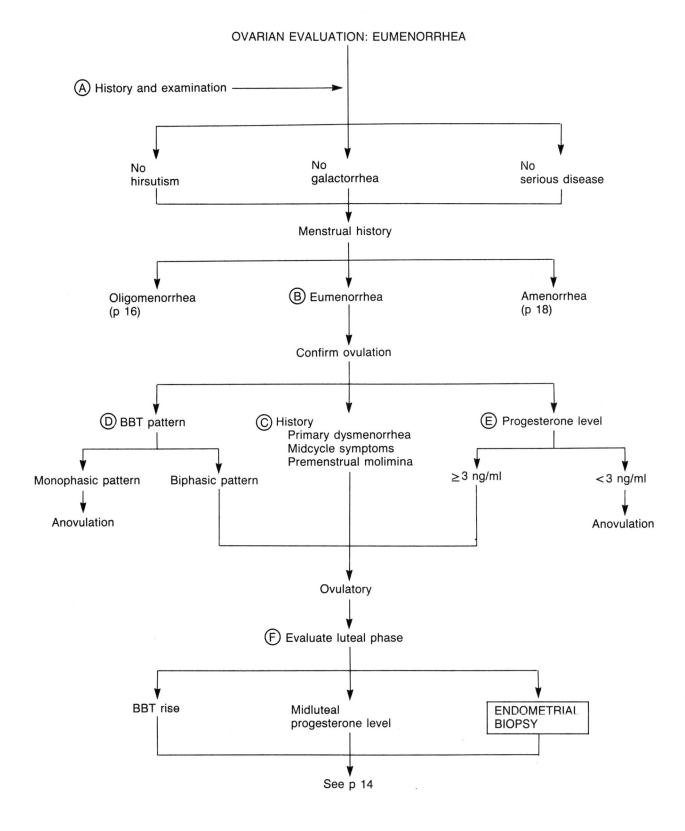

Ⓐ History and examination

No hirsutism | No galactorrhea | No serious disease

Menstrual history

Oligomenorrhea (p 16) | Ⓑ Eumenorrhea | Amenorrhea (p 18)

Confirm ovulation

Ⓓ BBT pattern | Ⓒ History Primary dysmenorrhea Midcycle symptoms Premenstrual molimina | Ⓔ Progesterone level

Monophasic pattern | Biphasic pattern | ≥3 ng/ml | <3 ng/ml

Anovulation | | | Anovulation

Ovulatory

Ⓕ Evaluate luteal phase

BBT rise | Midluteal progesterone level | ENDOMETRIAL BIOPSY

See p 14

OVARIAN EVALUATION: THE LUTEAL PHASE

Ervin E. Jones, M.D., Ph.D.
Stephen P. Boyers, M.D.

A. Both spontaneous and induced menstrual cycles may include an inadequate luteal phase. The incidence varies from 3 to 5 percent in spontaneous cycles to as high as 30 percent in habitual aborters or patients undergoing ovulation induction. Prior to initiating an evaluation of luteal phase adequacy, ovulation should be confirmed by the menstrual history and basal body temperature (BBT) pattern.

B. With few exceptions, the luteal phase should be evaluated by late luteal endometrial biopsy in all infertile ovulating patients. A thermal BBT rise maintained for less than 11 days or a midluteal serum progesterone level lower than 12.0 ng per milliliter is suggestive of a luteal phase defect, but luteal phase inadequacy can occur despite normal BBT and progesterone parameters (Fig. 1), and a late luteal endometrial biopsy with histologic dating is essential to distinguish between cycles with a normal or inadequate luteal phase. On the other hand, endometrial biopsy may produce considerable patient discomfort, and the combined costs of the biopsy, histologic processing, and pathologic interpretation are substantial. Occasionally the thermal shift and progesterone level are so abnormal that the diagnosis is obvious and the biopsy can be deferred until therapy has been initiated.

C. The late luteal endometrial biopsy is the definitive test of luteal phase adequacy. It should be done late in the cycle, 2 to 3 days before the anticipated onset of menstruation. It cannot be done at the onset of bleeding because menstrual endometrium presents a disrupted histologic pattern that defies reliable dating. Paracervical block may be used but is usually not necessary. After determining the uterine position by bimanual examination, the uterus is sounded and a strip of endometrial tissue is taken from the anterolateral fundal area using a Novak or Randall curette. Endometrium from the lower uterine segment is frequently insufficient for diagnosis. Bleeding is usually minimal. The risk of aborting when the endometrium is subjected to biopsy in a conception cycle appears to be no greater than the risk in nonbiopsied pregnant cycles.

D. Identification of an inadequate luteal phase requires that the endometrium be more than 2 days out of phase in two separate menstrual cycles. Endometrial dating is done according to the criteria of Noyes, Hertig, and Rock. The stage of endometrial maturation, as determined by histologic dating, is compared to the normalized cycle day on which the biopsy specimen was obtained. The onset of menstruation following the biopsy becomes, by convention, cycle day 28, and the cycle day of the biopsy is determined by counting back from day 28. Treatment of the inadequate luteal phase is outlined in a separate algorithm (p 38).

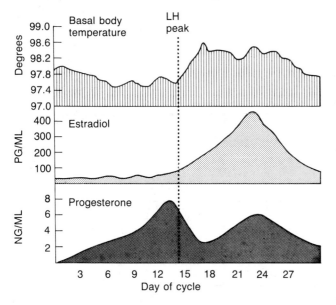

Figure 1 Basal body temperature, serum estradiol, and progesterone levels during the menstrual cycle.

References

Jones GE, Aksel S, Wentz AC. Serum progesterone values in the luteal phase defect: effects of chorionic gonadotropin. Obstet Gynecol 1974; 44:26–34.

Moghissi KS, Syner FN, Evans TN. A composite picture of the menstrual cycle. Am J Obstet Gynecol 1972; 114:405–418.

Murphy YS, Arronet GH, Parekh MC. Luteal phase inadequacy. Obstet Gynecol 1970; 36:758–761.

Noyes RW, Hertig AT, Rock J. Dating the endometrial biopsy. Fertil Steril 1950; 1:3–25.

Rosenfeld DL, Chudow S, Bronson RA. Diagnosis of luteal phase insufficiency. Obstet Gynecol 1980; 56:193–196.

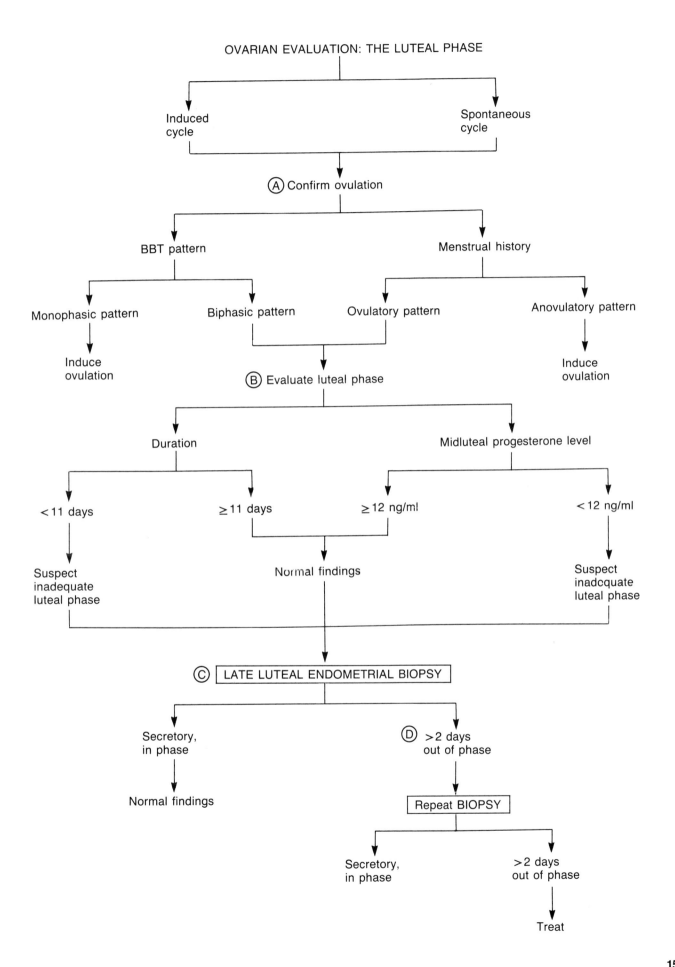

OVARIAN EVALUATION: THE LUTEAL PHASE

OVARIAN EVALUATION: OLIGOMENORRHEA

Ervin E. Jones, M.D., Ph.D.
Stephen P. Boyers, M.D.

A. Hirsutism or galactorrhea may be associated with diseases that cause disturbances of ovulation and menstruation. The evaluations of galactorrhea and hirsutism are discussed in separate algorithms (pp 24, 26). A variety of other serious diseases can also cause menstrual dysfunction and should be excluded early in the work-up for oligomenorrhea.

B. Oligomenorrhea is defined as menstrual cycles more than 36 days in length. Although some of these patients are anovulatory, the majority are irregular ovulators; in either case the chance to conceive is statistically decreased and these patients warrant an evaluation for infertility and therapy to induce regular ovulatory cycles.

C. Hypothyroidism may cause various disturbances of menstrual function, including oligomenorrhea and amenorrhea. It is important to exclude hypothyroidism in all oligomenorrheic women. The serum thyroid stimulating hormone (TSH) determination is the most useful laboratory test to detect intrinsic disease of the thyroid gland. A normal TSH value (less than 7 μU per milliliter) rules out primary hypothyroidism. Thyroid replacement restores normal menses and fertility in the majority of hypothyroid women. Thyroid replacement has no value in euthyroid patients.

D. Women who have hyperprolactinemia frequently present with menstrual dysfunction, including oligomenorrhea. The incidence of hyperprolactinemia in oligomenorrheic women without galactorrhea is less than 10 percent, but it is important to identify those patients because of the diagnostic and therapeutic implications of hyperprolactinemia. If the serum prolactin concentration is greater than 20 ng per milliliter, the test should be repeated. The evaluation of persistent hyperprolactinemia is outlined in another algorithm (p 36).

E. Once hyperprolactinemia, hypothyroidism, and other chronic underlying diseases have been excluded, patients with oligomenorrhea are candidates for a trial of ovulation induction. Clomiphene is the drug of choice in the treatment of these patients.

References

Bachman GA, Kemmann E. Prevalence of oligomenorrhea and amenorrhea in a college population. Am J Obstet Gynecol 1982; 144:98–102.

Davajan V, Kletzky O, March CM, Roy S, Mishell DR Jr. The significance of galactorrhea in patients with normal menses, oligomenorrhea and secondary amenorrhea. Am J Obstet Gynecol 1978; 130:894–900.

Hershman JM. Clinical application of thyrotropin-releasing hormone. Ann Intern Med 1971; 74:481–490.

Keye WR, Ho Yuen B, Knopf RF, Jaffe RB. Amenorrhea, hyperprolactinemia and pituitary enlargement secondary to primary hypothyroidism: successful treatment with thyroid replacement. Obstet Gynecol 1976; 48:697–702.

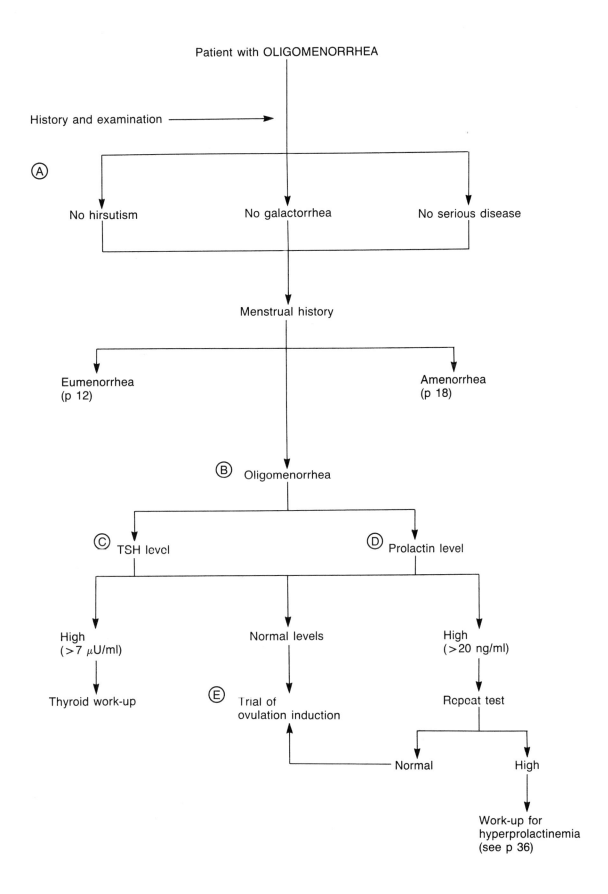

Patient with OLIGOMENORRHEA

History and examination ⟶

Ⓐ

No hirsutism   No galactorrhea   No serious disease

Menstrual history

Eumenorrhea   Amenorrhea
(p 12)   (p 18)

Ⓑ Oligomenorrhea

Ⓒ TSH level   Ⓓ Prolactin level

High   Normal levels   High
(>7 μU/ml)   (>20 ng/ml)

Thyroid work-up   Ⓔ Trial of   Repeat test
                    ovulation induction

                              Normal   High

                                         Work-up for
                                         hyperprolactinemia
                                         (see p 36)

OVARIAN EVALUATION: AMENORRHEA

Ervin E. Jones, M.D., Ph.D.
Stephen P. Boyers, M.D.

A. The work-up for amenorrhea depends on the presence or absence of coexisting abnormalities, such as galactorrhea and hirsutism, which are discussed in separate algorithms (pp 24, 26). A variety of chronic diseases may also cause menstrual dysfunction and should be excluded by history and physical examination early in the course of the evaluation of the amenorrheic patient.

B. Amenorrhea may be defined as primary or secondary. Primary amenorrhea is defined as failure to menstruate by age 16. In the absence of appropriate pubertal growth and secondary sexual development, or in the presence of obvious phenotypic abnormalities such as Turner's stigmata or vaginal agenesis, an evaluation should be initiated earlier. Secondary amenorrhea is defined as the absence of menstruation for 6 months in a woman who was previously menstruating regularly, or for an interval equal to three previous menstrual cycles in a patient who has been oligomenorrheic.

C. Pregnancy is the most common cause of amenorrhea in women of reproductive age, and the serum concentration of the beta subunit of human chorionic gonadotropin (β-hCG) should be measured early to identify these physiologically amenorrheic patients. When the β-hCG test is negative, the work-up should include measurements of the serum thyroid stimulating hormone (TSH) and prolactin levels and a progestin challenge test.

D. Although menstrual dysfunction is commonly seen in hypothyroid women, thyroid disease is an uncommon cause of amenorrhea. Nevertheless thyroid disease should be considered in the evaluation of amenorrhea. The best test of primary hypothyroidism is the serum TSH concentration. If the TSH level is elevated (greater than 7 μU per milliliter), a complete thyroid work-up is indicated. Hyperthyroidism also may be associated with menstrual dysfunction and should be excluded by measurements of the serum thyroxine (T_4) level and thyroxine binding capacity (resin T_3 uptake). The triiodothyronine (T_3) level is sometimes elevated in the presence of normal T_4 levels (T_3 toxicosis), but we reserve this assay for patients with clinical evidence of thyroid hyperfunction.

E. Hyperprolactinemia is found in up to one-third of amenorrheic women. The absence of galactorrhea does not exclude hyperprolactinemia, since the breast requires estrogen to respond to prolactin and many hyperprolactinemic patients are profoundly hypoestrogenic. Indeed galactorrhea occurs in only one-third of hyperprolactinemic patients. The evaluation and treatment of galactorrhea and hyperprolactinemia are discussed in accompanying algorithms (pp 24, 36).

F. The progestin challenge test provides valuable information about the endogenous estrogen level and the competency of the uterine outflow tract. Withdrawal bleeding following oral doses of medroxyprogesterone acetate (Provera, 10 mg per day for 7 days) or injectable progesterone in oil (150 mg intramuscularly) indicates a patent outflow tract and a responsive, estrogen primed endometrium. These patients are amenorrheic owing to anovulation and are usually responsive to ovulation induction. Failure to bleed after a progestin challenge indicates either hypoestrogenism, endometrial failure, or outflow tract obstruction.

G. A course of exogenous estrogen (Premarin, 2.5 mg per day for 25 days) and progestin (Provera, 10 mg per day, days 16 to 25) distinguishes patients with end organ failure (e.g., Asherman's syndrome) from those with hypoestrogenism. Failure to bleed should be further evaluated by endometrial biopsy, hysterosalpingography, and hysteroscopy. Bleeding indicates hypoestrogenism, either hypergonadotropic (ovarian failure) or hypogonadotropic (hypothalamic-pituitary). Measurement of the luteinizing hormone (LH) and follicle stimulating hormone (FSH) levels distinguishes between these two causes of hypoestrogenism. In practice, gonadotropins should be assayed before administering a course of exogenous estrogen with progestin, which partially suppresses LH-FSH secretion. The further evaluation of hypogonadotropic and hypergonadotropic hypogonadism is outlined in separate algorithms (pp 20, 22).

References

Hershman JM, Pittman JA. Utility of the radioimmunoassay of serum thyrotropin in man. Ann Intern Med 1971; 74:481–490.

Jacobs HS, Hull MGR, Murray MAF, Franks S. Therapy-oriented diagnosis of secondary amenorrhea. Horm Res 1975; 6:268–287.

Kletzky OA, Davajan V, Nakamura RM, Thorneycroft IH, Mishell DR Jr. Clinical categorization of patients with secondary amenorrhea using progesterone-induced uterine bleeding and measurement of serum gonadotropin levels. Am J Obstet Gynecol 1975; 121:695–703.

Philip J, Sele V, Trolle D. Primary amenorrhea: a study of 101 cases. Fertil Steril 1965; 16:795–804.

Schlechte J, Sherman B, Halmi N, et al. Prolactin secreting pituitary tumors. Endocr Rev 1980; 1:295.

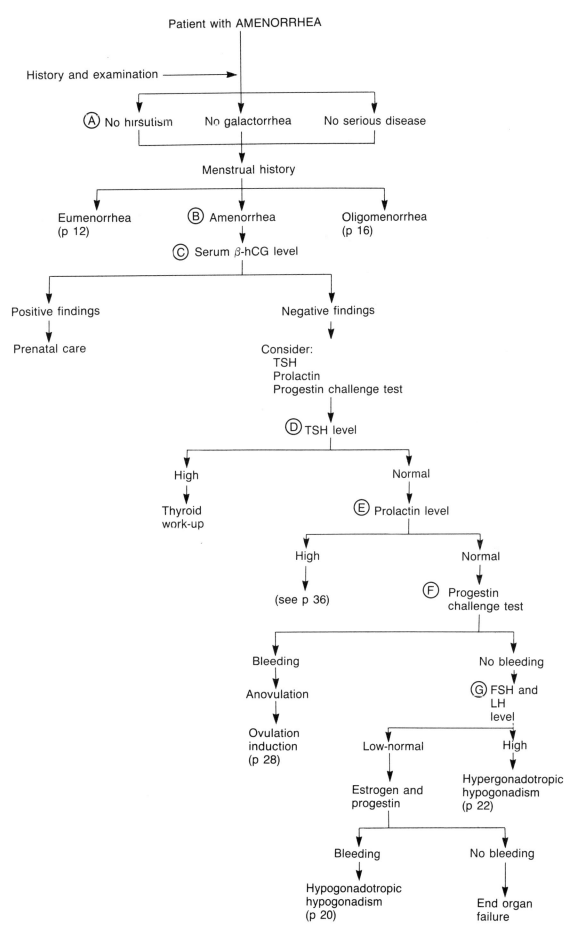

Patient with AMENORRHEA

History and examination →

Ⓐ No hirsutism   No galactorrhea   No serious disease

Menstrual history

Eumenorrhea
(p 12)

Ⓑ Amenorrhea

Oligomenorrhea
(p 16)

Ⓒ Serum β-hCG level

Positive findings

Prenatal care

Negative findings

Consider:
TSH
Prolactin
Progestin challenge test

Ⓓ TSH level

High

Thyroid
work-up

Normal

Ⓔ Prolactin level

High

(see p 36)

Normal

Ⓕ Progestin
challenge test

Bleeding

Anovulation

Ovulation
induction
(p 28)

No bleeding

Ⓖ FSH and
LH
level

Low-normal

Estrogen and
progestin

High

Hypergonadotropic
hypogonadism
(p 22)

Bleeding

Hypogonadotropic
hypogonadism
(p 20)

No bleeding

End organ
failure

HYPOGONADOTROPIC AMENORRHEA

Ervin E. Jones, M.D., Ph.D.
Stephen P. Boyers, M.D.

A. Prior to assessing gonadotropin levels during an evaluation for hypogonadotropic amenorrhea, several other causes of amenorrhea must be excluded. The most common cause of amenorrhea in women of reproductive age is pregnancy, and the beta human chorionic gonadotropin (β-hCG) level should be measured early. Patients with hirsutism, thyroid disease, and hyperprolactinemia should be identified and therapy instituted appropriately. A progestin challenge test should be done to exclude simple anovulation. Patients who fail to bleed following a progestin challenge either are hypoestrogenic or have endometrial failure or uterine outflow tract obstruction. The latter are identified by failure to bleed following a challenge with estrogen and progestin.

B. Amenorrheic patients who fail to bleed in response to a progestin challenge but bleed following exogenous estrogen with progestin are amenorrheic as a result of hypoestrogenism and an unstimulated endometrium. Measurement of the serum follicle stimulating hormone (FSH) and luteinizing hormone (LH) levels is necessary to distinguish between gonadal and hypothalamic-pituitary failure. For practical reasons we measure the FSH and LH levels before giving exogenous estrogen and progestin, which may partially suppress elevated gonadotropin levels and confuse the diagnosis of gonadal failure. Hypergonadotropic amenorrhea is discussed in a separate algorithm (p 22).

C. Hypogonadotropic amenorrhea indicates organic or functional hypothalamic-pituitary disease. Although the most common causes of hypogonadotropic hypogonadism are stress or weight related, organic central nervous system lesions may be life threatening and should be excluded. Hypothalamic lesions may cause amenorrhea by interfering with the control of gonadotropin or prolactin secretion. Pituitary lesions have similar effects. Both hypothalamic and pituitary lesions may be identified by computed tomography (CT) or magnetic resonance imaging (MRI) scan. Polytomography yields an unacceptably high incidence of false positive and false negative results and is no longer indicated. Abnormal CT or MRI scan results should be followed by a thorough neurologic assessment, visual field testing, and a Cortrosyn stimulation test to evaluate pituitary adrenal integrity. Even when amenorrhea seems clearly related to anorexia or changes in body weight, we recommend a CT or MRI scan, since organic central nervous system lesions may also affect the appetite and nutritional status.

D. The majority of women of reproductive age with hypogonadotropic hypogonadism have hypothalamic amenorrhea due to exercise stress, weight loss, anorexia nervosa, or other psychogenic disorders. The precise etiology of hypogonadotropism in these syndromes remains unclear, but it is probably the result of disturbances in gonadotropin releasing hormone. Weight gain or cessation of strenuous exercise usually restores normal gonadal function. When hypogonadotropism persists, ovulation induction with human menopausal gonadotropins (Pergonal) is indicated. We elect to perform a Cortrosyn stimulation test in these patients as well as in those with abnormal CT or MRI scan results, because pituitary insufficiency may be present even in the absence of a space occupying central nervous system lesion. Patients with pituitary adrenal insufficiency require corticosteroid replacement.

References

Baker ER. Menstrual dysfunction and hormonal status in athletic women: a review. Fertil Steril 1981; 36:691-696.

Haesslein HC, Lamb EJ. Pituitary tumors in patients with secondary amenorrhea. Am J Obstet Gynecol 1976; 125:759-767.

Kehlet H, Blichert-Toft M, Lindholm J. Short ACTH test in assessing hypothalamic-pituitary-adrenocortical function. Br Med J 1976; 1:249-251.

Klein SM, Garcia C-R: Asherman's syndrome: a critique and current review. Fertil Steril 1973; 24:722-735.

Vigersky RA, Andersen AE, Thompson RH, Loriaux DL. Hypothalamic dysfunction in secondary amenorrhea associated with simple weight loss. N Engl J Med 1977; 297:1141-1145.

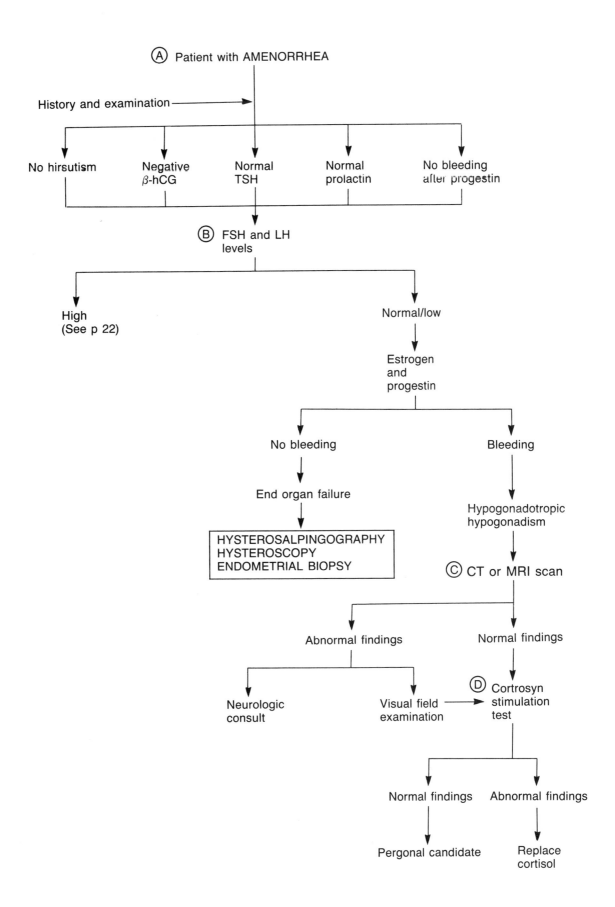

A Patient with AMENORRHEA

History and examination

No hirsutism | Negative β-hCG | Normal TSH | Normal prolactin | No bleeding after progestin

B FSH and LH levels

High (See p 22)

Normal/low

Estrogen and progestin

No bleeding

Bleeding

End organ failure

Hypogonadotropic hypogonadism

HYSTEROSALPINGOGRAPHY
HYSTEROSCOPY
ENDOMETRIAL BIOPSY

C CT or MRI scan

Abnormal findings

Normal findings

Neurologic consult

Visual field examination

D Cortrosyn stimulation test

Normal findings

Abnormal findings

Pergonal candidate

Replace cortisol

21

HYPERGONADOTROPIC AMENORRHEA

Ervin E. Jones, M.D., Ph.D.
Stephen P. Boyers, M.D.

A. As discussed in the section on hypogonadotropic amenorrhea, pregnancy, hirsutism, thyroid disease, and hyperprolactinemia must be excluded before initiating the work-up for hypergonadotropic amenorrhea. A progestin challenge test identifies well-estrogenized patients who are anovulatory and who are likely to respond to ovulation induction.

B. Hypergonadotropic hypogonadism is defined as hypoestrogenism and a serum follicle stimulating hormone (FSH) concentration of 45 mIU per milliliter or greater. A FSH concentration of 45 mIU per milliliter or greater indicates gonadal failure. In the patient with a high FSH level the test should be repeated in two weeks to exclude a midcycle gonadotropin surge as the etiology. Patients with FSH levels repeatedly of 45 mIU per milliliter or greater should be thoroughly evaluated to determine the cause of gonadal failure.

C. Although the mean age of physiologic menopause is 51 years, cessation of gonadal function as early as age 40 is within the range of onset of normal menopause. Beyond documentation of hypergonadotropism, an extensive evaluation is not indicated in these patients. Estrogen replacement is important for the prevention of osteoporosis, and adoption and even donor oocytes are options when fertility is a concern.

D. Premature ovarian failure is defined as hypergonadotropic hypogonadism occurring before age 40. The causes are several and generally may be divided into those with and without chromosomal abnormalities. A karyotype distinguishes between these two groups.

E. Although the majority of patients with gonadal dysgenesis and an abnormal karyotype present with primary amenorrhea and abnormal or absence of pubertal development, some initiate normal menstrual cycles and develop secondary amenorrhea, particularly those with mosaic forms of gonadal dysgenesis, either XX/XO or XX/XY. An abnormal karyotype in the absence of a Y chromosome establishes the diagnosis and directs therapy toward estrogen replacement. The most important function of a karyotype test in patients with premature ovarian failure, however, is to identify those with a Y chromosome, since these patients are at increased risk for gonadal neoplasia, and gonadectomy is indicated. The absence of genital ambiguity or virilization does not exclude the presence of a Y chromosome because only one third of the patients with Y carrying gonadal dysgenesis are clinically hyperandrogenized. Since it is rare for patients over age 30 to develop gonadoblastoma, gonadectomy is not indicated in this group.

F. Gonadal dysgenesis can occur in patients with a normal 46XX karyotype, but the majority of patients with normal karyotypes and premature ovarian failure have acquired rather than genetic ovarian failure. Gonadal x-irradiation, cytotoxic drugs, surgical removal, and gonadal infections such as mumps oophoritis are recognized causes of gonadal failure. Ovarian failure may occur as a component of a polyglandular autoimmune endocrine syndrome, which includes autoimmune thyroid, parathyroid, and adrenal failure. Although there are commercially available assays for antithyroid antibodies, tests for antiovarian and antiadrenal antibodies are still investigational and available on a limited basis. There are isolated reports of the return of ovarian function in patients with autoimmune ovarian failure following corticosteroid therapy.

G. Most patients with premature ovarian failure and a normal karyotype are diagnosed as having idiopathic hypergonadotropic hypogonadism. A few of these may have the insensitive oocyte syndrome, with elevated gonadotropin levels and hypoestrogenism despite a normal complement of oocytes, which are unresponsive to gonadotropin stimulation. The diagnosis requires ovarian tissue, which must be obtained by wedge resection at laparotomy, since laparoscopic biopsy may miss oocytes because of the small tissue sample. For the most part the diagnosis is of academic interest only and ovarian biopsy is not indicated. Patients likely to respond to an empiric trial of high dose Pergonal are best identified by weekly assays for FSH, luteinizing hormone (LH), and estradiol. Those showing no evidence of cyclic estradiol production are unlikely to respond to Pergonal. These patients are also candidates for estrogen replacement. Adoption or donor oocytes are options for couples desiring children.

References

Coulam CB, ed. Premature gonadal failure. Semin Reprod Endocrinol 1983; 1:79–178.

Goldenberg RL, Grodin JM, Rodbard D, Ross GT. Gonadotropins in women with amenorrhea: the use of plasma follicle-stimulating hormone to differentiate women with and without ovarian follicles. Am J Obstet Gynecol 1973; 116:1003–1012.

Rebar RW, Erickson GF, Yen SSC. Idiopathic premature ovarian failure: clinical and endocrine characteristics. Fertil Steril 1982; 37:35–41.

Sherman BM, Korenman SG. Hormonal characteristics of the human menstrual cycle throughout reproductive life. J Clin Invest 1975; 55:699–706.

Tan SL, Hague WM, Becker F, Jacobs HS. Autoimmune premature ovarian failure with polyendocrinopathy and spontaneous recovery of ovarian follicular activity. Fertil Steril 1986; 45:421–424.

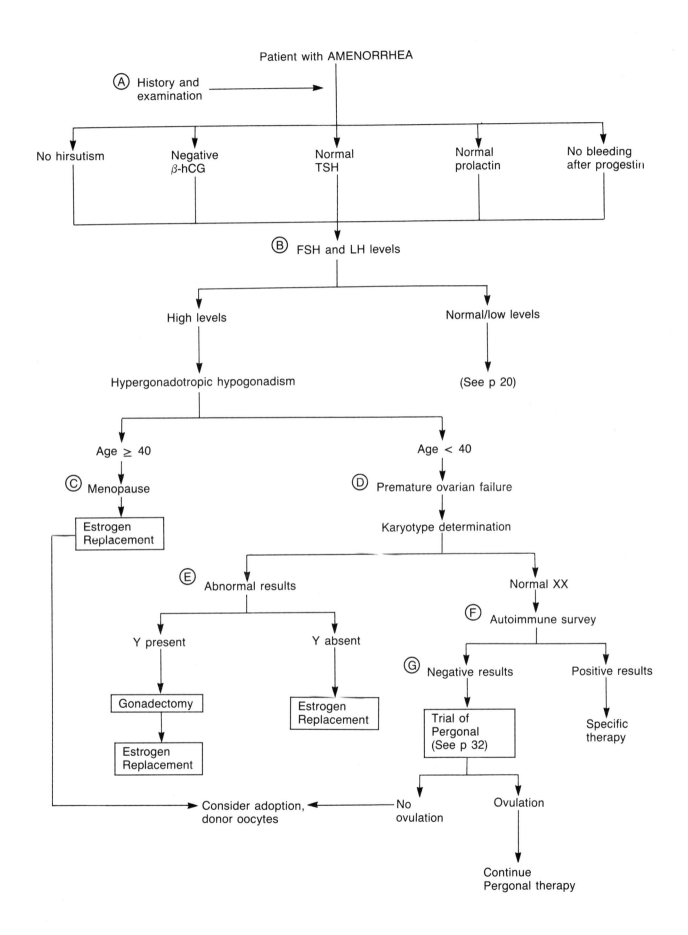

Patient with AMENORRHEA

(A) History and examination

No hirsutism Negative β-hCG Normal TSH Normal prolactin No bleeding after progestin

(B) FSH and LH levels

High levels Normal/low levels

Hypergonadotropic hypogonadism (See p 20)

Age ≥ 40 Age < 40

(C) Menopause (D) Premature ovarian failure

Estrogen Replacement Karyotype determination

(E) Abnormal results Normal XX

(F) Autoimmune survey

Y present Y absent

(G) Negative results Positive results

Gonadectomy Estrogen Replacement

Trial of Pergonal (See p 32) Specific therapy

Estrogen Replacement

Consider adoption, donor oocytes ← No ovulation Ovulation

Continue Pergonal therapy

23

OVARIAN EVALUATION: GALACTORRHEA

Ervin E. Jones, M.D.
Avi Lightman, M.D., M.Sc.
Stephen P. Boyers, M.D.

A. Galactorrhea warrants an evaluation regardless of the patient's menstrual status. Breast secretions may represent galactorrhea or another type of nipple discharge, including that from malignant disease. A sample of the secretion should be smeared on a clean glass slide and examined under the microscope for the presence of fat droplets. If fat is present, the secretion is galactorrhea. Secretions other than galactorrhea should be submitted for Papanicolaou staining to detect atypical cells. True galactorrhea may be caused by a variety of disorders, including infectious and traumatic lesions of the chest wall (herpes zoster, rib fracture, chest wall scar). Recent pregnancy must be ruled out, since galactorrhea in pregnancy is physiologic and does not require a work-up. Several classes of drugs may cause hyperprolactinemia and galactorrhea. The most common are neuroleptic drugs used to treat various mental disturbances, particularly those that act as dopamine receptor antagonists or those that interfere with dopamine function by other mechanisms.

B. One-third of the women with amenorrhea without an obvious etiology have hyperprolactinemia, and approximately one-third of the patients with elevated serum prolactin levels have galactorrhea. Whenever galactorrhea is identified, the serum prolactin level should be measured, preferably in a morning fasting sample. If the prolactin level is normal, bromocriptine may nevertheless be useful in suppressing galactorrhea. If the prolactin level is greater than 20 ng per milliliter, the serum thyroid stimulating hormone (TSH) level should be measured and the prolactin determination repeated. If the prolactin level is normal, observation or treatment with a dopamine receptor agonist is an option, since galactorrhea may occur in the presence of normoprolactinemia.

C. Because about 5 percent of the patients who have primary hypothyroidism also have hyperprolactinemia, it is important to exclude thyroid disease in patients with galactorrhea. An elevation of the serum TSH level (7 μU per milliliter or higher) is the most sensitive indicator of primary hypothyroidism. If the serum TSH level is higher than 7 μU per milliliter, the test should be repeated, and if the level is still elevated, a complete thyroid evaluation should be completed. With thyroid replacement, TSH and prolactin levels should return to normal.

D. One-third of the patients with secondary amenorrhea have evidence of pituitary adenoma; if galactorrhea is also present, the incidence increases to almost 50 percent. A pituitary adenoma should be suspected in every patient who has hyperprolactinemia, even those with relatively minor prolactin elevations, since a microadenoma has been reported in a patient with a prolactin level of only 23 ng per milliliter. Suprasellar lesions such as craniopharyngioma frequently cause only marginal hyperprolactinemia. The definitive diagnosis of pituitary or suprasellar lesions depends on the CT scan. The detection of a macroadenoma (larger than 10.0 mm) or a suprasellar lesion on a CT scan or magnetic resonance imaging (MRI) requires a formal neurologic consultation, visual field testing, and an adrenocorticotropic hormone (ACTH) stimulation test to exclude pituitary-adrenal insufficiency. Although macroadenomas may require neurosurgical management, the initial therapy for both macroadenomas and microadenomas should be bromocriptine. Tumor regression has been demonstrated repeatedly with bromocriptine. Prolonged suppression may be required to prevent tumor growth and the return of hyperprolactinemia, galactorrhea, and ovulatory dysfunction.

References

Chang RJ, Keye WR Jr, Young JR, Wilson CB, Jaffe RB. Detection, evaluation and treatment of pituitary microadenomas in patients with galactorrhea and amenorrhea. Am J Obstet Gynecol 1977; 128:356–363.

Davajan V, Kletzky O, March CM, Roy S, Mishell DR Jr. The significance of galactorrhea in patients with normal menses, oligomenorrhea, and secondary amenorrhea. Am J Obstet Gynecol 1979; 130:894–904.

Kleinberg DL, Noel GL, Frantz AG. Galactorrhea: a study of 235 cases, including 48 with pituitary tumors. N Engl J Med 1977; 296:589–600.

Molitch ME, Elton RL, Blackwell RE, et al. Bromocriptine as primary therapy for prolactin-secreting macroadenomas: results of a prospective multicenter study. J Clin Endocrinol Metab 1985; 60:698–705.

Turkington RW. Prolactin secretion in patients treated with various drugs. Arch Intern Med 1972; 130:349–354.

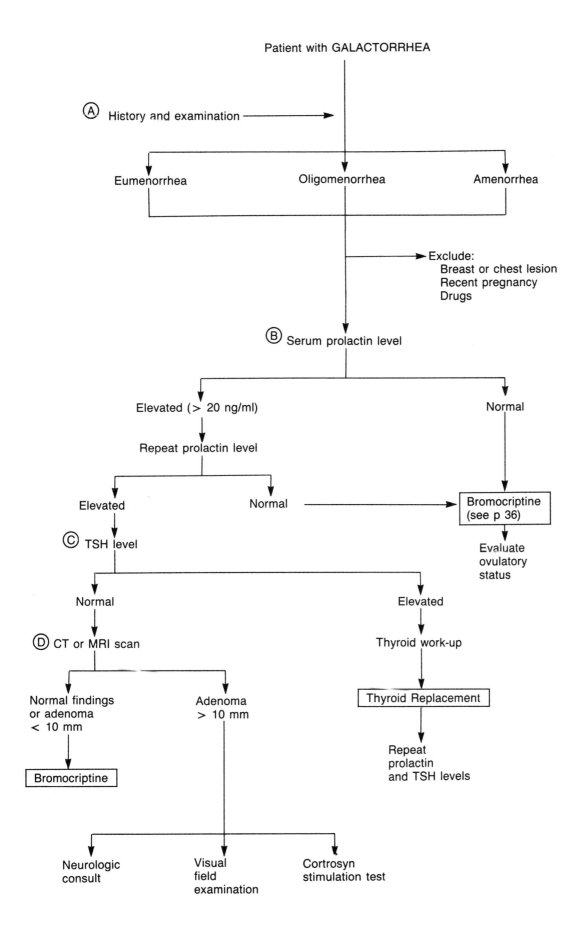

Patient with GALACTORRHEA

(A) History and examination ⟶

Eumenorrhea   Oligomenorrhea   Amenorrhea

⟶ Exclude:
   Breast or chest lesion
   Recent pregnancy
   Drugs

(B) Serum prolactin level

Elevated (> 20 ng/ml)   Normal

Repeat prolactin level

Elevated   Normal ⟶ Bromocriptine
                                   (see p 36)

(C) TSH level   Evaluate
                                           ovulatory
                                           status

Normal   Elevated

(D) CT or MRI scan   Thyroid work-up

Normal findings   Adenoma   Thyroid Replacement
or adenoma   > 10 mm
< 10 mm
                                Repeat
Bromocriptine   prolactin
                                and TSH levels

Neurologic   Visual   Cortrosyn
consult   field   stimulation test
               examination

OVARIAN EVALUATION: HIRSUTISM

Ervin E. Jones, M.D., Ph.D.
Stephen P. Boyers, M.D.

A. Hirsutism is characterized by the presence of coarse pigmented hair on the face, chest, upper back, or abdomen. Hirsutism is a sign of hyperandrogenism, and the degree of hirsutism correlates roughly with the free androgen concentration. Virilization represents the most advanced form of hyperandrogenization and is characterized by temporal balding, deepening of the voice, increased musculature and male body habitus, clitoromegaly, and hirsutism. Hirsutism may occur in women with eumenorrhea, oligomenorrhea, or amenorrhea and should be thoroughly investigated regardless of the menstrual status.

B. The causes of hirsutism and hyperandrogenism include androgen-producing ovarian or adrenal tumors, adrenal hyperplasia due to adrenal enzyme deficiencies, primary adrenocorticotropic hormone (ACTH) hypersecretion, exogenous drugs, and polycystic ovarian disease. The major reason for evaluating hirsutism is to distinguish functional disorders, which can be treated medically, from androgen-producing tumors, which require surgical intervention. The work-up hinges on measurement of the serum testosterone (T) and dehydroepiandrosterone sulfate (DHEA-S) concentrations. Testosterone is produced equally by ovarian and adrenal secretion; DHEA-S is produced almost exclusively by the adrenals.

C. High DHEA-S levels may be caused by both adrenal tumors and adrenal hyperplasia. These two are distinguished by the dexamethasone (DEX) suppression test. Dexamethasone, 2.0 mg, is given four times daily for 5 days. The DHEA-S level is measured by radioimmunoassay in fasting morning blood samples before and after 5 days of DEX. If the DHEA-S level fails to be suppressed to within the normal range, an adrenal tumor must be suspected.

D. With few exceptions, androgen-producing tumors are associated with testosterone levels of 200 ng per deciliter or higher or DHEA-S levels of 700 μg per deciliter or higher. If these levels are lower, a tumor is unlikely, especially when hirsutism has been long-standing and not rapidly progressive. Functional adrenal and ovarian disorders, especially polycystic ovarian disease, account for most cases of hirsutism.

E. When high dose dexamethasone fails to suppress the DHEA-S level, a CT scan of the adrenal glands is indicated. An adrenal mass warrants surgical exploration. When the CT scan findings are normal, bilateral retrograde adrenal vein catheterization should be performed to sample adrenal androgens. Adrenal venography may also be useful in delineating a tumor.

F. When the testosterone level alone is elevated, both adrenal and ovarian sources should be considered. An ovarian tumor may be detected by pelvic examination or ultrasound, and surgical exploration is required. The absence of ovarian enlargement by pelvic examination or ultrasound, however, does not exclude an androgen-producing ovarian tumor, which may be very small, and both the adrenals and the ovaries should be evaluated further. If the CT scan also fails to pinpoint an adrenal lesion, retrograde venous catheterization of both ovarian and adrenal veins should be considered. The procedure is technically difficult and not without risk and should be done only in centers with personnel experienced in catheter placement.

G. Fortunately androgen-producing tumors are rare, and most cases of hirsutism are caused by functional hyperandrogenism, which can be treated in a variety of ways. Oral contraceptive therapy is indicated in hirsute patients who desire contraception and have no contraindication to the use of oral contraceptives. Dexamethasone, 0.5 mg nightly, is effective in suppressing adrenal hyperfunction. Spironolactone may be useful in treating obese hirsute patients who are hypertensive when oral contraceptive therapy or DEX is contraindicated. Clomiphene is used when fertility is desired. None of these therapies can cause regression of existing hirsutism; electrolysis is the most effective cosmetic therapy and should be considered as an adjunct to androgen suppression.

References

Abraham GE. Ovarian and adrenal contribution to peripheral androgens during the menstrual cycle. J Clin Endocrinol Metab 1974; 39:340–346.

DeVane GW, Czekala NM, Judd HL, Yen SSC. Circulating gonadotrophins, estrogens, and adrogens in polycystic ovarian disease. Am J Obstet Gynecol 1975; 121:496–500.

Lachelin GCL, Barnett M, Hopper BR, Brink G, Yen SSC. Adrenal functions in normal women and women with the polycystic ovarian syndrome. J Clin Endocrinol Metab 1979; 49:892–898.

Meldrum DR, Abraham GE. Peripheral and ovarian venous concentrations of various steroid hormones in virilizing ovarian tumors. Obstet Gynecol 1979; 53:36–43.

Wentz AC, White RI, Migeon CJ, et al. Differential ovarian and adrenal vein catheterization. Am J Obstet Gynecol 1976; 125:1000–1007.

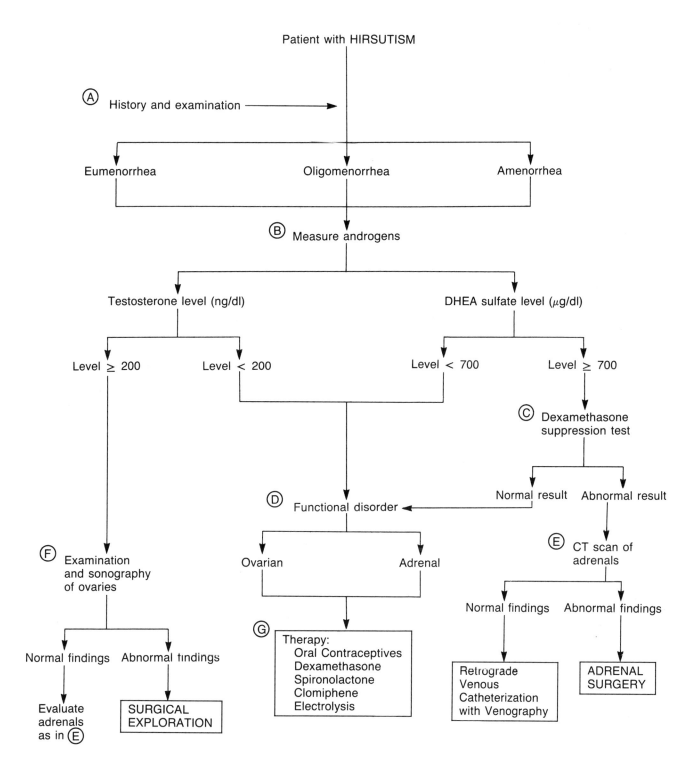

Patient with HIRSUTISM

Ⓐ History and examination

Eumenorrhea   Oligomenorrhea   Amenorrhea

Ⓑ Measure androgens

Testosterone level (ng/dl)   DHEA sulfate level (µg/dl)

Level ≥ 200   Level < 200   Level < 700   Level ≥ 700

Ⓒ Dexamethasone suppression test

Normal result   Abnormal result

Ⓓ Functional disorder

Ⓕ Examination and sonography of ovaries

Ovarian   Adrenal

Ⓔ CT scan of adrenals

Normal findings   Abnormal findings

Normal findings   Abnormal findings

Evaluate adrenals as in Ⓔ   SURGICAL EXPLORATION

Ⓖ Therapy:
Oral Contraceptives
Dexamethasone
Spironolactone
Clomiphene
Electrolysis

Retrograde Venous Catheterization with Venography   ADRENAL SURGERY

OVULATION INDUCTION

Stephen P. Boyers, M.D.
Ervin E. Jones, M.D., Ph.D.
Avi Lightman, M.D., M.Sc.

A. Patient selection is the most important determinant of success with ovulation induction. Clomiphene citrate has been called "one of the most abused drugs in gynecology." Clomiphene is not indicated in patients who are already ovulating regularly, except to treat a luteal phase defect. In patients who do not need clomiphene it may actually create problems when none existed before, inducing luteal phase defects or decreasing cervical mucus quantity and quality through its action as an antiestrogen. Ovarian failure is a contraindication to clomiphene. Patients with hyperprolactinemia should receive specific therapy with bromocriptine. A semen analysis should be done to exclude azoospermia and to identify subfertile males who need further evaluation.

B. Clomiphene citrate (Clomid, Serophene) therapy is usually started at a dose of 50 mg daily at either days 5 to 9 or days 3 to 7. The basal body temperature (BBT) chart is useful in following the patient's response. Once ovulatory cycles are established as judged by menstrual and BBT patterns, luteal phase adequacy should be documented by late luteal endometrial biopsy. The abnormal luteal phase requires further therapy. A postcoital test should also be done to document normal midcycle cervical mucus and sperm-mucus interaction, especially in view of clomiphene's antiestrogenic effects. Patients who fail to conceive after six ovulatory clomiphene cycles with normal postcoital test results and a normal luteal phase warrant further evaluation.

C. Although most patients respond to clomiphene at doses of 100 mg or less per day for 5 days, a minority require higher doses or an extended regimen to respond. Likewise some patients fail to respond to clomiphene alone but respond to clomiphene and 10,000 IU of human chorionic gonadotropin (hCG) administered intramuscularly at about day 15. Clomiphene failure has been defined as anovulation despite 250 mg of Clomid daily for 5 to 8 days combined with midcycle hCG administration. These patients are candidates for therapy with human menopausal gonadotropins (hMG, Pergonal).

D. Compared with Clomid, Pergonal is expensive, is tedious to administer and monitor, and is accompanied by increased risks of multiple gestation and ovarian hyperstimulation. Therefore, it should not be used in the patient with significant tubal disease. Hysterosalpingography (HSG) should be completed before considering a trial of hMG. Patients with a normal uterus and tubal patency are candidates for a trial of Pergonal. Those with abnormal HSG findings and those who fail to conceive after three to six ovulatory Pergonal cycles should undergo laparoscopy before starting or continuing hMG therapy.

E. Failure to ovulate with clomiphene alone is an indication for combined clomiphene and hMG-hCG, or hMG-hCG alone. The use of clomiphene with hMG may increase ovulatory responsiveness and decreases the total hMG requirement. Once ovulation has been secured, the luteal phase and postcoital test results should be evaluated, just as with ovulation induced with clomiphene. Failure to ovulate with Clomid and Pergonal requires re-evaluation for hyperprolactinemia or early ovarian failure. Poor responders who have normal serum prolactin and gonadotropin levels are candidates for a trial of ovulation induction with gonadotropin releasing hormone by pulsatile intravenous or subcutaneous administration.

References

Kistner RW. Induction of ovulation with clomiphene citrate. In: Behrman SJ, Kistner RW, eds. Progress in infertility. 2nd ed. Boston: Little, Brown, 1975:509.

Kistner RW. Sequential use of clomiphene citrate and human menopausal gonadotropin in ovulation induction. Fertil Steril 1976; 27:72–82.

March CM, Tredway DR, Mishell DR Jr. Effect of clomiphene citrate upon amount and duration of human menopausal gonadotropin therapy. Am J Obstet Gynecol 1976; 125:699–704.

Pepperell RJ. A rational approach to ovulation induction. Fertil Steril 1983; 40:1–14.

Rust LA, Israel R, Mishell DR Jr. An individualized graduated therapeutic regimen for clomiphene citrate. Am J Obstet Gynecol 1974; 120:785–790.

OVULATION INDUCTION: CLOMIPHENE CITRATE

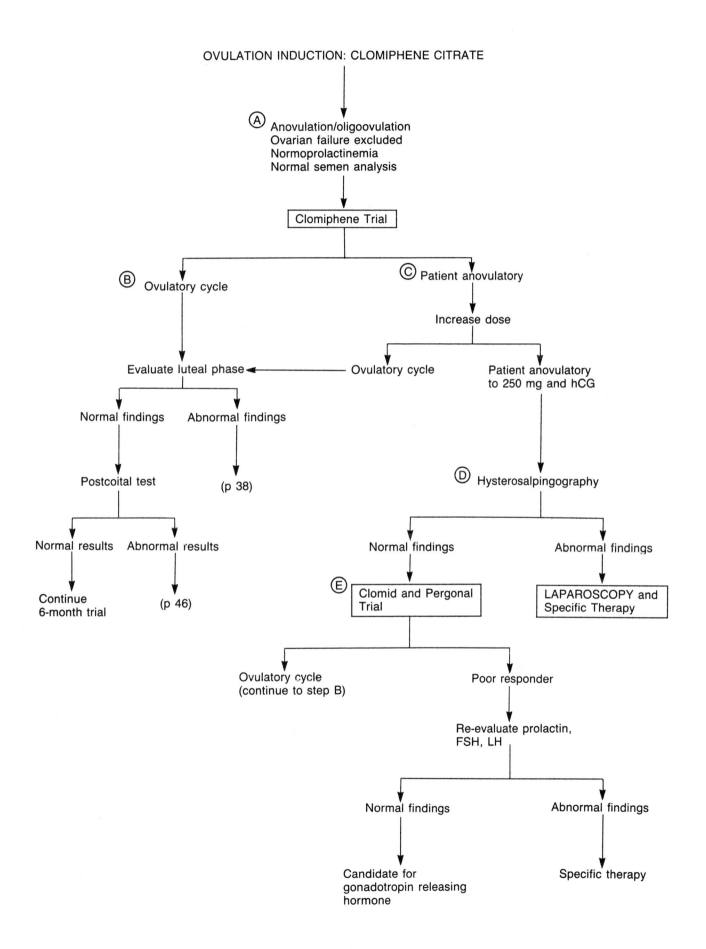

Ⓐ Anovulation/oligoovulation
Ovarian failure excluded
Normoprolactinemia
Normal semen analysis

Clomiphene Trial

Ⓑ Ovulatory cycle

Ⓒ Patient anovulatory

Increase dose

Evaluate luteal phase ◄— Ovulatory cycle

Patient anovulatory to 250 mg and hCG

Normal findings   Abnormal findings

Postcoital test   (p 38)

Ⓓ Hysterosalpingography

Normal results   Abnormal results

Continue 6-month trial   (p 46)

Normal findings   Abnormal findings

Ⓔ Clomid and Pergonal Trial   LAPAROSCOPY and Specific Therapy

Ovulatory cycle (continue to step B)   Poor responder

Re-evaluate prolactin, FSH, LH

Normal findings   Abnormal findings

Candidate for gonadotropin releasing hormone   Specific therapy

OVULATION INDUCTION: CLOMIPHENE CITRATE

Avi Lightman, M.D., M.Sc.
Stephen P. Boyers, M.D.

A. Between 10 and 25 percent of all cases of infertility are caused by ovulatory failure. An individualized regimen of ovulation induction with clomiphene citrate results in ovulation in 80 to 90 percent of these patients. Conception incidences of 40 to 50 percent are generally reported, but incidences as high as 85 percent can be achieved in selected women with pure anovulatory infertility. The key to success is patient selection. Clomiphene is not indicated in patients who are already ovulating regularly, except to treat an inadequate luteal phase. Patients with ovarian or hypothalamic-pituitary failure are unlikely to respond to clomiphene. Hyperprolactinemic anovulation should be treated specifically with bromocriptine. Evaluation of both partners should proceed in parallel, and male factors should be excluded before embarking on a trial of clomiphene ovulation induction.

B. Therapy with clomiphene citrate (Clomid, Serophene) is usually started at a dose of 50 mg daily for 5 days. Both day 5–9 and day 3–7 regimens have been successful (Fig. 1). Once ovulation has been established, as judged by basal body temperature and menstrual patterns, luteal phase adequacy should be documented. We have outlined the luteal phase evaluation in another algorithm (p 14).

C. In clomiphene induced cycles, ovulation usually occurs 10 to 15 days after clomiphene initiation. A postcoital test (PCT) should be done during this period to document normal midcycle cervical mucus and normal sperm-mucus interaction. In previously anovulatory patients ovulation induction is a prerequisite to the PCT. In oligoovulators or women receiving clomiphene as therapy for an inadequate luteal phase, a PCT may already have been done. Nevertheless the PCT should be repeated during a clomiphene cycle because clomiphene's antiestrogenic action may compromise cervical mucus quality. If both the PCT and the luteal phase are normal in ovulatory cycles induced with clomiphene, a trial of ovulation induction should continue for at least six cycles. In patients who still fail to conceive, other factors should be evaluated further before continuing clomiphene.

D. Failure to ovulate after treatment with 50 mg of clomiphene for 5 days is an indication for increasing the dose to 100 mg per day. Most patients ovulate in response to 50 or 100 mg per day, and 80 percent of conceptions occur in the first three ovulatory cycles. Success is maximized by individualizing the clomiphene regimen, increasing the dose in a stepwise fashion to as high as 200 to 250 mg per day for 5 to 8 days. With this regimen fully one-third of the patients conceived with clomiphene treatment at doses above 100 mg, and half of these required more than 150 mg per day.

E. Patients who fail to ovulate after 150 mg of clomiphene daily for 5 days may ovulate with the addition of 10,000 IU of human chorionic gonadotropin (hCG) between days 13 and 15 if clomiphene has been given on days 3 to 7, or between days 15 and 17 if the day 5–9 clomiphene regimen has been used. The timing of hCG therapy may be empiric or may be based on cervical score or follicle size, as for in vitro fertilization. Five to 10 percent of the patients fail to ovulate despite clomiphene doses up to 250 mg daily for 5 days with the addition to hCG 10,000 IU. In these women an extended regimen of clomiphene, consisting of 250 mg for 8 days followed by 10,000 IU of hCG, has been successful and should be considered before beginning a trial of human menopausal gonadotropin (hMG).

F. The dehydroepiandrosterone sulfate (DHEA-S) level is frequently increased in infertile women with ovulatory dysfunction, and elevated DHEA-S levels may interfere with the response to clomiphene. The combination of dexamethasone (DEX) 0.5 mg nightly and clomiphene has been successful in patients with elevated DHEA-S levels who failed to respond to clomiphene alone. Indeed, in women with DHEA-S levels of 200 μg per deciliter or higher, one randomized trial demonstrated significantly higher incidences of ovulation and pregnancy in patients treated initially with clomiphene and dexamethasone than with clomiphene alone. We have generally reserved DEX for patients failing to ovulate with clomiphene alone. When DEX is added, the clomiphene dose is started back at 50 mg per day and increased in a stepwise fashion as needed.

References

Daly DC, Walters CA, Soto-Albors CE, Tohan N, Riddick DH. A randomized study of dexamethasone in ovulation induc-

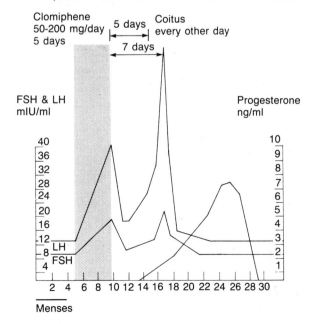

Figure 1 Ovulation induction using clomiphene citrate.

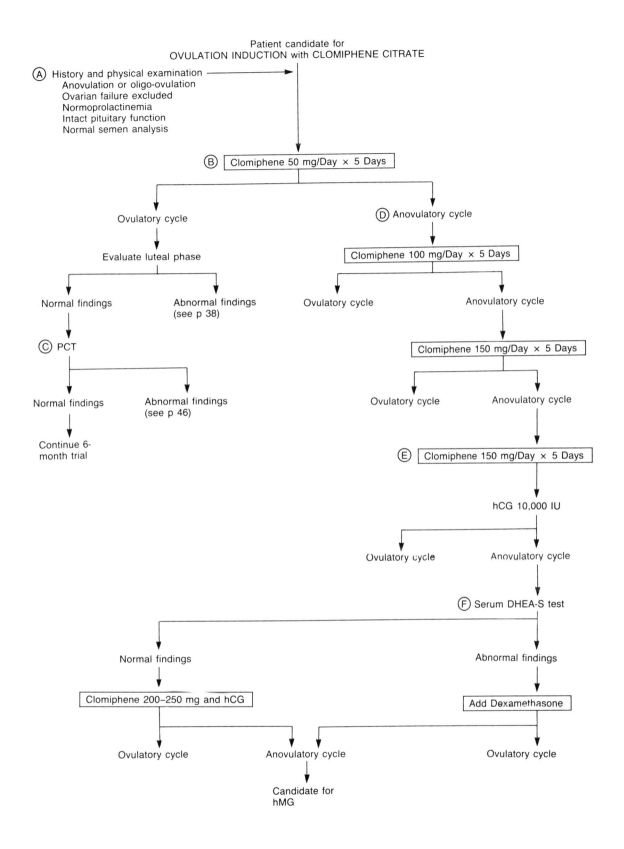

Patient candidate for
OVULATION INDUCTION with CLOMIPHENE CITRATE

(A) History and physical examination
Anovulation or oligo-ovulation
Ovarian failure excluded
Normoprolactinemia
Intact pituitary function
Normal semen analysis

(B) Clomiphene 50 mg/Day × 5 Days

Ovulatory cycle

Evaluate luteal phase

Normal findings

Abnormal findings
(see p 38)

(C) PCT

Normal findings

Abnormal findings
(see p 46)

Continue 6-month trial

(D) Anovulatory cycle

Clomiphene 100 mg/Day × 5 Days

Ovulatory cycle   Anovulatory cycle

Clomiphene 150 mg/Day × 5 Days

Ovulatory cycle   Anovulatory cycle

(E) Clomiphene 150 mg/Day × 5 Days

hCG 10,000 IU

Ovulatory cycle   Anovulatory cycle

(F) Serum DHEA-S test

Normal findings   Abnormal findings

Clomiphene 200–250 mg and hCG   Add Dexamethasone

Ovulatory cycle   Anovulatory cycle   Ovulatory cycle

Candidate for
hMG

tion with clomiphene citrate. Fertil Steril 1984; 41:844–848.

Gysler M, March CM, Mishell DR Jr, Bailey EJ. A decade's experience with an individualized clomiphene treatment regimen including its effect on the postcoital test. Fertil Steril 1982; 37:161–167.

Hoffman D, Lobo RA. Serum dehydroepiandrosterone sulfate and the use of clomiphene citrate in anovulatory women. Fertil Steril 1985; 43:196–199.

Lobo RA, Granger LR, Davajan V, Mishell DR Jr. An extended regimen of clomiphene citrate in women unresponsive to standard therapy. Fertil Steril 1982; 37:762–766.

Lobo RA, Wellington P, March CM, Granger L, Kletzky OA. Clomiphene and dexamethasone in women unresponsive to clomiphene alone. Obstet Gynecol 1982; 60:497–501.

OVULATION INDUCTION: HUMAN MENOPAUSAL GONADOTROPINS

Avi Lightman, M.D., M.Sc.
Ervin E. Jones, M.D., Ph.D.
Stephen P. Boyers, M.D.

A. Human menopausal gonadotropin (hMG), (75 mIU follicle stimulating hormone and 75 mIU luteinizing hormone per ampule, Pergonal, Serono Laboratories, Inc., Randolph, MA) is indicated for the treatment of anovulation or luteal phase inadequacy when other simpler methods have failed, and for controlled hyperstimulation for in vitro fertilization and embryo transfer. Because Pergonal therapy is complex and expensive, other causes of infertility should be excluded prior to its use. Patients with ovarian failure do not respond to Pergonal, and these patients should be identified by serum gonadotropin assays and excluded from hMG therapy. Hyperprolactinemia should also be identified; bromocriptine is indicated for hyperprolactinemic anovulation.

B. We usually start hMG at a dose of two ampules per day, beginning on cycle day 3. Couples are instructed in the use and intramuscular administration of hMG during a "Pergonal class," which is held weekly. The first dose of hMG is given the evening of cycle day 3 and is continued every evening from days 3 through 7 (five doses). On the morning of day 8 a blood sample is drawn for rapid estradiol (E_2) assay. Results are available by 4 PM. The dose of hMG on day 8 is determined by the morning E_2 level.

C. When the day 8 morning serum E_2 level is less than 100 pg per milliliter, indicating no response to hMG, the dose is increased to three ampules per day and the serum E_2 level is measured again in 48 hours. If there is still no response, the hMG dose is further increased to four ampules per day, and again to five ampules per day if the E_2 level remains low. When the E_2 level fails to rise despite 48 hours of treatment with five ampules per day, the cycle is discontinued. Following a canceled cycle, the next hMG cycle would be started at a dose of four to five ampules per day on days 3 to 7 following a spontaneous or induced menses.

D. When the day 8 E_2 concentration exceeds 100 pg per milliliter (indicating a response to hMG), the dose is held constant and morning serum E_2 levels are monitored every 24 to 48 hours, depending on the E_2 levels. Below 300 pg per milliliter, we wait 48 hours before the next E_2 assay, but between 300 and 800 pg per milliliter, we request daily E_2 monitoring.

E. When the E_2 concentration is greater than 800 pg per milliliter, we perform ovarian ultrasonography to assess the number of preovulatory follicles, those with a diameter greater than or equal to 15 mm. Our goal is to decrease the risk for multiple gestation, and we have advised the withholding of human chorionic gonadotropin (hCG) when there are more than four large follicles. When there are less than two large follicles and the E_2 level is less than 1,500 pg per milliliter, we continue hMG and repeat the ultrasonography and E_2 assay 24 hours later. If the E_2 level is 1,500 or higher, see step F. When there are two to four mature follicles, the decision to give hCG again depends on the E_2 level.

F. The risk of hyperstimulation increases as the preovulatory E_2 level increases, although hyperstimulation does not develop if hCG is withheld. We do not give hCG when the E_2 level exceeds 2,000 pg per milliliter or when it is between 1,500 and 2,000 pg per milliliter and a steep rise (more than 50 percent higher than the previous day's level) is seen.

G. Because ovulation generally occurs 36 hours after hCG administration, couples should be instructed to have intercourse 24 and 48 hours after hCG.

References

Berquist C, Nillius SJ, Wide L. Human gonadotropin therapy. Serum estradiol and progesterone patterns during conceptual cycles. Fertil Steril 1983; 39:761–765.

Dor J, Itzkowic DJ, Mashiach S, Lunenfeld B, Serr DM. Cumulative conception rates following gonadotropin therapy. Am J Obstet Gynecol 1980; 136:102–105.

Hack M, Brish M, Serr M, Insler V, Lunenfeld B. Outcome of pregnancy after induced ovulation: follow-up of pregnancies and children born after gonadotropin therapy. JAMA 1970; 211:791–797.

Karafiol PE, Rosenfeld DL, Pek H, Goldman MA, Bronson RA. Prediction of multiple gestation in hMG-induced ovulation: a case report. J Reprod Med 1982; 27:367–370.

Oelsner G, Serr DM, Mashiach S, et al. The study of induction of ovulation with menotropins: analysis of results of 1897 treatment cycles. Fertil Steril 1978; 30:538–544.

Seibel MM, McArdle CR, Thompson IE, Berger MJ, Taymor ML. The role of ultrasound in ovulation induction: a critical appraisal. Fertil Steril 1981; 36:573–577.

Treadway DR, Goebelsmann U, Thorneycroft IH, Mishell DR Jr. Monitoring induction of ovulation with human menopausal gonadotropin by a rapid estrogen radioimmunoassay. Am J Obstet Gynecol 1974; 120:1035–1040.

Wang CF, Gemzell C. The use of human gonadotropins for the induction of women with polycystic ovarian disease. Fertil Steril 1980; 33:479–486.

Wilson EA, Jawad MJ, Hayden TL. Rates of exponential increase of serum estradiol concentration in normal and human menopausal gonadotropin-induced cycles. Fertil Steril 1982; 37:46–49.

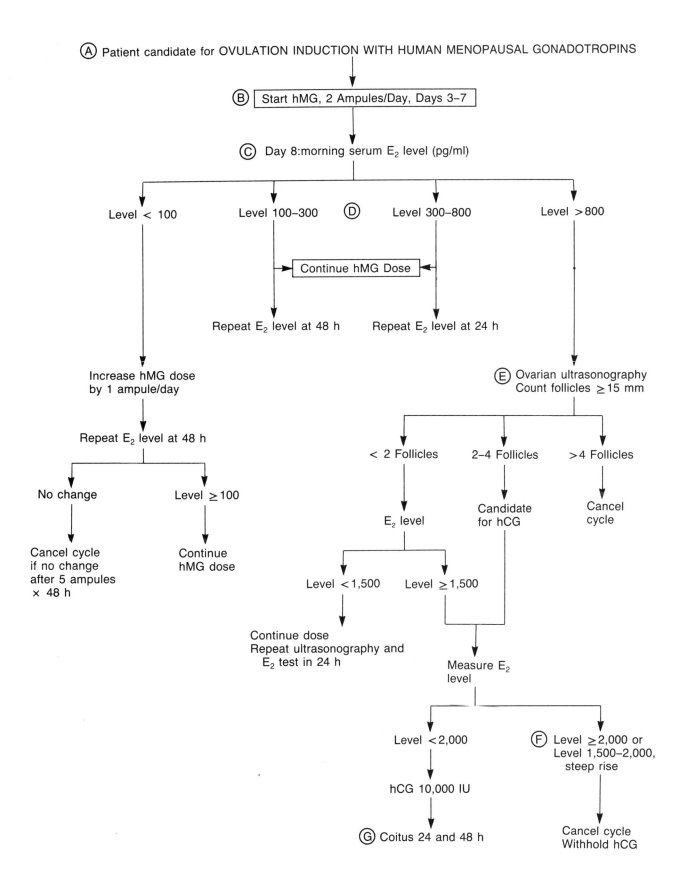

(A) Patient candidate for OVULATION INDUCTION WITH HUMAN MENOPAUSAL GONADOTROPINS

(B) Start hMG, 2 Ampules/Day, Days 3–7

(C) Day 8:morning serum E_2 level (pg/ml)

Level < 100   Level 100–300   (D)   Level 300–800   Level >800

Continue hMG Dose

Repeat E_2 level at 48 h   Repeat E_2 level at 24 h

Increase hMG dose
by 1 ampule/day

Repeat E_2 level at 48 h

No change   Level ≥ 100

Cancel cycle
if no change
after 5 ampules
× 48 h

Continue
hMG dose

(E) Ovarian ultrasonography
Count follicles ≥ 15 mm

< 2 Follicles   2–4 Follicles   >4 Follicles

E_2 level   Candidate
for hCG   Cancel
cycle

Level <1,500   Level ≥1,500

Continue dose
Repeat ultrasonography and
E_2 test in 24 h

Measure E_2
level

Level <2,000   (F) Level ≥2,000 or
Level 1,500–2,000,
steep rise

hCG 10,000 IU   Cancel cycle
Withhold hCG

(G) Coitus 24 and 48 h

OVULATION INDUCTION: GONADOTROPIN RELEASING HORMONE

Ervin E. Jones, M.D., Ph.D.
Stephen P. Boyers, M.D.

A. Failure to ovulate in response to clomiphene, human menopausal gonadotropin–human chorionic gonadotropin (hMG-hCG), or clomiphene-hMG-hCG is an indication for a trial of gonadotropin releasing hormone (GnRH). Anovulatory patients with hypogonadotropic hypogonadism of hypothalamic origin usually respond to GnRH and its analogues. If the pituitary gland is functionally intact, GnRH induces an endogenous release of luteinizing hormone (LH) and follicle stimulating hormone (FSH). These two gonadotropins stimulate follicular growth and development and, eventually, ovulation. Multiple follicular maturation has been achieved with GnRH in normally cycling women, making this method of ovarian stimulation potentially useful for patients requiring in vitro fertilization. The efficacy and safety of GnRH for ovulation induction have been demonstrated in several studies.

B. We administer GnRH subcutaneously via an infusion pump that is programed to release a 20 to 40 μg bolus of the hormone at 120 minute intervals. Therapy is begun on day 3 of a spontaneous or induced cycle. The ovarian response to GnRH is monitored by daily serum estradiol assays and ovarian ultrasound examination to follow follicular development. Monitoring is initiated on day 8 of the cycle.

C. Monitoring of ovulation induction with GnRH is essentially the same as for hMG. Serum estradiol levels are expected to rise progressively to 500 pg per milliliter or higher as follicles grow. Ultrasound should reveal progressive follicular development, and the dominant follicle should reach a diameter of 15 mm or greater, at which time 10,000 IU of hCG is given. If a satisfactory response does not occur within 30 days, the cycle is discontinued.

References

Leyendecker G, Wildt L, Hansmann M. Pregnancies following chronic intermittent (pulsatile) administration of GnRH by means of a portable pump (Zyklomat): a new approach in the treatment of infertility in hypothalamic amenorrhea. J Clin Endocrinol Metab 1980; 51:1214–1216.

Liu JH, Durfee R, Musa K, Yen SSC. Induction of multiple ovulation by pulsatile administration of gonadotropin-releasing hormone. Fertil Steril 1983; 40:18–22.

Miller DS, Reid R, Cetel N, Yen SSC. Pulsatile administration of low dose gonadotropin-releasing hormone (GnRH) for the induction of ovulation and pregnancy in patients with hypothalamic amenorrhea. JAMA 1983; 250:2937–2941.

Reid RL, Leopold GR, Yen SSC. Induction of ovulation and pregnancy with pulsatile luteinizing hormone releasing factor: dosage and mode of delivery. Fertil Steril 1981; 36:553–559.

Schoenmaker JA, Simmons HM, Von Osuabrugge GJC, Lugtenburg C, Van Kessel H. Pregnancy after prolonged pulsatile administration of luteinizing hormone-releasing hormone in a patient with clomiphene-resistant secondary amenorrhea. J Clin Endocrinol Metab 1981; 52:882–885.

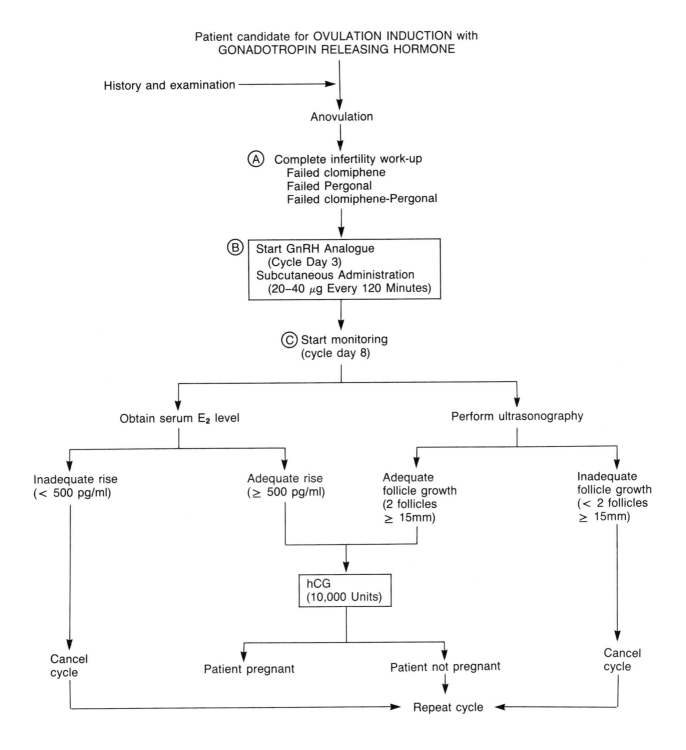

Patient candidate for OVULATION INDUCTION with
GONADOTROPIN RELEASING HORMONE

History and examination ⟶

Anovulation

(A) Complete infertility work-up
    Failed clomiphene
    Failed Pergonal
    Failed clomiphene-Pergonal

(B) Start GnRH Analogue
    (Cycle Day 3)
    Subcutaneous Administration
    (20–40 μg Every 120 Minutes)

(C) Start monitoring
    (cycle day 8)

Obtain serum E₂ level

Perform ultrasonography

Inadequate rise
(< 500 pg/ml)

Adequate rise
(≥ 500 pg/ml)

Adequate
follicle growth
(2 follicles
≥ 15mm)

Inadequate
follicle growth
(< 2 follicles
≥ 15mm)

hCG
(10,000 Units)

Cancel
cycle

Patient pregnant

Patient not pregnant

Cancel
cycle

Repeat cycle

OVULATION INDUCTION: BROMOCRIPTINE

Ervin E. Jones, M.D., Ph.D.
Stephen P. Boyers, M.D.

A. Hyperprolactinemia causes a spectrum of ovulatory disorders, from the inadequate luteal phase to oligo-ovulation to complete anovulation and amenorrhea. Approximately one-third of hyperprolactinemic women also have galactorrhea. The incidence of hyperprolactinemia in amenorrhea alone is about 30 percent, increasing to 60 to 70 percent when amenorrhea and galactorrhea occur together.

B. The cause of hyperprolactinemia should be thoroughly investigated before initiating therapy. A variety of drugs, especially psychotropic and antihypertensive drugs, increase prolactin levels by interfering with dopamine function. Hyperprolactinemia occurs in 5 percent of the women who have primary hypothyroidism. Pregnancy and lesions of the breast or chest wall must be excluded. As many as 90 percent of the women with persistent hyperprolactinemia not caused by drugs, thyroid or other disease, or pregnancy have radiographic evidence (by CT or magnetic resonance imaging scanning) of a pituitary microadenoma or macroadenoma, which should be completely investigated before beginning therapy.

C. Bromocriptine mesylate (Parlodel) is a dopamine receptor agonist. Since dopamine inhibits prolactin secretion, bromocriptine has become the drug of choice to treat hyperprolactinemia, including that caused by prolactin-secreting adenomas of the anterior pituitary gland. The usual dose of bromocriptine is 2.5 mg twice daily, but tolerance to the drug should be tested by initiating therapy at a dose of half a tablet (1.25 mg) twice daily for the first week to reduce the unpleasant side effects of nausea and syncope. Rarely are side effects so severe that bromocriptine cannot be continued. Usually side effects are mild and the dose can be increased gradually to achieve normoprolactinemia.

D. The serum prolactin determination should be repeated about 4 weeks after starting bromocriptine. If the prolactin concentration remains elevated, the dose of bromocriptine should be increased in 2.5 mg increments until a normal prolactin level is achieved. Once the prolactin level is normal, that dose is continued and the patient is instructed to use a barrier method of contraception until menstrual function returns. At the resumption of menstruation, basal body temperatures should be charted. If anovulation continues despite the restoration of normal prolactin levels, clomiphene may be added to induce ovulatory cycles. Once ovulation is established, whether by bromocriptine alone or by bromocriptine and clomiphene, luteal phase adequacy should be assessed as outlined in a separate algorithm (p 14). When conception occurs, bromocriptine should be discontinued.

References

Cuellar FG. Bromocriptine mesylate (Parlodel) in the management of amenorrhea/galactorrhea associated with hyperprolactinemia. Obstet Gynecol 1980; 55:278–281.

Del Pozo E, Wyss H, Tolis J, et al. Prolactin and deficient luteal function. Obstet Gynecol 1979; 53:282–286.

Keye WR, Chang RJ, Wilson CB, Jaffe RB. Prolactin-secreting pituitary adenomas in women. III. Frequency and diagnosis in amenorrhea-galactorrhea. JAMA 1980; 244:1329–1332.

Keye WR, Ho Yuen B, Knopf RF, Jaffe RB. Amenorrhea, hyperprolactinemia and pituitary enlargement secondary to primary hypothyroidism: successful treatment with thyroid replacement. Obstet Gynecol 1976; 48:697–702.

Turksoy RN, Biller BJ, Farber M, Cetrulo C, Mitchell GW Jr. Ovulatory response to clomiphene citrate during bromocriptine-failed ovulation in amenorrhea-galactorrhea and hyperprolactinemia. Fertil Steril 1982; 37:441–444.

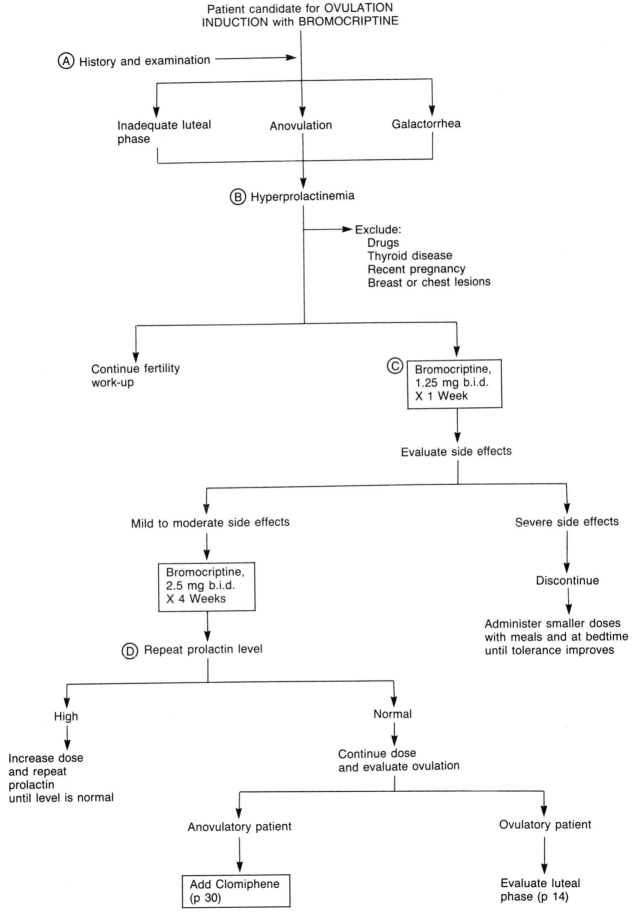

Patient candidate for OVULATION INDUCTION with BROMOCRIPTINE

Ⓐ History and examination

Inadequate luteal phase   Anovulation   Galactorrhea

Ⓑ Hyperprolactinemia

Exclude:
Drugs
Thyroid disease
Recent pregnancy
Breast or chest lesions

Continue fertility work-up

Ⓒ Bromocriptine, 1.25 mg b.i.d. X 1 Week

Evaluate side effects

Mild to moderate side effects   Severe side effects

Bromocriptine, 2.5 mg b.i.d. X 4 Weeks

Discontinue

Administer smaller doses with meals and at bedtime until tolerance improves

Ⓓ Repeat prolactin level

High   Normal

Increase dose and repeat prolactin until level is normal

Continue dose and evaluate ovulation

Anovulatory patient   Ovulatory patient

Add Clomiphene (p 30)

Evaluate luteal phase (p 14)

INADEQUATE LUTEAL PHASE: TREATMENT

Avi Lightman, M.D., M.Sc.
Stephen P. Boyers, M.D.

A. An inadequate luteal phase occurs in 3 to 5 percent of infertile women and in up to 35 percent of patients with recurrent first trimester abortions. Identification of an inadequate luteal phase requires that the histologic development (Fig. 1), shown by late luteal endometrial biopsy, be more than 2 days out of phase in two different cycles. Hyperprolactinemia and hypothyroidism may cause luteal phase inadequacy and should be excluded before further treatment. An inadequate luteal phase associated with hyperprolactinemia should be treated with bromocriptine and the endometrial biopsy repeated after prolactin levels have returned to normal.

B. Corpus luteum function probably reflects the quality of the follicle that preceded it. Follicle growth is in turn dependent on follicle stimulating hormone (FSH) stimulation. Cycles with inadequate luteal function are associated with significantly lower early follicular phase FSH levels than cycles with normal luteal function. Clomiphene citrate stimulates gonadotropin secretion and folliculogenesis and is therefore a logical first choice therapy. The details of clomiphene ovulation induction are outlined separately (p 30).

C. The midluteal progesterone concentration in normal ovulatory cycles is 12 ng per milliliter or higher. We monitor clomiphene cycles with measurement of the basal body temperature and do not repeat the endometrial biopsy until the response to clomiphene appears adequate by basal body temperature and progesterone criteria. Once a normal response is documented, luteal phase adequacy following therapy should be documented by a repeat late luteal endometrial biopsy. When the endometrial biopsy is normal, therapy is continued for at least six cycles. If pregnancy still fails despite luteal phase adequacy, other fertility factors should be reviewed.

D. When the endometrial biopsy findings remain abnormal, or midluteal serum progesterone levels remain below 12 ng per milliliter despite clomiphene, we add exogenous progesterone in the form of 25 mg vaginal suppositories, two to three times daily, beginning on the second day of the basal body temperature rise, continued until menses. An alternative is to use vaginal progesterone only, without clomiphene. Again it is essential to evaluate the adequacy of therapy by a repeat late luteal endometrial biopsy. Therapy is continued once a normal in-phase late secretory endometrium has been documented.

E. When neither clomiphene nor vaginal progesterone alone or in combination is successful in restoring luteal phase adequacy, a trial of human menopausal gonadotropin–human chorionic gonadotropin (hMG-hCG) is warranted. The details of hMG-hCG therapy are outlined separately (p 32). An ovulatory response to hMG is not a guarantee of normal luteal function, however, and luteal adequacy should be tested again by endometrial biopsy. Indeed the high estradiol levels seen with hMG, although reflecting adequate folliculogenesis, may actually be luteolytic, and it has been suggested that combination clomiphene-hMG-hCG therapy may be more effective, the antiestrogenic action of clomiphene ameliorating the effects of hyperestrogenism on the corpus luteum.

F. The success of these therapies varies according to patient selection criteria. Pregnancy incidences as high as 85 percent have been reported in couples with pure luteal phase inadequacy who comply with the therapy outlined.

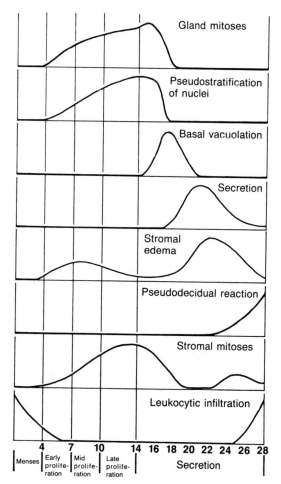

Figure 1 Morphologic criteria used to determine the menstrual status of the endometrium.

References

Daly DC, Walters CA, Soto-Albors CE, Riddick DH. Endometrial biopsy during treatment of luteal phase defects is predictive of therapeutic outcome. Fertil Steril 1983; 40:305-310.

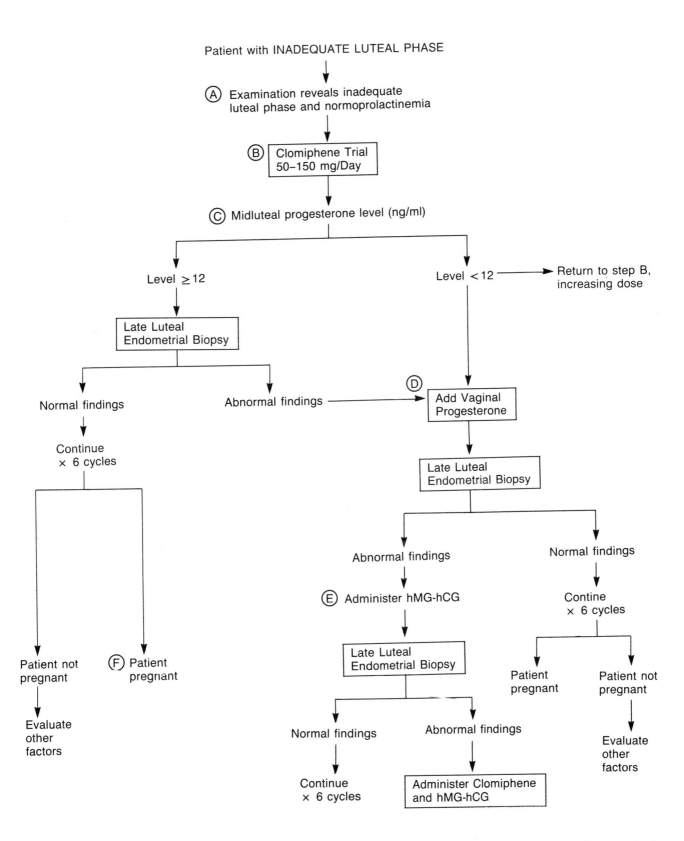

Patient with INADEQUATE LUTEAL PHASE

(A) Examination reveals inadequate
luteal phase and normoprolactinemia

(B) Clomiphene Trial
50–150 mg/Day

(C) Midluteal progesterone level (ng/ml)

Level ≥ 12

Level < 12 → Return to step B,
increasing dose

Late Luteal
Endometrial Biopsy

Normal findings

Abnormal findings →

(D) Add Vaginal
Progesterone

Continue
× 6 cycles

Late Luteal
Endometrial Biopsy

Abnormal findings

Normal findings

(E) Administer hMG-hCG

Contine
× 6 cycles

Patient not
pregnant

(F) Patient
pregnant

Late Luteal
Endometrial Biopsy

Patient
pregnant

Patient not
pregnant

Evaluate
other
factors

Normal findings

Abnormal findings

Evaluate
other
factors

Continue
× 6 cycles

Administer Clomiphene
and hMG-hCG

DiZerega GS, Hodgen GD. Luteal phase dysfunction infertility: a sequel to aberrant folliculogenesis. Fertil Steril 1981; 35:489-499.

Jones GS, Maffezzoli RD, Strott CA, Ross GT, Kaplan G. Pathophysiology of reproductive failure after clomiphene-induced ovulation. Am J Obstet Gynecol 1970; 108:847-867.

Olson JL, Rebar RW, Schreiber JR, Vaitukaitis JL. Shortened luteal phase after ovulation induction with human menopausal gonadotropin and human chorionic gonadotropin. Fertil Steril 1983; 39:284-291.

Shangold M, Berkeley A, Gray J. Both midluteal serum progesterone levels and late luteal endometrial histology should be assessed in all infertile women. Fertil Steril 1983; 40:627-630.

Wentz AC, Herbert CM, Maxson WS, Garner CH. Outcome of progesterone treatment of luteal phase inadequacy. Fertil Steril 1984; 41:856–862.

HYPERSTIMULATION SYNDROME: DIAGNOSIS

Robert G. Brzyski, M.D.
Ervin E. Jones, M.D., Ph.D.
Stephen P. Boyers, M.D.

A. The ovarian hyperstimulation syndrome is a potentially life threatening complication of ovulation induction therapy. The diagnosis is made and the severity of the syndrome is determined by a combination of the history, physical examination, ultrasonography, and laboratory data. This syndrome is rare unless human chorionic gonadotropin (hCG) is administered to trigger ovulation. Most cases occur with pre-hCG serum estradiol levels greater than 2,000 pg per milliliter, but lower estrogen levels do not exclude development of the syndrome. Symptoms commonly develop 3 to 10 days after hCG administration. Abdominal pain, distention, and nausea are universal in all but the mildest cases.

B. Ovarian hyperstimulation has been classified as mild, moderate, or severe on the basis of ovarian size, determined by pelvic examination and ultrasonography. Patient management, however, is based on both the degree of ovarian enlargement and the presence or absence of associated problems, including ascites, pleural effusion, postural hypotension, vomiting, dyspnea, hemoconcentration, hyperkalemia, and abnormal renal function. A major decision is whether to hospitalize patients who have the hyperstimulation syndrome. Although most patients with mild hyperstimulation can be managed at home, all those with ovaries larger than 12.0 cm should be hospitalized. Patients who have moderate hyperstimulation also may require hospitalization in the presence of ancillary problems.

C. Mild hyperstimulation is defined as ovarian enlargement less than 7.0 cm. In the absence of ascites, pulmonary or gastrointestinal symptoms, or other problems these patients are candidates for outpatient management. Moderate hyperstimulation, with ovarian enlargement 7.0 to 12.0 cm, is most frequently associated with other problems requiring hospitalization, but in the absence of ascites, pleural effusion, hypovolemia, vomiting, dyspnea, hemoconcentration, or electrolyte or renal abnormalities, these patients also may be cautiously managed at home. Patients with severe hyperstimulation usually have ancillary problems as well as marked ovarian enlargement, and all these women, regardless of symptoms, should be hospitalized. The details of therapy for hyperstimulation syndrome are discussed separately (p 42).

References

Engel T, Jewelewicz R, Dyrenfurth I, Speroff L, Vande Wiele RL. Ovarian hyperstimulation syndrome. Am J Obstet Gynecol 1972; 112:1052–1060.

Radwanska E. Induction of ovulation. Obstet Gynecol Annu 1983; 12:227–257.

Schenker JG, Weinstein D. Ovarian hyperstimulation syndrome: a current study. Fertil Steril 1978; 30:255–268.

Shapiro AJ, Thomas T, Epstein M. Management of hyperstimulation syndrome. Fertil Steril 1977; 28:237–240.

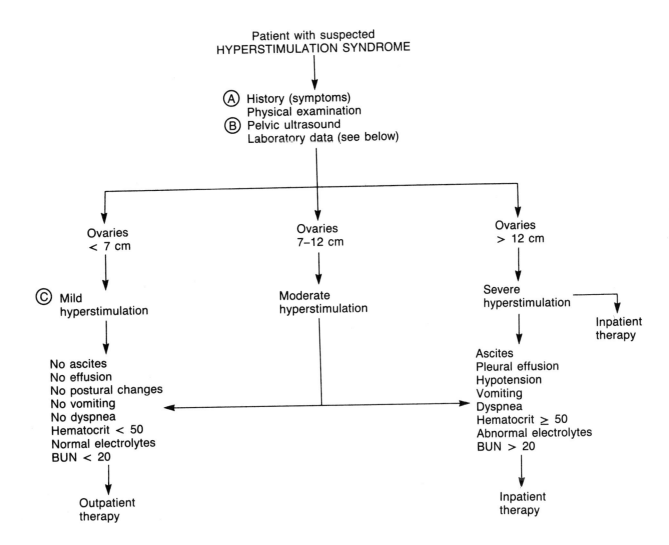

Patient with suspected
HYPERSTIMULATION SYNDROME

Ⓐ History (symptoms)
Physical examination
Ⓑ Pelvic ultrasound
Laboratory data (see below)

Ovaries
< 7 cm

Ovaries
7–12 cm

Ovaries
> 12 cm

Ⓒ Mild
hyperstimulation

Moderate
hyperstimulation

Severe
hyperstimulation

Inpatient
therapy

No ascites
No effusion
No postural changes
No vomiting
No dyspnea
Hematocrit < 50
Normal electrolytes
BUN < 20

Ascites
Pleural effusion
Hypotension
Vomiting
Dyspnea
Hematocrit ≥ 50
Abnormal electrolytes
BUN > 20

Outpatient
therapy

Inpatient
therapy

HYPERSTIMULATION SYNDROME: THERAPY

Robert G. Brzyski, M.D.
Ervin E. Jones, M.D., Ph.D.
Stephen P. Boyers, M.D.

A. The first decision to be made in the management of ovarian hyperstimulation is whether hospitalization is required. All patients with severe hyperstimulation should be hospitalized regardless of ancillary findings. Most patients with mild hyperstimulation and many with moderate hyperstimulation can be managed at home, but in either group the development of ancillary problems requires hospitalization.

B. The natural conclusion of ovarian hyperstimulation is spontaneous resolution. Therefore, management of patients with the ovarian hyperstimulation syndrome centers on supportive measures. All patients require bed rest and daily weight measurements. Serial human chorionic gonadotropin (hCG) measurements are used to detect pregnancy and predict the severity of the syndrome. In addition, hospitalized patients should be monitored with serial hematocrit, electrolyte, blood urea nitrogen (BUN), and creatinine levels. The fluid status should be carefully monitored. Clinical resolution usually occurs within 7 to 14 days in nonpregnant women but may require 30 days when pregnancy occurs and endogenous hCG provides additional ovarian stimulation.

C. With progression of the syndrome, oliguria is common although tolerable if the BUN and creatinine levels are stable and the urine sodium level is low. Controversy exists about the management of persistent severe oliguria. Volume expanders, such as dextran, albumin, or normal saline, contribute to third space volume, but withholding them in a patient with hypovolemia can lead to renal damage secondary to hypoperfusion. Salt and fluid restriction should be the initial approach to management, with attempts at volume expansion reserved for patients with previously compromised renal function or with marked hypotension. Appropriate consultation should be sought in these circumstances.

D. Electrolyte disturbances reflect renal responses to a decrease in intravascular volume. Hyperkalemia is potentially most serious and should be treated with exchange resins if electrocardiographic changes occur. However, the sodium content of exchange resins may stimulate ascites formation. As in the case of rising BUN and creatinine levels, medical consultation should be obtained.

E. Hemoconcentration combined with extremely high circulating estrogen levels may lead to a state of hypercoagulability, and thrombosis can occur. Prophylactic heparin use has not been advocated, despite its theoretic attractiveness. A fall in the hematocrit level may herald resolution of the syndrome if accompanied by diuresis but may also reflect intraperitoneal hemorrhage secondary to ovarian rupture or torsion. If there is clinical deterioration, laparotomy with conservative surgery to attain hemostasis may be required.

F. In a severe case of the ovarian hyperstimulation syndrome, ascites and pleural effusions may compromise respiratory function. Patients with hyperstimulation who experience dyspnea should be evaluated by chest x-ray examination for the presence of pleural fluid. Pleural effusions usually resolve with fluid and salt restriction, although thoracentesis also provides temporary relief. Routine paracentesis should be avoided in the presence of large cystic ovaries because the risk of rupture and hemorrhage is significant. Prevention of ovarian hyperstimulation requires the judicious use of ultrasonography and serum estradiol measurements during ovulation induction. Therapy with hCG should be withheld if serum estradiol levels reach 2,000 pg per milliliter. Severe ovarian hyperstimulation is rare with estradiol levels lower than 2,000 pg per milliliter.

References

Eugel T, Jewelewicz R, Dyrenfurth I, Speroff L, Vande Wiele RL. Ovarian hyperstimulation syndrome. Am J Obstet Gynecol 1972; 112:1052–1060.

Nuosu UC, Corson SL, Bolognese RJ. Hyperstimulation and multiple side effects of menotropin therapy: a case report. J Reprod Med 1974; 12:117–120.

Radwanska E. Induction of ovulation. Obstet Gynecol Annu 1983; 12:227–257.

Shapiro AJ, Thomas T, Epstein M. Management of hyperstimulation syndrome. Fertil Steril 1977; 28:237–240.

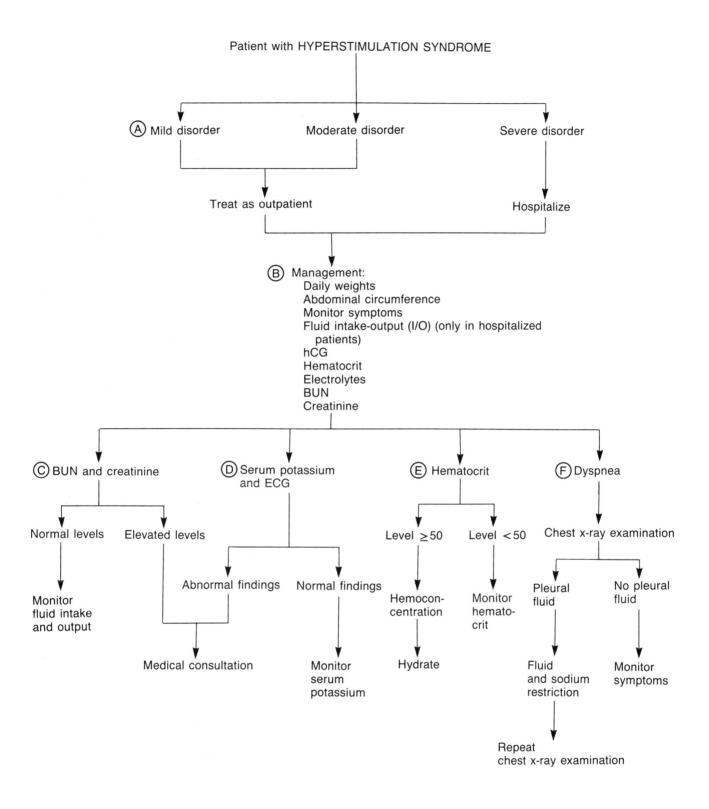

Patient with HYPERSTIMULATION SYNDROME

Ⓐ Mild disorder   Moderate disorder   Severe disorder

Treat as outpatient   Hospitalize

Ⓑ Management:
  Daily weights
  Abdominal circumference
  Monitor symptoms
  Fluid intake-output (I/O) (only in hospitalized
    patients)
  hCG
  Hematocrit
  Electrolytes
  BUN
  Creatinine

Ⓒ BUN and creatinine   Ⓓ Serum potassium   Ⓔ Hematocrit   Ⓕ Dyspnea
                               and ECG

Normal levels   Elevated levels   Level ≥ 50   Level < 50   Chest x-ray examination

                     Abnormal findings   Normal findings

Monitor   Hemocon-   Monitor   Pleural   No pleural
fluid intake   centration   hemato-   fluid   fluid
and output   crit

                Medical consultation   Monitor   Hydrate   Fluid   Monitor
                                        serum   and sodium   symptoms
                                        potassium   restriction

                                                                                  Repeat
                                                                                  chest x-ray examination

CERVICAL FACTOR EVALUATION

Stephen P. Boyers, M.D.
Romaine B. Bayless, M.D.

A. Cervical factors account for about 10 percent of the cases of female infertility. A history of cervical surgery such as conization, cryotherapy, or cautery may increase the suspicion of a cervical factor, although there is good evidence that these procedures do not necessarily impair fertility. Regardless of the history, the postcoital test (PCT) is the mainstay of any cervical factor evaluation. To be meaningful the postcoital test must be done during the preovulatory phase of an ovulatory cycle.

B. A normal postcoital test, defined as good quality cervical mucus and more than 10 progressively motile sperm per high power field, is reassuring, implying good semen quality, ejaculatory potency, and receptive cervical mucus. When infertility continues, the postcoital test should be repeated every 6 months to insure that no change has occurred. The significance of cervical steno-sis with a normal PCT is unclear, but if infertility persists, treatment may be considered.

C. The significance of an abnormal PCT is controversial, since intraperitoneal sperm have been recovered at laparoscopy following a poor PCT. Although some patients conceive despite a poor PCT, we still believe that an abnormal test result deserves attention, especially if infertility continues and other factors are eliminated. The definition of an abnormal PCT is also controversial. The complete absence of motile sperm or the finding of less than five motile sperm per high power field warrants concern and further evaluation.

D. Poor quality cervical mucus despite optimal preovulatory timing and normal results on semen analysis indicates a cervical cause of the abnormal PCT. Cervical cultures for *Chlamydia* and Ureaplasma may be helpful in directing antibiotic therapy.

E. When the PCT is abnormal despite the presence of good quality midcycle cervical mucus, an in vitro test of sperm-mucus penetration is helpful in distinguishing cervical from male causes. The semen analysis gives additional information. When the results of semen analysis and in vitro mucus penetration testing point to male factors, attention is focused away from the cervix. When semen analysis results are normal and in vitro testing indicates a cervical factor, immunologic testing by the immuno-bead test is indicated. In the absence of antisperm anti-bodies, the diagnosis of idiopathic cervical factor infertility is made. Husband artificial insemination may be beneficial.

F. When cultures are negative, poor quality mucus may improve with estrogen, Pergonal, or cryotherapy. If these empiric and unproven treatments fail to normalize mucus quality, husband artificial insemination, using an intrauterine technique with washed, migrated sperm, may be worthwhile.

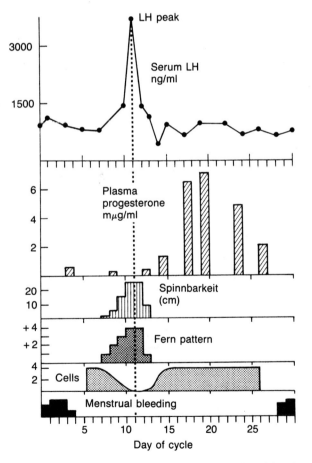

Figure 1 Properties of cervical mucus in relation to the mid-cycle luteinizing hormone peak. Spinnbarkeit and ferning are maximal and cellularity is minimal immediately prior to ovulation.

References

Alexander NJ. Antibodies to human spermatozoa impede sperm penetration of cervical mucus or hamster eggs. Fertil Steril 1984; 41:433–439.

Asch RH. Laparoscopic recovery of sperm from peritoneal fluid in patients with negative or poor Sims-Huhner test. Fertil Steril 1976; 27:1111–1114.

Buller RE, Jones HW III. Pregnancy following cervical coniza-tion. Am J Obstet Gynecol 1982; 142:506–512.

Davajan V, Nakamura RM, Kharma K. Spermatozoan transport in cervical mucus. Obstet Gynecol Surv 1970; 25:1–43.

Katz DF, Overstreet JW, Hanson FW. A new quantitative test for sperm penetration into cervical mucus. Fertil Steril 1980; 33:179–186.

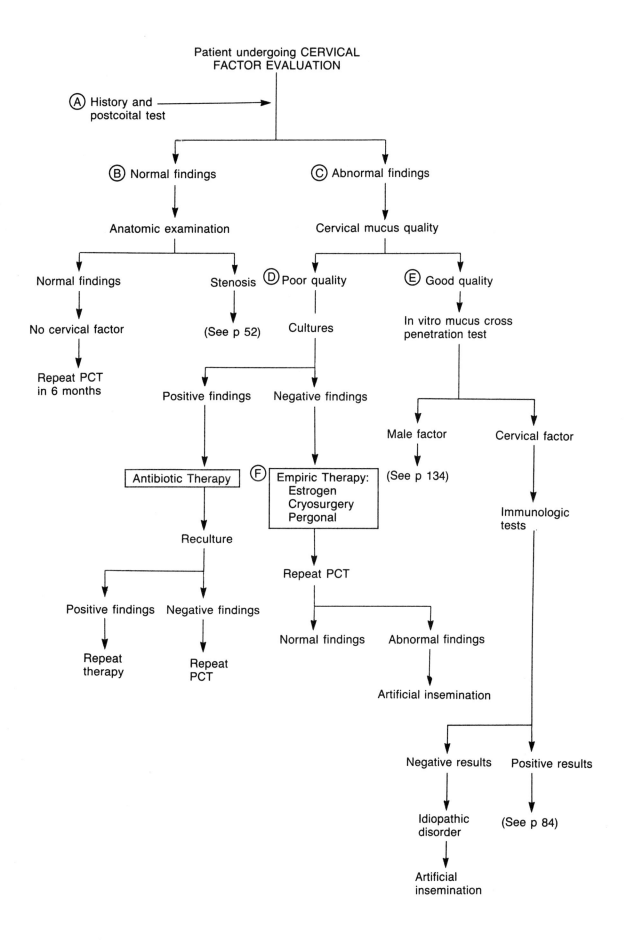

Patient undergoing CERVICAL
FACTOR EVALUATION

(A) History and
postcoital test

(B) Normal findings

(C) Abnormal findings

Anatomic examination

Cervical mucus quality

Normal findings

Stenosis

(D) Poor quality

(E) Good quality

No cervical factor

(See p 52)

Cultures

In vitro mucus cross
penetration test

Repeat PCT
in 6 months

Positive findings

Negative findings

Male factor

Cervical factor

Antibiotic Therapy

(F) Empiric Therapy:
Estrogen
Cryosurgery
Pergonal

(See p 134)

Reculture

Repeat PCT

Immunologic
tests

Positive findings

Negative findings

Normal findings

Abnormal findings

Repeat
therapy

Repeat
PCT

Artificial insemination

Negative results

Positive results

Idiopathic
disorder

(See p 84)

Artificial
insemination

POSTCOITAL TEST: CERVICAL COMPONENT

Romaine B. Bayless, M.D.
Stephen P. Boyers, M.D.

A. This algorithm and its companion on the sperm component offer a stepwise approach to the postcoital test (PCT) for the evaluation of cervical factor infertility. The postcoital or Sims-Huhner test should be done during the preovulatory portion of the menstrual cycle. The timing is identical to that for scheduling artificial insemination, by a combination of the basal body temperature (BBT) pattern, urinary luteinizing hormone (LH) level, and cervical score. The couple should abstain from intercourse for 2 days prior to the test, since it takes 48 hours to replete sperm reserves. The optimal interval is controversial, with recommendations ranging from 1 to 12 hours. We try to do the test within 6 hours after coitus. Patients should be cautioned to avoid lubricant creams, jellies, or ointments and not to douche after coitus.

B. When the cervical score is abnormal, with a closed cervical os and scant, cloudy, thick, cellular cervical mucus, the first thought should be to evaluate timing. Patients should be charting BBTs, and many will be following urinary LH with home monitoring kits. If timing is late and ovulation has already occurred, a change in BBT pattern or urinary LH levels should be apparent.

C. An accurate assessment of sperm factors after intercourse can be made only in the presence of optimal midcycle cervical mucus. Even the healthiest, hardiest sperm do poorly in the scant, thick, cellular mucus found at times other than midcycle. The cervical score quantitates cervical mucus volume, spinnbarkeit, cellularity, ferning, and the state of the cervical os (Fig. 1). Under normal circumstances the cervical os at midcycle is open, and there is an abundant amount of clear, thin, stretchy cervical mucus cascading from the cervical os. Microscopically, midcycle mucus is acellular and demonstrates pronounced ferning.

D. In the absence of these changes it can be assumed either that timing is early or that there is a cervical factor. Serial PCT measurements every 48 hours are helpful. If the cervical score is normal on repeat testing, the first test was indeed early. If the score remains abnormal, timing should be re-evaluated. If the phase is still preovulatory, the PCT should be repeated. If it is postovulatory, the earlier test 48 hours before was optimally timed and the problem is with the cervix itself, either an anatomic problem, such as cervical stenosis or cervicitis, or idiopathic "hostile" cervical mucus. Those topics are each addressed separately in the following pages.

References

Collins JA, So Y, Wilson EH, Wrixon W, Casper RF. The postcoital test as a predictor of pregnancy among 355 infertile couples. Fertil Steril 1984; 41:703-708.

Davajan V, Kunitake GM. Fractional in-vivo and in-vitro examination of postcoital cervical mucus in the human. Fertil Steril 1969; 20:197–210.

Harrison RF. The diagnostic and therapeutic potential of the postcoital test. Fertil Steril 1981; 36:71-75.

Insler V, Melmed H, Serr D, Lunenfeld B. The cervical score. Int J Gynecol Obstet 1972; 10:223–228.

Moghissi KS. Postcoital test: physiologic basis, technique and interpretation. Fertil Steril 1976; 27:117–129.

Scott JZ, Nakamura RM, Mutch J, Davajan V. The cervical factor in infertility: diagnosis and treatment. Fertil Steril 1977; 28:1289–1294.

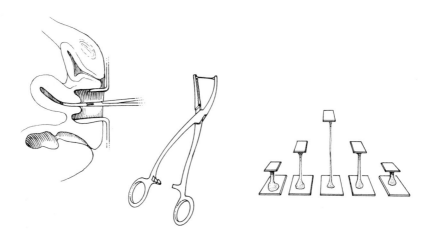

Figure 1 Evaluation of cervical mucus one day before ovulation. Mucus is removed from the cervix and evaluated for color, clarity, stretchability and drying pattern on glass slides.

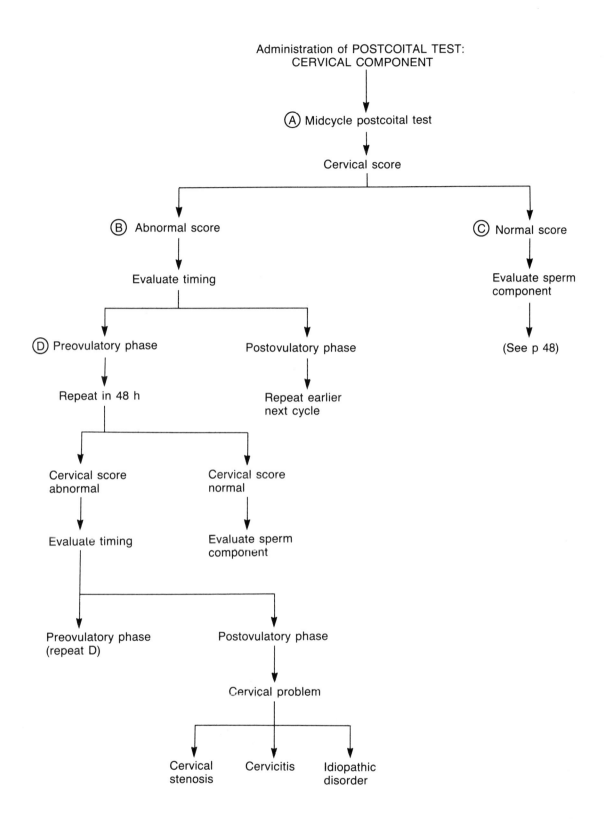

Administration of POSTCOITAL TEST:
CERVICAL COMPONENT

Ⓐ Midcycle postcoital test

Cervical score

Ⓑ Abnormal score

Ⓒ Normal score

Evaluate timing

Evaluate sperm
component

Ⓓ Preovulatory phase

Postovulatory phase

(See p 48)

Repeat in 48 h

Repeat earlier
next cycle

Cervical score
abnormal

Cervical score
normal

Evaluate timing

Evaluate sperm
component

Preovulatory phase
(repeat D)

Postovulatory phase

Cervical problem

Cervical
stenosis

Cervicitis

Idiopathic
disorder

POSTCOITAL TEST: SPERM COMPONENT

Romaine B. Bayless, M.D.
Stephen P. Boyers, M.D.

A. The most difficult and most important aspect of the post-coital test (PCT) is midcycle timing, as judged by the basal body temperature pattern, urinary luteinizing hormone level, and cervical score.

B. Poorly timed tests should be repeated. Persistently poor quality cervical mucus, despite optimal timing, identifies a cervical factor.

C. Good quality midcycle mucus in a patient with a normal cervical score allows an evaluation of sperm penetration and sperm-mucus interaction. The first step should be microscopic examination of a sample of mucus placed on a clean glass slide and covered with a coverslip. Mucus should be taken from within the cervical canal rather than from the exocervix by first wiping away exocervical mucus with a cotton swab. In a couple with a normal semen analysis and good quality cervical mucus (Fig. 1), the absence of sperm in mucus at microscopic examination implies either a coital problem or a problem with sperm-mucus interaction. The next step is evaluation of sperm in the vaginal pool.

D. When initial microscopic examination of cervical mucus reveals the presence of sperm, their motility should be evaluated. The quality of the test is judged by the number of progressively motile sperm per high power field (hpf), not the total number of sperm. Motile sperm with only motility-in-place, or "shaking" motility, are abnormal and should arouse a suspicion of antisperm antibodies. The definition of a normal postcoital test is con-troversial. Certainly the absence of motile sperm is abnormal and deserves follow-up with repeat testing and an in vitro mucus cross penetration test. A normal PCT, defined as good quality cervical mucus and 10 or more progressively motile sperm per hpf, is reassuring and implies good semen quality, ejaculatory potency, and receptive cervical mucus. Intermediate quality test results, with one to nine motile sperm per hpf, are less reassuring and warrant follow-up and consideration of in vitro mucus cross penetration testing.

E. When sperm are present in the vaginal pool but absent in cervical mucus, the postcoital test should be repeated. A similar picture on repeat PCT suggests either a sperm factor or "impenetrable" cervical mucus, either of which may be associated with antisperm antibodies. An in vitro mucus cross penetration test can be used to distinguish between cervical and sperm problems. When motile sperm are present in mucus on repeat examination, their numbers and progressive motility should be quantitated.

F. The absence of sperm in both the cervical mucus and the vaginal fluid samples suggests a coital problem. The husband may have been impotent owing to the stress of scheduled intercourse. Couples may be embarrassed to volunteer this information and should be reassured that the problem is a common and transient one. Uninformed couples may have had "sex" without having had vaginal intercourse, unaware of the importance of intravaginal ejaculation. Retrograde ejaculation may present the same picture, as may azoospermia. The latter is evident from semen analysis, and retrograde ejaculation is apparent on examination of a postcoital urine sample.

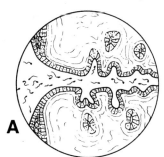

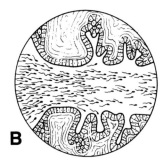

Figure 1 Cervical canal: *A*, a narrow cervical canal with scant mucus impedes sperm migration; *B*, a broad cervical canal with thin watery mucus enhances sperm migration.

References

Davajan V, Kunitake GM. Fractional in-vivo and in-vitro examination of postcoital cervical mucus in the human. Fertil Steril 1969; 20:197.

Giner J, Merino G, Luna J, Aznar R. Evaluation of the Sims-Huhner postcoital tests in fertile couples. Fertil Steril 1974; 25:145-148.

Glass RH, Mroueh A. The postcoital test and semen analysis. Fertil Steril 1967; 18:314-317.

Jette NT, Glass RH. Prognostic value of the postcoital test. Fertil Steril 1972; 23:29-32.

MacLeod J, Martens F, Silberman C, Sobrero AJ. The postcoital and postinsemination cervical mucus and semen quality. Stud Fertil 1958; 10:41-51.

Moghissi KS. Postcoital test: physiologic basis, technique and interpretation. Fertil Steril 1976; 27:117–129.

Scott JZ, Nakamura RM, Mutch J, Davajan V. The cervical factor in infertility: diagnosis and treatment. Fertil Steril 1977; 28:1289–1294.

Tredway DR. The interpretation and significance of the fractional postcoital test. Am J Obstet Gynecol 1976; 124:352–355.

Tredway DR, Buchanan GC, Drake TS. Comparison of the fractional postcoital tests and semen analysis. Am J Obstet Gynecol 1978; 130:647–652.

Tredway DR, Settlage DS, Nakamura RM, et al. The significance of timing for the postcoital evaluation of cervical mucus. Am J Obstet Gynecol 1975; 121:387–393.

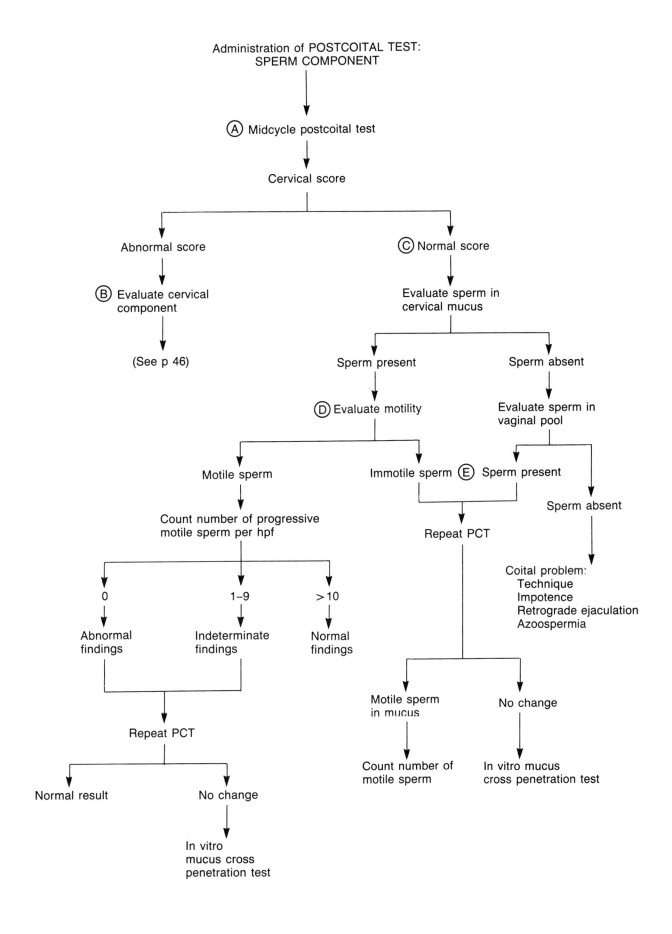

IN VITRO MUCUS CROSS PENETRATION TEST

Romaine B. Bayless, M.D.
Bruce S. Shapiro, M.D.
Stephen P. Boyers, M.D.

A. An abnormal postcoital test (PCT) in an ovulatory patient with optimal midcycle timing, a normal cervical score, and a husband with normal semen analysis could be caused by either sperm or cervical factors. The in vitro mucus cross penetration test is designed to distinguish between sperm and cervical factors and to direct further testing. The test is done at midcycle and requires the availability of periovulatory donor mucus and donor sperm. An active artificial insemination by donor (AID) program provides access to both.

B. Two different techniques have been used for in vitro testing of sperm-mucus interaction: the slide method and the capillary tube technique. The slide method, originally described by Miller and Kurzrok, is more qualitative and less quantifiable (Fig. 1). It involves placing a drop of cervical mucus and a drop of semen next to one another on a glass slide. A coverslip placed gently over the adjacent drops brings them into contact without mixing. Sperm penetrate the semen-mucus interface. The capillary tube method, as originally described by Kremer and modified by Overstreet, requires a flat, optically true glass capillary tube and a small reservoir for semen (Fig. 2). Cervical mucus is drawn into the capillary tube and semen is placed in the reservoir. The base of the capillary tube is placed into the sperm reservoir. Movement of sperm into the mucus column can be observed directly under the microscope. The distance and density of linear sperm penetration are recorded at fixed time intervals. The capillary tube method is preferred because it is more quantitative.

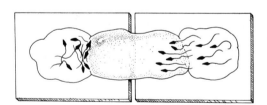

Figure 1 In vitro slide penetration test.

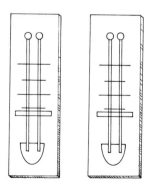

Figure 2 Capillary tube techniques for in vitro testing of sperm-mucus interaction.

C. As controls, donor sperm are tested with donor mucus. Poor penetration requires new controls and scrutiny of the testing procedure. Normal penetration of donor sperm into donor mucus insures a valid test.

D. Normal penetration of donor mucus by donor sperm and abnormal penetration of patient mucus by husband sperm set the stage for a crossover test to check donor mucus with husband sperm and patient mucus with donor sperm.

E. If the husband's sperm penetrate the patient's mucus normally in vitro but not after intercourse, a vaginal factor should be considered and the postcoital test repeated. A normal PCT requires no further testing. Persistence of an abnormal PCT suggests an unexplained vaginal factor. Low semen volume may also be related. To test the vaginal factor hypothesis, we perform intra-cervical insemination with a Milex cervical cup and do a postinsemination PCT. If sperm-mucus interaction is normal, artificial insemination by husband (AIH) should be continued. If there are still no sperm or very few sperm in the cervical mucus, the discrepancy between in vitro and in vivo tests remains unexplained. A trial of intrauterine insemination (IUI) may be worthwhile.

F. Normal penetration of donor mucus by husband sperm suggests a cervical factor. Failure of husband sperm to penetrate donor mucus points to a sperm factor. An immunobead test is indicated to look for antisperm antibodies.

G. Normal penetration of patient mucus by donor sperm confirms the existence of a sperm factor. Failure of donor sperm to penetrate patient mucus confirms the existence of a cervical factor. Immunologic testing is directed appropriately.

References

Hanson FW, Overstreet JW. The interaction of human spermatozoa with cervical mucus in vivo. Am J Obstet Gynecol 1981; 140:173–178.

Katz DF, Overstreet JW, Hanson FW. A new quantitative test for sperm penetration into cervical mucus. Fertil Steril 1980; 33:179–186.

Kremer J. A simple sperm penetration test. Int J Fertil 1965; 10:209.

Miller EG Jr, Kurzrok R. Biochemical studies of human semen. III. Factors affecting migration of sperm through the cervix. Am J Obstet Gynecol 1932; 24:19–26.

Moghissi KS, Sacco AG, Borin K. Immunologic infertility. I. Cervical mucus antibodies and postcoital test. Am J Obstet Gynecol 1980; 136:941–950.

World Health Organization: Sperm-cervical mucus interaction. In: Belsey MA, Eliasson R, Gallegos AJ, et al, eds. Laboratory manual for the examination of human semen and semen-cervical mucus interaction. Singapore: Press Concern, 1980:33.

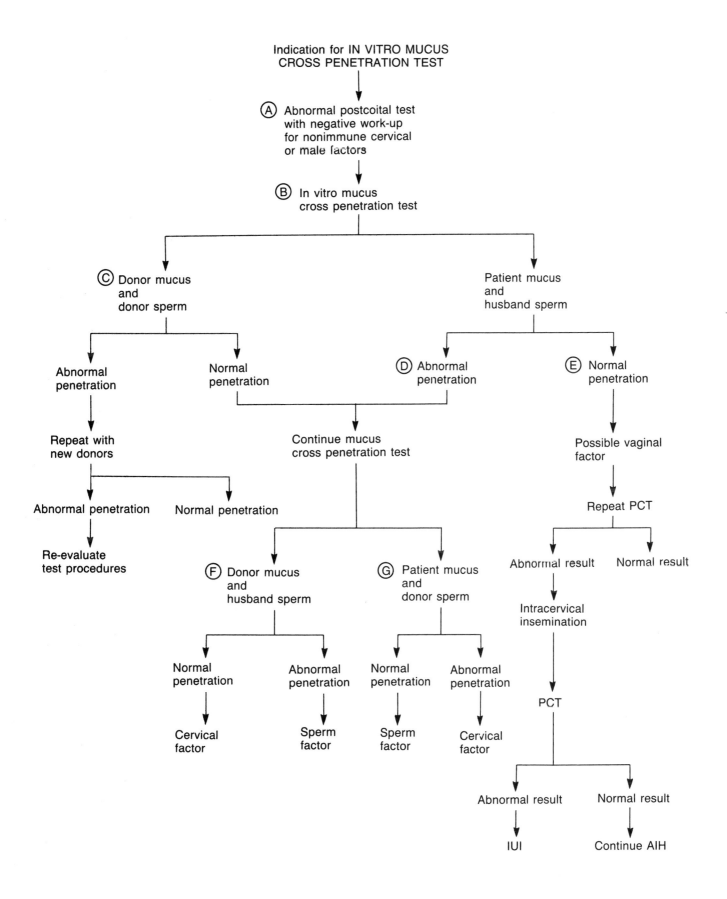

Indication for IN VITRO MUCUS CROSS PENETRATION TEST

Ⓐ Abnormal postcoital test with negative work-up for nonimmune cervical or male factors

Ⓑ In vitro mucus cross penetration test

Ⓒ Donor mucus and donor sperm

Patient mucus and husband sperm

Abnormal penetration

Normal penetration

Ⓓ Abnormal penetration

Ⓔ Normal penetration

Repeat with new donors

Continue mucus cross penetration test

Possible vaginal factor

Abnormal penetration

Normal penetration

Repeat PCT

Re-evaluate test procedures

Ⓕ Donor mucus and husband sperm

Ⓖ Patient mucus and donor sperm

Abnormal result

Normal result

Normal penetration

Abnormal penetration

Normal penetration

Abnormal penetration

Intracervical insemination

Cervical factor

Sperm factor

Sperm factor

Cervical factor

PCT

Abnormal result

Normal result

IUI

Continue AIH

ANATOMIC CERVICAL FACTOR

Romaine B. Bayless, M.D.
Stephen P. Boyers, M.D.

A. An abnormal postcoital test (PCT) with scant cervical mucus, a poor cervical score, cervical stenosis, or an endocervix that is friable and bleeds in response to gentle manipulation may indicate cervical factor infertility with an anatomic basis. Cervical stenosis may be congenital, but most frequently it is the result of prior cervical conization, cautery, or cryosurgery. Although these procedures may compromise the endocervix, cervical surgery does not necessarily impair fertility. Acquired dysmenorrhea following cervical surgery supports a diagnosis of cervical stenosis. Cervical friability and a history of postcoital bleeding may indicate an endocervical polyp or varicosities. A high index of suspicion for cervical neoplasia is essential. A Papanicolaou smear should be evaluated and colposcopy and directed biopsies performed whenever indicated.

B. When the external cervical os appears stenotic, we attempt to pass a small, 2 to 4 mm, curved cervical dilator. Frequently the dilator passes easily, there being no true cervical stenosis, and the external os deagglutinates with little resistance. Bleeding is usually minimal, and endocervical mucus frequently flows from the os when the procedure is done at midcycle. In this case we repeat the postcoital test and proceed accordingly.

C. When the dilator passes easily but stimulates bleeding, we suspect an endocervical polyp or varicosities. Colposcopy is done with an endocervical speculum. The cryoprobe or laser may be useful in treating these endocervical lesions. The postcoital test should be repeated in the second or third cycle following treatment.

D. When the small dilator does not readily pass the internal os, a diagnosis of true cervical stenosis is made. In the absence of a history of cervical trauma or neoplasia a congenital origin is suspected. Tight cervical stenosis is a difficult problem, which is not easily overcome, but it is important to try to establish a cervical opening that is at least sufficient to perform hysterosalpingography and endometrial biopsy and to allow for a trial of intrauterine insemination (IUI).

E. Application of estrogen vaginal cream (Premarin or Dienestrol) twice daily for 3 to 4 weeks may soften a stenotic cervix and allow the small dilator to pass. In this case we sometimes have been able to dilate the cervix with Lamicel or *Laminaria* without operative dilation. Repeated office dilation is usually necessary to prevent restenosis, and the result is often disappointing. When office attempts to overcome cervical stenosis fail, operative dilation combined with hysteroscopy-laparoscopy, endometrial biopsy, and tubal dye study is required. These patients also may have intrauterine synechiae involving the lower uterine segment. We have treated these patients with lysis of synechiae, insertion of an intrauterine Foley catheter, and high doses of estrogen with some success, at least in re-establishing a patent cervical os that allows intrauterine insemination.

F. The postcoital test seldom reverts to normal following such procedures. A trial of intrauterine insemination is warranted when cervical mucus continues to be of poor quality.

References

Bjerre B, Eliasson G, Linell F, Soderberg H, Sjoberg N-O. Conization as only treatment of carcinoma in situ of the uterine cervix. Am J Obstet Gynecol 1976; 125:143-152.

Darney PD. Dilatation—old and new techniques. Contemp Obstet Gynecol 1985; 26:41-54.

Davajan V, Nakamura RM. The cervical factor. In: Behrman SJ, Kistner RW, eds. Progress in infertility. 2nd ed. Boston: Little, Brown, 1975:37.

Jones HW III, Buller RE. The treatment of cervical intraepithelial neoplasia by cone biopsy. Am J Obstet Gynecol 1980; 137:882–886.

Pittaway DE, Daniell J, Maxson W, Boehm F. Reconstruction of the cervical canal after complete postconization obstruction: a case report. J Reprod Med 1984; 29:339-340.

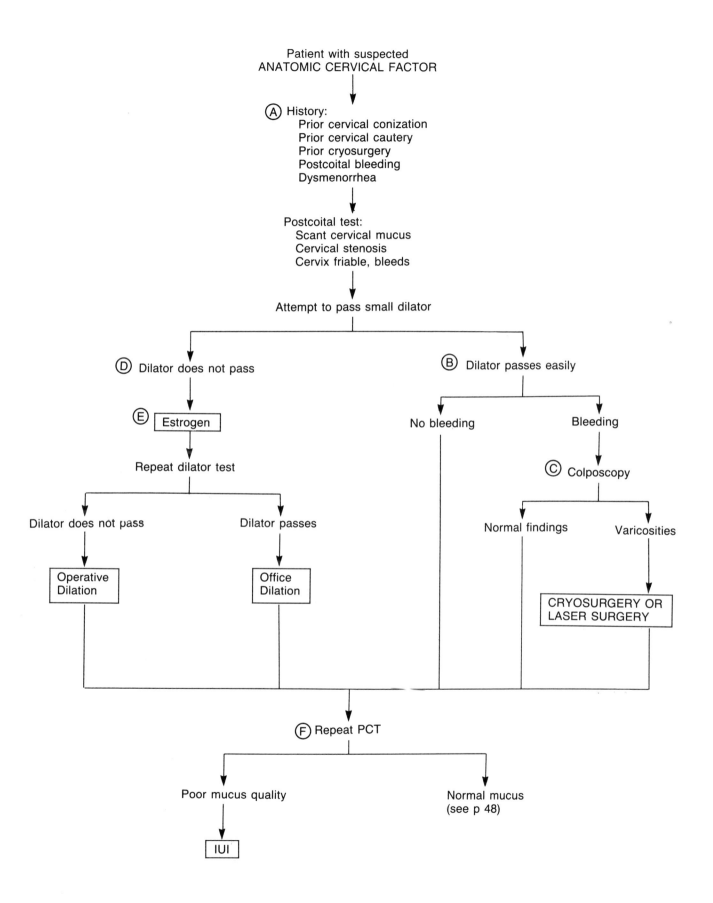

Patient with suspected
ANATOMIC CERVICAL FACTOR
↓

(A) History:
    Prior cervical conization
    Prior cervical cautery
    Prior cryosurgery
    Postcoital bleeding
    Dysmenorrhea
↓

Postcoital test:
    Scant cervical mucus
    Cervical stenosis
    Cervix friable, bleeds
↓

Attempt to pass small dilator

(D) Dilator does not pass

(E) Estrogen

Repeat dilator test

Dilator does not pass

Dilator passes

Operative Dilation

Office Dilation

(B) Dilator passes easily

No bleeding

Bleeding

(C) Colposcopy

Normal findings

Varicosities

CRYOSURGERY OR LASER SURGERY

(F) Repeat PCT

Poor mucus quality

Normal mucus (see p 48)

IUI

CERVICITIS

Romaine B. Bayless, M.D.
Stephen P. Boyers, M.D.

A. An abnormal postcoital test (PCT) with thick, purulent, cellular cervical mucus, with or without a vulvovaginal discharge, erythema, or lesions, despite optimal midcycle timing may indicate cervical factor infertility with an infectious etiology. The cervix may be red or granular. Nabothian cysts may form as the result of occlusion of endocervical glands.

B. Both primary cervical disease and disease secondary to primary vaginal infection can produce leukorrhea of cervical origin. Therefore, the vaginal discharge should be examined microscopically for organisms causing vaginitis. At the same time the cervix should be cultured for organisms. If dilution of a small amount of vaginal discharge with 10 percent potassium hydroxide reveals oval budding cells with pseudomycelia, a diagnosis of candidiasis may be made. Treatment with one of the several antifungal drugs (e.g., clotrimazole, miconazole, or nystatin) should be instituted. Trichomoniasis, diagnosed by observing motile flagellated organisms in a drop of vaginal discharge mixed with normal saline, should be treated with metronidazole in both partners. The presence of clue cells, vaginal squamous epithelial cells that appear granular owing to organisms on the cell surface, is associated with *Gardnerella vaginalis* infection. The drug of choice in this infection is ampicillin or metronidazole for both the patient and her partner.

C. Positive cervical cultures should direct specific therapy—doxycycline for *Chlamydia* or Ureaplasma infection and an appropriate Center for Disease Control (CDC) protocol for gonorrhea. An alternate approach is to culture for gonococcus only and to empirically treat all patients who have a mucopurulent cervical discharge with doxycycline and culture for *Chlamydia* and Ureaplasma only when the PCT remains abnormal after therapy. Although *Chlamydia's* role in tubal infertility seems well established, its effect on the cervix is less clear and the role of genital mycoplasmas in infertility is in doubt. Controlled trials of doxycycline have failed to significantly improve fertility.

D. When there is no evidence of vaginitis and cervical cultures are completely negative, yet the PCT remains abnormal with poor quality cervical mucus, the diagnosis is idiopathic "hostile" cervical mucus.

References

Friberg J, Gnarpe H. Mycoplasma and human reproductive failure. III. Pregnancies in "infertile" couples treated with doxycycline for T-mycoplasmas. Am J Obstet Gynecol 1973; 116:23–26.

Gump DW, Gibson M, Ashikaga T. Lack of association between genital mycoplasmas and infertility. N Engl J Med 1984; 310:937-941.

Harrison RF, de Louvois J, Blades M, Hurley R. Doxycycline treatment and human infertility. Lancet 1975; 1:605–607.

Novy MJ. Infections as a cause of infertility. In: Sciarra JJ, ed. Gynecology and obstetrics. Vol. 5. Hagerstown: Harper & Row, 1985.

Sweet RL, Schachter J, Landers DV. Chlamydial infections in obstetrics and gynecology. Clin Obstet Gynecol 1983; 26:143–164.

Patient with suspected
INFECTIOUS CERVICAL FACTOR

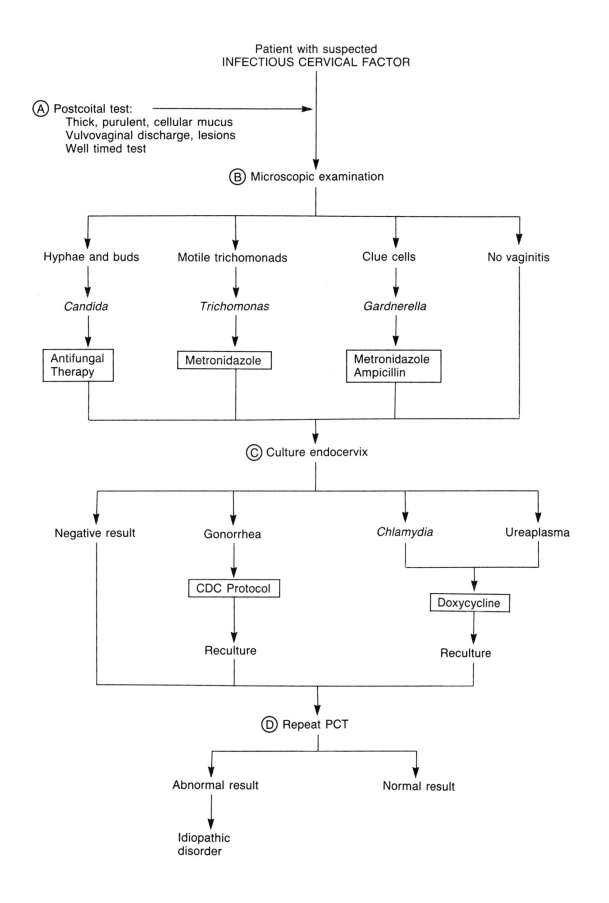

Ⓐ Postcoital test:
    Thick, purulent, cellular mucus
    Vulvovaginal discharge, lesions
    Well timed test

Ⓑ Microscopic examination

| Hyphae and buds | Motile trichomonads | Clue cells | No vaginitis |

Candida   *Trichomonas*   *Gardnerella*

| Antifungal Therapy | Metronidazole | Metronidazole Ampicillin |

Ⓒ Culture endocervix

Negative result   Gonorrhea   *Chlamydia*   Ureaplasma

CDC Protocol

Doxycycline

Reculture   Reculture

Ⓓ Repeat PCT

Abnormal result   Normal result

Idiopathic
disorder

IDIOPATHIC CERVICAL FACTOR

Romaine B. Bayless, M.D.
Stephen P. Boyers, M.D.

A. Periovulatory cervical mucus that is abnormal in quantity or quality without evidence of an infectious or anatomic etiology may be the result of inadequate stimulation of the endocervical mucus-producing cells due to low levels of estrogen or failure of endocervical cells to respond to normal levels of estrogen. If clomiphene citrate has been used to induce ovulation, its antiestrogenic effects may result in decreased mucus production. The rationale, albeit unproven, for much of the empiric approach to therapy for idiopathic hostile cervical mucus is that higher levels of estrogen may improve cervical mucus quantity and quality. There have been no controlled studies to test the effectiveness of this approach.

B. Exogenous estrogen should be given only in the second half of the follicular phase, at a time when endogenous estradiol levels are beginning to rise to the preovulatory peak. Estrogen given earlier in the cycle may suppress gonadotropins prematurely and block or delay ovulation. We have used ethinyl estradiol, 0.01 mg per day on days 6 to 9, increased to 0.02 mg per day on days 10 to 13 of a 28-day cycle. The postcoital test (PCT) is repeated on day 13 and the cervical score is evaluated. If the cervix responds with an improvement in cervical mucus quality, we repeat this regimen monthly for a 6-month trial.

C. Cryosurgery has been used to treat cervical infertility when chronic cervicitis is suspected despite negative cultures or a failure to respond to doxycycline. It is applicable primarily when cervical mucus is present but chronically cellular rather than when scant or absent. There are only anecdotal reports of its efficacy.

D. Pergonal is given as for ovulation induction in anovulatory infertility or in in vitro fertilization (IVF). The rationale for its use in cervical infertility is to stimulate endocervical glands through hyperestrogenism. The risks of multiple gestation and ovarian hyperstimulation and the expense and tedium of daily injections and monitoring should be carefully reviewed with the patient and tubal patency documented before beginning such a trial.

E. If Pergonal fails to normalize the cervical mucus, a trial of intrauterine insemination, with or without Pergonal, may be initiated to bypass the cervical barrier to sperm transport.

References

Check JH, Adelson HG. Improvement of cervical factor by high-dose estrogen and human menopausal gonadotropin therapy with ultrasound monitoring. Obstet Gynecol 1984; 63:179-181.

Check JH, Wu CH, Dietterich C, Lauer CC, Liss J. The treatment of cervical factor with ethinyl estradiol and human menopausal gonadotropins. Int J Fertil 1986; 31:148-152.

Insler V, Melmed H, Serr D, Lunenfeld B. The cervical score. Int J Gynecol Obstet 1972; 10:223-228.

Scott JZ, Nakamura RM, Mutch J, Davajan V. The cervical factor in infertility: diagnosis and treatment. Fertil Steril 1977; 28:1289-1294.

Sher G, Katz M. Inadequate cervical mucus—a cause of "idiopathic" infertility. Fertil Steril 1976; 27:886-891.

Suspected IDIOPATHIC CERVICAL FACTOR

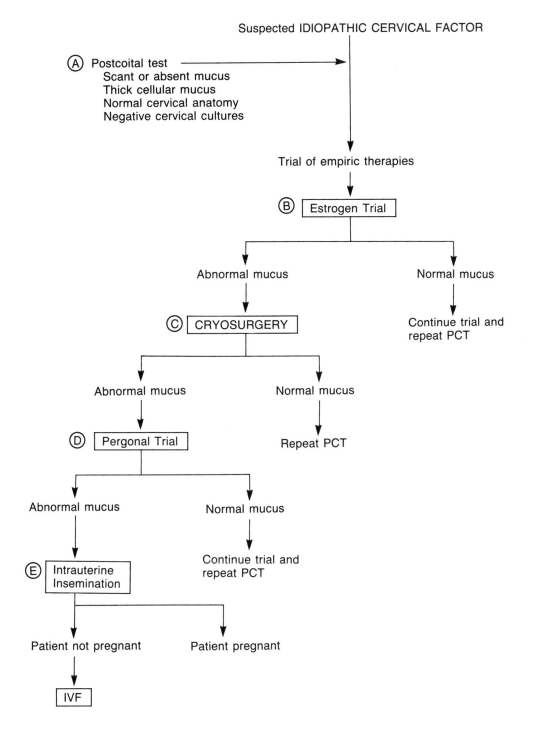

(A) Postcoital test
    Scant or absent mucus
    Thick cellular mucus
    Normal cervical anatomy
    Negative cervical cultures

Trial of empiric therapies

(B) Estrogen Trial

Abnormal mucus

Normal mucus

(C) CRYOSURGERY

Continue trial and
repeat PCT

Abnormal mucus

Normal mucus

(D) Pergonal Trial

Repeat PCT

Abnormal mucus

Normal mucus

(E) Intrauterine
Insemination

Continue trial and
repeat PCT

Patient not pregnant

Patient pregnant

IVF

ENDOMETRIAL FACTORS

Lawrence Grunfeld, M.D.
Mary Lake Polan, M.D., Ph.D.

A. Infection is a predisposing factor in most cases of endometrial damage. The infection can be acute and may resolve without permanent sequelae or can lead to chronic endometritis. It is only when chronic endometritis occurs that impairment of fertility results.

B. The endometrium is most susceptible to trauma in the first 4 weeks post partum. At other times the basalis layer is capable of regeneration. When the endometrium heals with fusion of the anterior and posterior walls, Asherman's syndrome results. This is discussed further on p 64.

C. Endometrial biopsy is important in diagnosing chronic endometritis. The presence of plasma cells in a background of abnormal appearing glands and stroma is diagnostic. When endometritis is suspected, it is best to obtain a biopsy specimen of the endometrium at midcycle so that the normal inflammatory response to menses does not obscure the diagnosis.

D. Hysterosalpingography is usually performed as the initial diagnostic tool in evaluation of the endometrial cavity. When a filling defect is detected, hysteroscopy is usually performed to identify the nature of the disorder. The disorder can often be corrected at the time of hysteroscopy.

E. When the endometrial biopsy reveals chronic endometritis, a course of antibiotics is suggested. Rarely can a definitive organism be identified, as in tuberculosis, which requires specific therapy. In most cases the infection is presumed to be caused by *Chlamydia* or *Mycoplasma*. Both of these organisms are susceptible to doxycycline.

F. Uterine filling defects can be caused by air bubbles, polyps, myomas, septa, or intrauterine synechiae. Hysteroscopy is usually performed after hysterosalpingography to elucidate the nature of the filling defect. Most of these pathologic entities can be treated through the hysteroscope. A detailed discussion of the therapy of Asherman's syndrome is presented on p 66.

References

Czernobelski B. Endometritis and infertility. Fertil Steril 1978; 30:119–140.

Schenker J, Margolioth E. Intrauterine adhesions: an updated appraisal. Fertil Steril 1982; 37:593–610.

Valle R. Clinical management of uterine factors in infertile patients. Semin Reprod Endocrinol 1985; 3:149.

Vasudeva K, Thrasher T, Richart R. Chronic endometritis: clinical and electron microscopic study. Am J Obstet Gynecol 1972; 112:749–758.

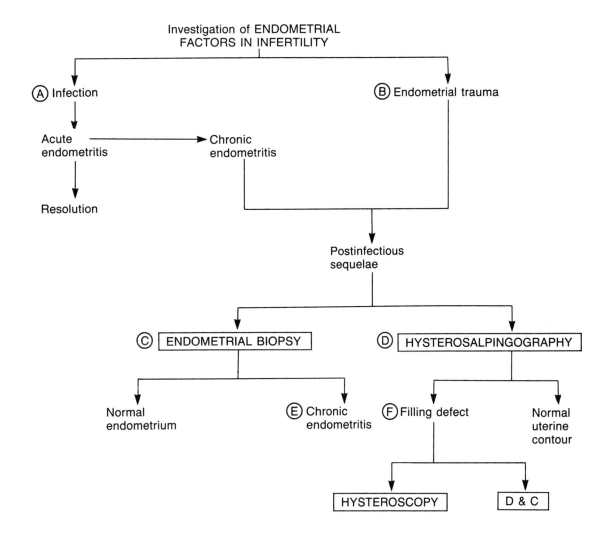

Investigation of ENDOMETRIAL FACTORS IN INFERTILITY

(A) Infection

(B) Endometrial trauma

Acute endometritis → Chronic endometritis

Resolution

Postinfectious sequelae

(C) ENDOMETRIAL BIOPSY

(D) HYSTEROSALPINGOGRAPHY

Normal endometrium

(E) Chronic endometritis

(F) Filling defect

Normal uterine contour

HYSTEROSCOPY

D & C

ACUTE ENDOMETRITIS

Lawrence Grunfeld, M.D.
Mary Lake Polan, M.D., Ph.D.

A. Puerperal acute endometritis is most often limited to the endometrium. Infection of the endometrium is most commonly seen following cesarean section, in prolonged labor with ruptured membranes, and following multiple pelvic examinations. A lower socioeconomic status is an additional risk factor for the development of postpartum endometritis. This type of infection is effectively treated with antibiotics and rarely progresses to chronic endometritis. Acute endometritis is not a common cause of infertility.

B. Acute salpingitis is often associated with endometritis. The endometritis is self-limiting, and infertility is usually secondary to tubal disease. Gonococcal endometritis can develop into chronic endometritis. It is only when chronic endometritis occurs that abnormal implantation results. Resolution of the acute infection is associated with normal conception unless tubal damage has occurred.

C. Instrumentation of the uterus can permit the entry of bacteria into the endometrial cavity. A flare-up of endometritis or salpingitis following instrumentation is sometimes seen. Following hysterosalpingography, approximately 1 to 3 percent of the patients develop upper genital tract infections.

D. Appropriate therapy of acute endometritis results in the resolution of symptoms. The endometrial infection usually resolves without permanent damage to the endometrium. Normal conception can occur unless damage to the fallopian tubes follows the endometrial infection.

E. Chronic endometritis rarely develops after acute endometritis. However, when it does, it occurs most frequently with gonococcal infection, tuberculosis, and viral infections. The management of chronic endometritis is discussed on p 62.

References

Czernobilsky B. Endometritis and infertility. Fertil Steril 1978; 30:119–130.

Duff P. Pathophysiology and management of postcesarean endomyometritis. Obstet Gynecol 1986; 67:269–276.

Stumpf P, March CM. Febrile morbidity following hysterosalpingography: identification of risk factors and recommendations for prophylaxis. Fertil Steril 1980; 33:487–492.

Valle R. Clinical management of uterine factors in infertile patients. Semin Reprod Endocrinol 1985; 3:149.

Patient with ACUTE ENDOMETRITIS

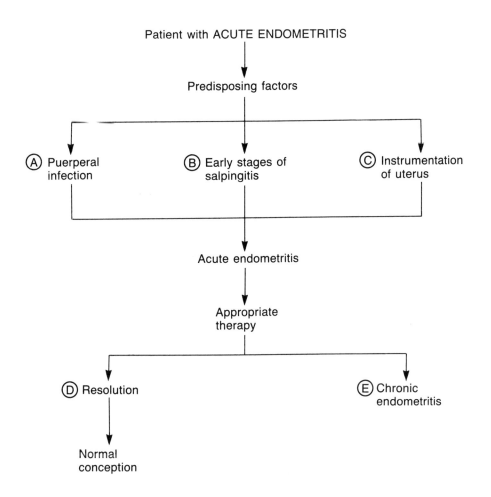

CHRONIC ENDOMETRITIS

Lawrence Grunfeld, M.D.
Mary Lake Polan, M.D., Ph.D.

A. Endometritis is suspected in patients with profuse irregular bleeding, pelvic pain, vaginal discharge, or infertility. Cadena found that 16 percent of the patients with chronic endometritis were asymptomatic.

B. Endometrial biopsy for dating is best performed premenstrually. This is not appropriate for diagnosing endometritis because the inflammatory infiltrate that normally accompanies the premenstrual endometrium can obscure the diagnosis of endometritis. Biopsy performed on days 12 to 14 is suggested for this diagnosis. It is best to obtain at least two samples, since endometritis can be focal in distribution.

C. The highest yield in tuberculous granulomas is obtained from menstrual endometrium. Tuberculous endometritis is seen following hematogenous spread of mycobacteria from another primary locus. It is most common in patients of low socioeconomic backgrounds who reside in regions where tuberculosis is endemic. Culture of menstrual blood can also confirm the diagnosis. If the suspicion is great, a formal curettage during menses should be performed, since the disease can be focal.

D. Chronic endometrial infection can be caused by foreign bodies, bacteria, viruses, and parasites. This is seen in patients with intrauterine devices and may be the mechanism of contraceptive action. Although, *Mycoplasma* has been implicated as a cause of infertility and habitual abortion, this association has been disputed. Chronic endometritis rarely follows acute infection. When chronic endometritis is found in endometrial biopsy specimens, a course of doxycycline, 100 mg twice daily for at least 14 days, is suggested.

E. *Herpesvirus hominis* has not been demonstrated in the endometrium. Cytomegalovirus has been found in the endometrium of patients with spontaneous abortions. Characteristic intranuclear inclusions are seen in this disorder.

F. Tuberculous endometritis is diagnosed with either histologic examination or culture of the menstrual blood. A formal dilation and curettage during menses yields the highest incidence of recovery of tuberculous granulomas. This disease carries a very poor prognosis for fertility and may obliterate the endometrium. If the tubes are involved, surgical correction of adhesions is very rarely successful.

References

Cadena D, Cavanzo F, Leone C, et al. Chronic endometritis. A comparative and clinicopathologic study. Obstet Gynecol 1973; 41:733–738.

Czernobilsky B. Endometritis and infertility. Fertil Steril 1978; 30:119–130.

Gnarp H, Friberg J. Mycoplasma and human reproductive failure. Am J Obstet Gynecol 1972; 114:727–731.

Henderson D, Harkins J, Stitt J. Pelvic tuberculosis. Am J Obstet Gynecol 1966; 94:630–636.

McCracken A, D'Agostino A, Brucks A, et al. Acquired cytomegalovirus infection presenting as viral endometritis. Am J Clin Pathol 1974; 61:556–560.

Patient with CHRONIC ENDOMETRITIS

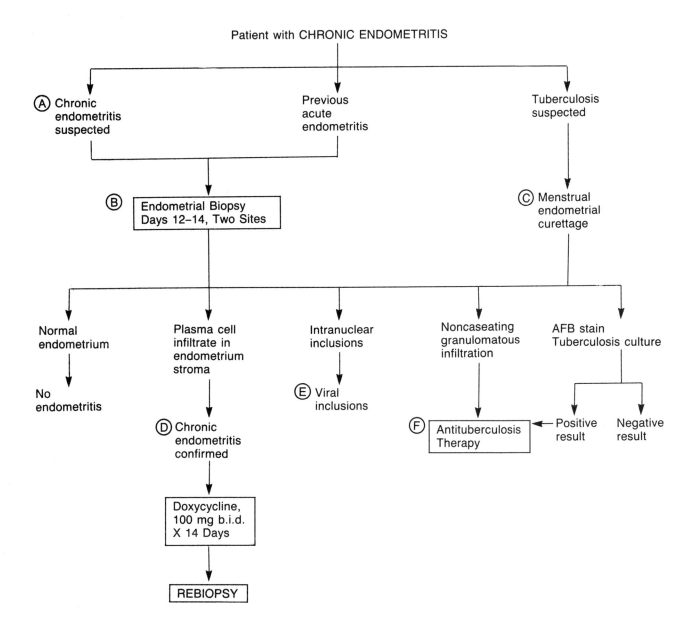

ASHERMAN'S SYNDROME: DIAGNOSIS

Lawrence Grunfeld, M.D.
Mary Lake Polan, M.D., Ph.D.

A. Menstrual disturbance is the most common complaint in Asherman's syndrome, with only 6 percent of the patients having normal menses. Of the menstrual disturbances, amenorrhea and hypomenorrhea are the most common. Prior to proceeding with examination of the uterus, pregnancy and endocrinologic causes of amenorrhea should be investigated.

B. Infertility is a common complaint in patients with endometrial synechiae. In a review of the world literature, Schenker found that 43 percent of the patients with Asherman's syndrome were infertile. Abnormal implantation may occur because of distortion of the endometrial cavity. If the adhesions are in the lower uterine segment, obstruction to penetration by spermatozoa may occur.

C. Habitual abortion is also a common presenting complaint in this syndrome. Fourteen percent of the patients with this diagnosis presented with habitual abortion. Other pregnancy abnormalities include placenta accreta, placenta previa, and premature labor. This is presumably the result of abnormal placentation because of the restriction in the endometrial surface.

D. Pregnancy is a predisposing factor in 90 percent of the cases of Asherman's syndrome. The endometrium is most susceptible to adhesion formation in the first 4 weeks post partum. Schenker's review of the world literature found that 66 percent of the cases occurred after induced abortion or curettage after spontaneous abortion, 20 percent after late postpartum curettage, 2 percent after cesarean section, and 0.6 percent after evacuation of a molar pregnancy. Only 1 percent occurred secondary to trauma in nonpregnant patients. Genital tuberculosis accounted for 4 percent of the cases.

E. Hysterosalpingography is the principal procedure for establishing this diagnosis. In the presence of a normal uterine contour, other causes of infertility or amenorrhea should be investigated. Filling defects do not necessarily correspond to synechiae. The differential diagnosis includes air bubbles, myomas, polyps, and septae, as well as synechiae.

F. When the hysterosalpingogram reveals a filling defect, hysteroscopy should be performed. Hysteroscopy provides a definitive diagnosis as well as the possibility of correction of the defect. Polyps can be removed through the hysteroscope or by curettage. Myomas can often be resected with the hysteroscope if a resectoscope is available. The management of synechiae is discussed on p 66.

References

DeCherney A, Polan ML. Hysteroscopic management of intrauterine lesions and intractable uterine bleeding. Obstet Gynecol 1983; 61:392–397.

Foix A, Bruno R, Davison T, et al. The pathology of postcurettage intrauterine adhesions. Am J Obstet Gynecol 1966; 96:1027–1033.

Jensen P, Stromme W. Amenorrhea secondary to puerperal curettage. Am J Obstet Gynecol 1972; 113:150–157.

Klein ST, Garcia C. Asherman's syndrome: a critique and current review. Fertil Steril 1973; 24:722–735.

Schenker J, Margolioth E. Intrauterine adhesions: an updated appraisal. Fertil Steril 1982; 37:593–610.

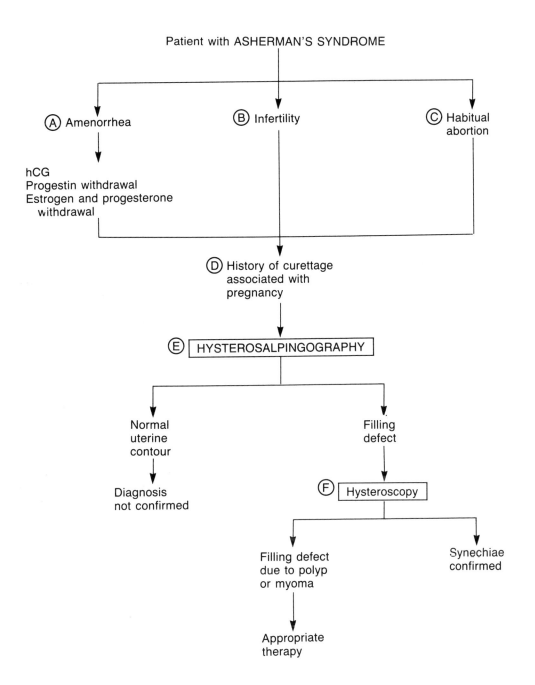

Patient with ASHERMAN'S SYNDROME

(A) Amenorrhea   (B) Infertility   (C) Habitual abortion

hCG
Progestin withdrawal
Estrogen and progesterone
    withdrawal

(D) History of curettage
    associated with
    pregnancy

(E) HYSTEROSALPINGOGRAPHY

Normal
uterine
contour

Filling
defect

Diagnosis
not confirmed

(F) Hysteroscopy

Filling defect
due to polyp
or myoma

Synechiae
confirmed

Appropriate
therapy

ASHERMAN'S SYNDROME: TREATMENT

Lawrence Grunfeld, M.D.
Mary Lake Polan, M.D., Ph.D.

A. Expectant management is associated with a 45 percent incidence of conception and a 73 percent incidence of resumption of menses. Nonintervention is appropriate in patients who do not desire resumption of menses or fertility. It is important to note that the diagnostic maneuvers such as hysterosalpingography can be therapeutic in effecting removal of adhesions near the cervical os.

B. The treatment of choice for uterine synechiae is hysteroscopic lysis of adhesions. The hysteroscope is important as both a diagnostic and a therapeutic tool. Occasionally complete obliteration of the endometrial cavity is encountered when hysteroscopy is unsuccessful, and it can result in uterine perforation. For this reason hysteroscopy is often performed under laparoscopic guidance when Asherman's syndrome is suspected. When hysteroscopic resection is unsuccessful, abdominal lysis of adhesions may be necessary. This carries a poor prognosis for conception or normalization of menses.

C. Mild synechiae should be treated through the hysteroscope. In occasional patients attempts at lysing adhesions vaginally are unsuccessful. Hysterotomy can be offered, but the prognosis is poor. In four patients treated at Hadassah University, no pregnancies were achieved. Three of the four had recurrence of symptoms.

D. The incidence of cure is similar whether a Foley catheter or an intrauterine device (IUD) is used. The duration of treatment varies from 1 to 8 weeks. Those utilizing Foley catheters usually remove them earlier because of fear of infection. Most authors suggest that prophylactic antibiotic treatment be used during the interval that a foreign device is left in the endometrium.

E. Estrogen therapy has improved the results following lysis of adhesions. Several different regimens have been suggested. Doses of Premarin range from 1.25 to 7.5 mg per day. Resumption of menses is expected in nearly all patients, and conception occurs in 50 to 80 percent of treated patients.

References

Klein S, Garcia CR. Asherman's syndrome: a critique and current review. Fertil Steril 1973; 24:722–735.

Schenker J, Margolioth E. Intrauterine adhesions: an updated appraisal. Fertil Steril 1982; 37:593–610.

Sugimoto O. Diagnostic and therapeutic hysteroscopy for traumatic intrauterine adhesions. Am J Obstet Gynecol 1978; 131:539–547.

Valle R. Clinical management of uterine factors in infertile patients. Semin Reprod Endocrinol 1985; 3:149.

Valle R. Hysteroscopy in the evaluation of female infertility. Am J Obstet Gynecol 1980; 137:425–431.

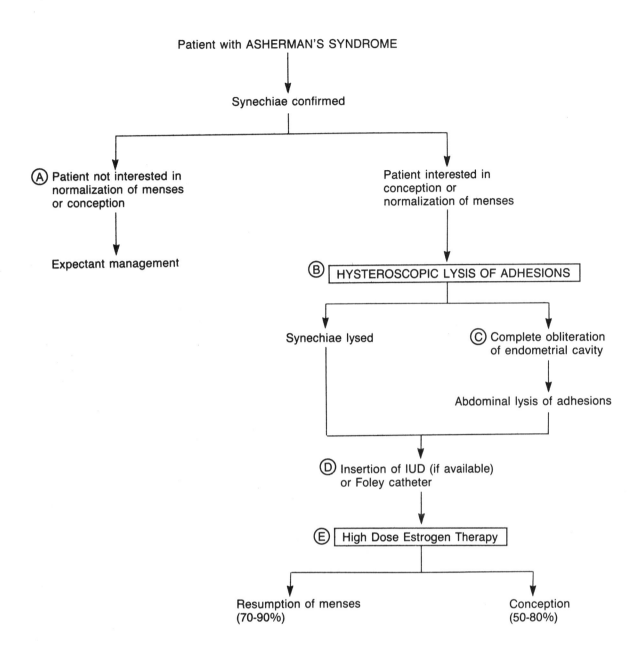

ENDOMETRIAL SAMPLING

Michael P. Diamond, M.D.
Mary Lake Polan, M.D., Ph.D.

A. Endometrial sampling is primarily performed by endometrial biopsy or by dilatation and curettage (D & C) of the uterus. Prior to introducing an instrument into the uterine cavity, the cervix should be cleansed with Betadine or some other antiseptic. The procedures to be described are often facilitated by placement of a tenaculum on the cervix.

B. For endometrial dating to establish ovulation and rule out a luteal phase defect, endometrial biopsy can be performed as an office procedure (Fig. 1). It also can be per-

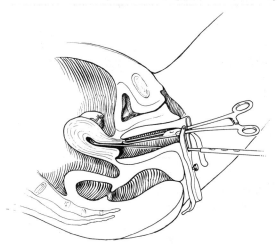

Figure 1 Endometrial biopsy using a Duncan curette. Samples are taken from both the anterior and the posterior surfaces of the uterine cavity.

formed as an office procedure for the diagnosis of endometritis.

C. For individuals who have potential uterine malignant diseases, initial parts of the evaluation can be performed in the office. This involves an endocervical curetting followed by a four quadrant endometrial biopsy. If the biopsy study is positive for malignant disease, the patient can be referred for appropriate therapy. If uterine malignant disease is considered to be highly likely but the biopsy study is negative for malignant disease, dilatation and curettage of the uterus are necessary for further evaluation.

D. Dysfunctional uterine bleeding unresponsive to hormonal therapy can be treated by dilatation and curettage of the uterus. If this is successful, control of the bleeding with restoration of the preceding menstrual pattern is established. If it is unsuccessful, the patient is considered to have intractable uterine bleeding and should be treated as described on p 70.

E. A woman presenting with an incomplete spontaneous miscarriage or desiring abortion can also be treated by uterine curettage; this is usually performed using a suction curette as well as sharp curettage and tissue forceps. Cervical dilatation is often required.

Reference

Noyes RW, Hertig AT, Rock J. Dating the endometrial biopsy. Fertil Steril 1950; 1:3–25.

Patient undergoing ENDOMETRIAL SAMPLING

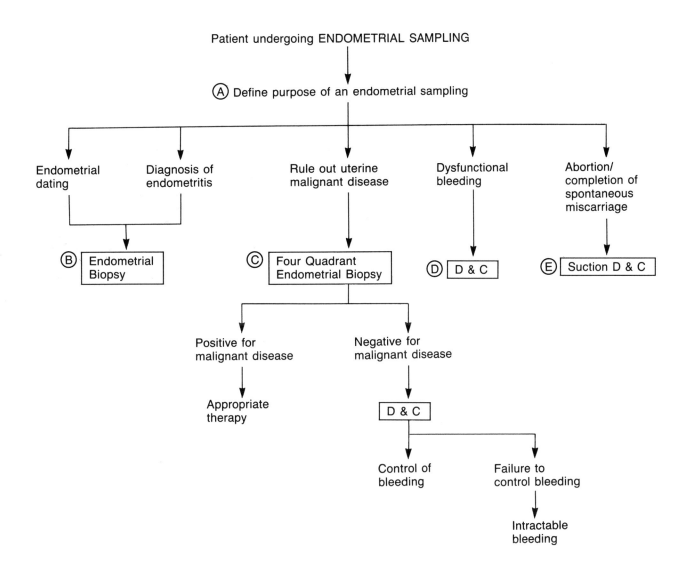

Ⓐ Define purpose of an endometrial sampling

| Endometrial dating | Diagnosis of endometritis | Rule out uterine malignant disease | Dysfunctional bleeding | Abortion/ completion of spontaneous miscarriage |

Ⓑ Endometrial Biopsy

Ⓒ Four Quadrant Endometrial Biopsy

Ⓓ D & C

Ⓔ Suction D & C

Positive for malignant disease → Appropriate therapy

Negative for malignant disease → D & C → Control of bleeding / Failure to control bleeding → Intractable bleeding

INTRACTABLE UTERINE BLEEDING

Michael P. Diamond, M.D.
Mary Lake Polan, M.D., Ph.D.

A. Patients with intractable uterine bleeding have failed to benefit from conservative therapy for the control of bleeding, including the oral and parenteral administration of estrogen and progesterone as well as intravenous Premarin therapy. Dilation and curettage (D&C) of the uterus also have failed to control bleeding in such patients. The tissue obtained from curettage must be submitted for pathologic study to rule out malignant disease.

B. The clinical presentation determines the appropriate course of therapy. The history should reveal any contraindications to general anesthesia or concomitant medical problems. Therapy also depends in part on the patient's feelings about undergoing a hysterectomy.

C. In women with intractable uterine bleeding in whom there are contraindications to general anesthesia or prolonged surgery, bleeding can be controlled by radiation therapy or ablation of the endometrial cavity.

D. Radiation therapy to control intractable uterine bleeding often takes 2 to 3 days to become effective. Complications can arise from radiation damage to the bladder or bowel.

E. Resectoscopic ablation of the uterine cavity, when absolutely essential, can be performed without concomitant laparoscopy. This procedure has been successful in the control of such bleeding, and causes the development of an Asherman-like syndrome.

F. In women who desire to keep the uterus, endometrial ablation can be considered. This procedure has been performed using either a urologic resectoscope or the Nd:Yag laser. Each of these methods has been clinically successful, although long term follow-up data are not yet available. Each leaves the uterus with an Asherman-like appearance, although foci of endometrial tissue can develop into endometrial cancer. Because of the risk of uterine perforation with damage to the bowel, bladder, and blood vessels, elective endometrial ablation should be performed concomitantly with diagnostic laparoscopy.

G. Hysterectomy can be performed by the vaginal or abdominal route. The method is determined in part by coexisting disease or the likelihood that disease is present. Thus evaluation of uterine size is necessary as well as consideration of the likelihood of pelvic adhesions or history of endometriosis.

References

DeCherney AH, Diamond MP, Lavy G, Polan ML. Endometrial ablation for intractable uterine bleeding: hysteroscopic resection. Obstet Gynecol (in press).

Goldrath MH, Fuller TA, Segal S. Laser photovaporization of endometrium for the treatment of menorrhagia. Am J Obstet Gynecol 1981; 140:14–19.

Patient with INTRACTABLE UTERINE BLEEDING

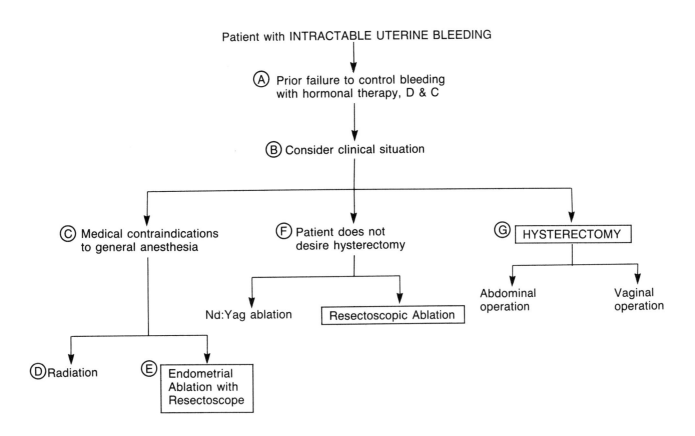

(A) Prior failure to control bleeding
with hormonal therapy, D & C

(B) Consider clinical situation

(C) Medical contraindications
to general anesthesia

(F) Patient does not
desire hysterectomy

(G) HYSTERECTOMY

Nd:Yag ablation

Resectoscopic Ablation

Abdominal
operation

Vaginal
operation

(D) Radiation

(E) Endometrial
Ablation with
Resectoscope

HABITUAL ABORTION

Mary Lake Polan, M.D., Ph.D.

A. Conventional pregnancy tests reveal that 15 percent of all pregnancies end in spontaneous abortion. Newer, more sensitive radioreceptor assays suggest that the incidence of miscarriage may be even higher. The strict definition of habitual abortion requires three consecutive pregnancy losses before 20 weeks' gestation with fetuses weighing under 500 grams. This definition excludes an incompetent cervix as an etiology.

B. An estimated 10 to 15 percent of habitual abortors have a uterine abnormality (Fig. 1) with a visible septum or bicornuate uterus on hysterosalpingography (HSG). Although 50 percent of the women with these anomalies do not experience pregnancy wastage, the other half should be evaluated with hysteroscopy and simultaneous laparoscopy. Surgical removal of the septum either through the hysteroscope or by abdominal metroplasty results in term pregnancy in 75 percent of the cases.

C. Hypothyroidism is a questionable cause of habitual abortion, but replacement is indicated if thyroid function is depressed. A short luteal phase with inadequate progesterone production documented by endometrial biopsy may also be a cause of habitual abortion. Treatment with either progesterone vaginal suppositories or ovulation inducing drugs such as clomiphene citrate or human menopausal gonadotropin (Pergonal) is effective.

D. Approximately 50 to 60 percent of first trimester miscarriages involve genetic defects, compared with a 7 percent incidence of chromosomal abnormalities in therapeutically aborted conceptuses. Nearly one-fourth of the cases of habitual abortion have a genetic cause. In cases of a parental balanced translocation, 50 percent of the progeny will be viable. The only therapy currently available is for a paternal abnormality, in which case donor insemination is required.

E. Infectious agents such as *Toxoplasma, Mycoplasma, Listeria,* and *Chlamydia* have been suggested as causes of recurrent miscarriage. Treatment with Vibramycin or erythromycin has resulted in increased term pregnancy rates.

F. Collagen vascular disease such as systemic lupus erythematosus has been associated with a 40 percent incidence of abortion, presumably because of compromised blood flow. In addition, couples with shared HLA-B antigens may be at higher risk for repetitive pregnancy loss. Maternal therapy with leukocyte transfusions may decrease pregnancy wastage.

G. Cases in which there is a hormonal etiology for habitual abortion have the best chance of success with therapy (90 percent), with an anatomic etiology second (60 percent), and a genetic cause third (32 percent). However, 40 percent of the couples evaluated have no demonstrable etiology for the pregnancy loss. They must be counseled that they too have a good prognosis; nearly 70 percent of the couples with no known etiology eventually have term births without therapy.

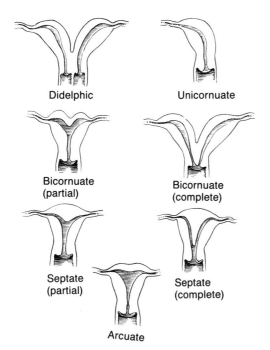

Didelphic

Unicornuate

Bicornuate (partial)

Bicornuate (complete)

Septate (partial)

Septate (complete)

Arcuate

Figure 1 Uterine anomalies.

References

Beer AE, Quebbeman JF, Ayers JWT, et al. Major histocompatibility complex antigens, maternal and paternal immune responses, and chronic habitual abortions in humans. Am J Obstet Gynecol 1981; 141:987–997.

Glass RH, Golbus MH. Habitual abortion. Fertil Steril 1978; 29:257–265.

Jones WS. Obstetric significance of female genital anomalies. Obstet Gynecol 1957; 10:113–127.

Taylor C, Faulk WP. Prevention of recurrent abortion with leukocyte transfusions. Lancet 1981; 2:68–69.

Tho Thi P, Byrd JR, McDonough PG. Etiologies and subsequent reproductive performance of 100 couples with recurrent abortion. Fertil Steril 1979; 32:389–395.

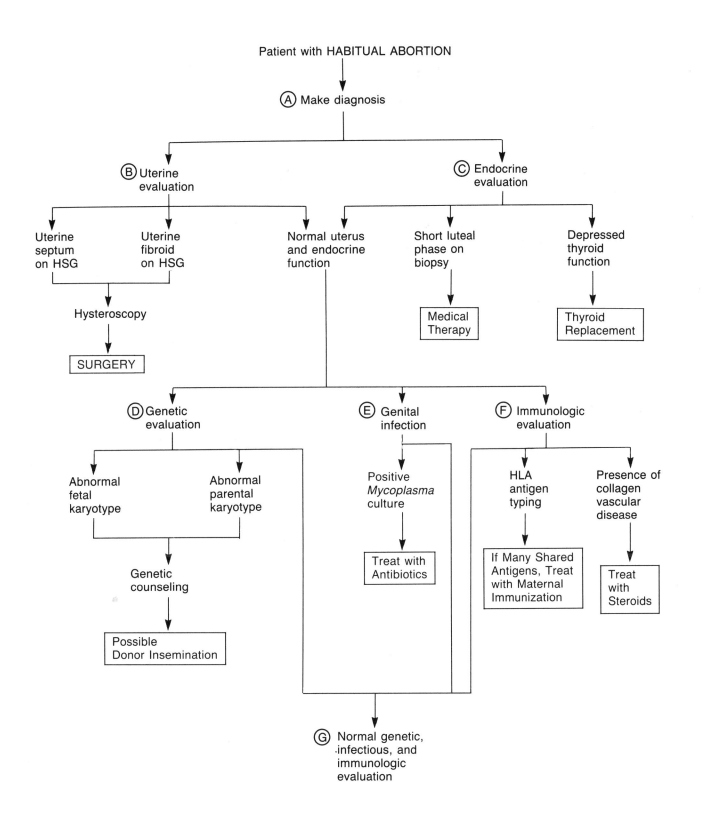

Patient with HABITUAL ABORTION

Ⓐ Make diagnosis

Ⓑ Uterine evaluation

Ⓒ Endocrine evaluation

Uterine septum on HSG

Uterine fibroid on HSG

Normal uterus and endocrine function

Short luteal phase on biopsy

Depressed thyroid function

Hysteroscopy

Medical Therapy

Thyroid Replacement

SURGERY

Ⓓ Genetic evaluation

Ⓔ Genital infection

Ⓕ Immunologic evaluation

Abnormal fetal karyotype

Abnormal parental karyotype

Positive *Mycoplasma* culture

HLA antigen typing

Presence of collagen vascular disease

Genetic counseling

Treat with Antibiotics

If Many Shared Antigens, Treat with Maternal Immunization

Treat with Steroids

Possible Donor Insemination

Ⓖ Normal genetic, infectious, and immunologic evaluation

DIAGNOSTIC CRITERIA

Robert A. Graebe, M.D.
Mary Lake Polan, M.D., Ph.D.

A. Fifteen percent of clinical pregnancies end in miscarriage, usually because of lethal nonrecurrent embryonic abnormalities. A thorough history is helpful in distinguishing pregnancy loss due to an incompetent cervix.

B. Pregnancy loss occurring in the second trimester with painless cervical dilation, especially in a patient with an anatomically abnormal cervix, points to the diagnosis of incompetent cervix. Patients with such a history should be followed closely and considered for cerclage.

C. Pregnancy loss occurring in the first trimester, preceded by bleeding and pain, points to a diagnosis of spontaneous abortion. Diethylstilbestrol (DES) exposed daughters have a higher incidence of müllerian abnormalities and are at greater risk for pregnancy loss.

D. The relatively high incidence of spontaneous miscarriage makes the possibility of two miscarriages in succession more likely. Most of these couples have no identifiable maternal or paternal cause for repeated pregnancy loss. Although a full evaluation of the causes of habitual abortion reveals little in these couples, such an evaluation may be indicated nonetheless to alleviate anxiety and to provide reassurance.

E. A complete evaluation for habitual abortion is indicated after the third miscarriage. In up to 30 percent of women there is an inadequate luteal phase, in another 30 percent there are uterine abnormalities, and 10 to 15 percent of habitual abortions involve genetic factors. The remaining patients have infectious, immunologic, or other medical causes of the recurrent pregnancy losses. Those with a normal evaluation can be reassured of a 70 percent chance of carrying the next pregnancy to term.

References

DeCherney AH, Polan ML. Helping habitual aborters. Contemp Obstet Gynecol 1982; 20:241–248.

Glass RH, Globus MS. Habitual abortion. Fertil Steril 1978; 29:257–265.

Richard RM, Sortle BE. Correcting cervical incompetence after habitual abortions. Contemp Obstet Gynecol 1986; 27:147–166.

Rock JA, Zacur HA. The clinical management of repeated early pregnancy wastage. Fertil Steril 1983; 39:123–140.

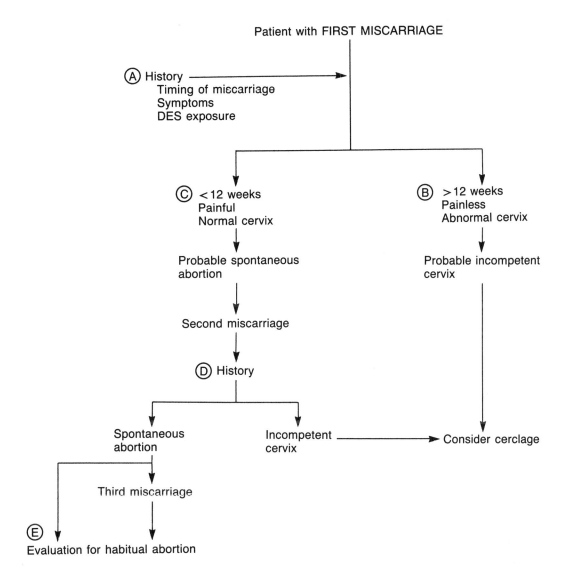

Patient with FIRST MISCARRIAGE

Ⓐ History
  Timing of miscarriage
  Symptoms
  DES exposure

Ⓒ < 12 weeks
   Painful
   Normal cervix

Ⓑ > 12 weeks
   Painless
   Abnormal cervix

Probable spontaneous abortion

Probable incompetent cervix

Second miscarriage

Ⓓ History

Spontaneous abortion

Incompetent cervix

Consider cerclage

Third miscarriage

Ⓔ
Evaluation for habitual abortion

UTERINE EVALUATION

Robert A. Graebe, M.D.
Mary Lake Polan, M.D., Ph.D.

A. The major diagnostic procedure used in evaluating the uterus is hysterosalpingography performed with a water soluble, iodinated, radio-opaque dye. The procedure is done on an outpatient basis and gives information about tubal patency as well as intrauterine contour.

B. If a normal intrauterine contour is seen, the uterine evaluation is considered negative. Abnormalities that may be seen include isolated discrete filling defects or an intrauterine septum. However, such radiographic abnormalities are not always associated with habitual abortion, and many women with uterine malformations do not experience fetal loss.

C. It is impossible to identify a simple intrauterine septum solely on the basis of the intrauterine contour in a hysterosalpingogram. Diagnostic laparoscopy and hysteroscopy should be performed to verify that the external uterine contour is normal in order to make the firm identification of an intrauterine septum. Even in the case of filling defects, laparoscopy is helpful, since therapeutic surgery with the hysteroscope is most safely performed under direct laparoscopic visualization.

D. If at the time of surgery a polyp, submucous myoma, and/or synechiae are visualized, they can be resected using the urologic resectoscope, resulting in a smooth and normal intrauterine contour. If synechiae are seen, it is advisable to leave a pediatric Foley catheter in the uterus for several days following surgery and to give the patient estrogen to prevent recurrence of adhesions.

E. If the extrauterine contour is normal and a small septum is well visualized, it can be resected using the urologic resectoscope. This transvaginal procedure results in term pregnancy incidences equivalent to those following abdominal metroplasty.

F. If the extrauterine contour is normal but the septum is either large or poorly visualized, abdominal metroplasty by either the Tomkins or Jones method is recommended rather than trying to utilize hysteroscopic resection.

G. If an abnormal extrauterine contour is seen at laparoscopy and the uterus is bicornuate, an abdominal metroplasty is the procedure of choice. However, a bicornuate uterus frequently results in premature labor at 32 to 36 weeks with an abnormally positioned infant rather than in habitual abortion.

References

Gray SE, Roberts DK, Franklin RR. Fertility after metroplasty of the septate uterus. J Reprod Med 1984; 29:185–188.

Mercer CA, Long WN, Thompson JD. Uterine unification: indications and technique. Clin Obstet Gynecol 1981; 24:1199–1216.

Rock JA, Zacur HA. The clinical management of repeated early pregnancy wastage. Fertil Steril 1983; 39:123–140.

Russell JB, DeCherney AH, Graebe RA, Polan ML. Resectoscopic management of müllerian fusion defects. Fertil Steril 1986; 45:726–728.

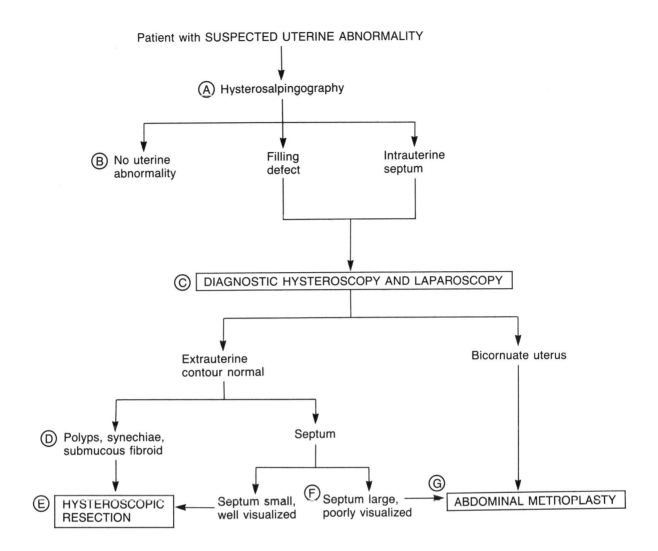

Patient with SUSPECTED UTERINE ABNORMALITY

Ⓐ Hysterosalpingography

Ⓑ No uterine abnormality

Filling defect

Intrauterine septum

Ⓒ DIAGNOSTIC HYSTEROSCOPY AND LAPAROSCOPY

Extrauterine contour normal

Bicornuate uterus

Ⓓ Polyps, synechiae, submucous fibroid

Septum

Ⓔ HYSTEROSCOPIC RESECTION

Septum small, well visualized

Ⓕ Septum large, poorly visualized

Ⓖ ABDOMINAL METROPLASTY

ENDOCRINE EVALUATION

Robert A. Graebe, M.D.
Mary Lake Polan, M.D., Ph.D.

A. Uncontrolled diabetes mellitus has been associated with higher than usual incidences of pregnancy wastage, although the association is controversial, with some investigators reporting that repetitive pregnancy loss is not higher than in nondiabetic women. Fasting blood sugar and 2 hour postprandial blood glucose levels are sufficient for screening. Diabetics who wish to become pregnant should achieve optimal control both before and after conception, since hyperglycemia may be teratogenic.

B. Successful implantation requires adequate luteal function with sufficient progesterone to stimulate a normal uterine secretory response. Assessment of luteal function includes the basal body temperature (BBT) pattern, midluteal serum progesterone level, and late luteal endometrial biopsy for histologic dating. Both hyperandrogenism and hyperprolactinemia may be causally related to inadequate luteal function. Dehydroepiandrosterone sulfate (DHEA-S) and prolactin levels should be evaluated.

C. Hyperprolactinemia is associated with a spectrum of ovulatory disorders, from anovulation to inadequate luteal phase. Hyperprolactinemia is present when a morning fasting prolactin level exceeds 20 ng per milliliter. A CAT scan should be done to rule out a pituitary microadenoma. Hypothyroidism should also be considered as a cause of hyperprolactinemia, since thyrotropin releasing hormone (TRH) stimulates the pituitary production of prolactin as well as thyroid stimulating hormone (TSH).

D. Thyroid dysfunction is an uncommon cause of anovulation. Thyroid evaluation should include serum thyroxine (T_4), thyroxine binding capacity (RT_3 uptake), and TSH determinations. The serum T_3 level may be useful if hyperthyroidism is suspected. Empiric thyroid replacement therapy has no value.

E. Luteal inadequacy should be suspected when the basal body temperature fails to show a sustained temperature rise for more than 10 days or the midluteal serum progesterone level is less than 12 ng per milliliter. The diagnosis is confirmed when endometrial biopsies performed in two separate cycles in the late luteal phase demonstrate developmental lags greater than 2 days by histologic dating criteria. The therapy for luteal inadequacy may include progesterone vaginal suppositories, 25 mg twice daily beginning on the third day of the BBT rise, clomiphene citrate in doses of 50 to 200 mg per day on days 5 to 9 of the cycle, or Pergonal when luteal inadequacy persists despite clomiphene or progesterone therapy. During therapy the endometrial biopsy should be repeated to insure that the defect has been corrected.

F. Hypothyroidism should be treated with thyroid replacement and thyroid function followed. Elevated prolactin levels accompanying hypothyroidism return to normal when adequate thyroid replacement is given.

G. Hyperthyroidism may be present without the classic tachycardia and hypermetabolism. Antithyroid drugs such as propylthiouracil are effective for suppression. Although hypothyroidism has been implicated primarily in infertility, hyperthyroidism has been more closely associated with pregnancy wastage.

H. The medical therapy for hyperprolactinemia is bromocriptine (Parlodel), 2.5 mg orally twice daily. The prolactin level usually returns to normal within a few days. In most cases ovulatory menses resume and luteal defects are corrected.

References

Crane JP, Wahl N. The role of maternal diabetes in repetitive spontaneous abortion. Fertil Steril 1981; 36:477–479.

Glass RH, Golbus MS. Habitual abortion. Fertil Steril 1978; 29:257–265.

Horta JLH, Fernandez JG, deLeon BS, Cortes-Gallegos V. Direct evidence of luteal insufficiency in women with habitual abortion. Obstet Gynecol 1977; 49:705–708.

Montoro M, Collea JV, Frasier D, Mestman JH. Successful outcome of pregnancy in women with hypothyroidism. Ann Intern Med 1981; 94:31–34.

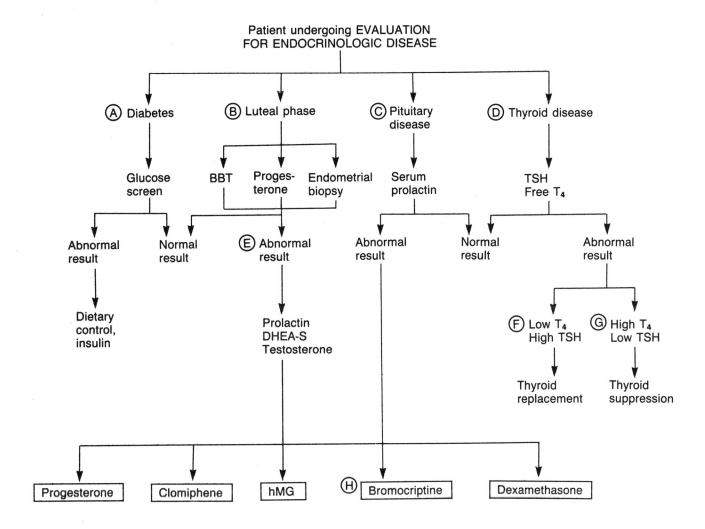

Patient undergoing EVALUATION
FOR ENDOCRINOLOGIC DISEASE

(A) Diabetes   (B) Luteal phase   (C) Pituitary disease   (D) Thyroid disease

Glucose screen   BBT   Progesterone   Endometrial biopsy   Serum prolactin   TSH Free T$_4$

Abnormal result   Normal result   (E) Abnormal result   Abnormal result   Normal result   Abnormal result

Dietary control, insulin

Prolactin DHEA-S Testosterone

(F) Low T$_4$ High TSH   (G) High T$_4$ Low TSH

Thyroid replacement   Thyroid suppression

Progesterone   Clomiphene   hMG   (H) Bromocriptine   Dexamethasone

GENETIC EVALUATION

Robert A. Graebe, M.D.
Mary Lake Polan, M.D., Ph.D.

A. A karyotype with banding is the standard diagnostic procedure for genetic evaluation in general and for evaluation of habitual abortion in particular. Although it is an expensive and rather sophisticated test with no therapy available when the karyotype is abnormal, it does provide couples with an answer to questions about their genetic normalcy.

B. When three successive miscarriages have occurred, or when there have been one or more miscarriages with an abnormal child, both parents should be karyotyped. In most cases parental karyotypes are normal, and only 4 percent of couples with a history of habitual abortion exhibit an abnormal karyotype.

C. Fetal tissue, including placenta, from early miscarriages should be karyotyped whenever possible. It has been estimated that at least 50 percent of spontaneous abortions are the result of some chromosomal abnormality.

D. There is increasing awareness of chromosomal damage secondary to radiation or environmental toxins. This type of damage is often permanent, resulting in repetitive abnormalities in the offspring.

E. The most common genetic abnormality found in couples is a balanced translocation. In such a situation 25 percent of the offspring have an abnormal karyotype that is expressed, 25 percent have a normal chromosomal composition, and 50 percent of the offspring have a balanced translocation but are functionally normal.

F. In situations involving permanent, repetitive genetic abnormalities, genetic counseling should be obtained. Alternatives include midtrimester amniocentesis to insure a normal chromosomal complement in the fetus, adoption, donor ovum or donor sperm depending on which parent carries the chromosomal abnormality, and the use of a surrogate parent.

G. Nonrepetitive abnormal fetal karyotypes are the most common finding. In such a situation, when parents have normal karyotypes, they should be reassured that a chance event has occurred. In such a situation genetic counseling helps the couple to understand that a nonrepetitive event of low statistical probability has occurred and is unlikely to occur again. The next conception carries the same risk of miscarriage as any other pregnancy (approximately 15 to 20 percent).

References

Boue J, Boue A, Lazer P. Retrospective and prospective epidemiologic studies of 1500 karyotyped spontaneous human abortions. Teratology 1975; 12:11–26.

Davis JR, Weinstein L, Veomett IC, et al. Balanced translocation karyotypes in patients with repetitive abortion. Am J Obstet Gynecol 1982; 144:229–233.

Elias S, Simpson JL. Evaluation and clinical management of patients at apparent increased risk for spontaneous abortion. In: Porter I, Hook EB, eds. Human embryonic and fetal death. New York: Academic Press, 1980:331.

Simpson JL. What causes chromosomal abnormalities and gene mutations? Contemp Obstet Gynecol 1981; 17:99–114.

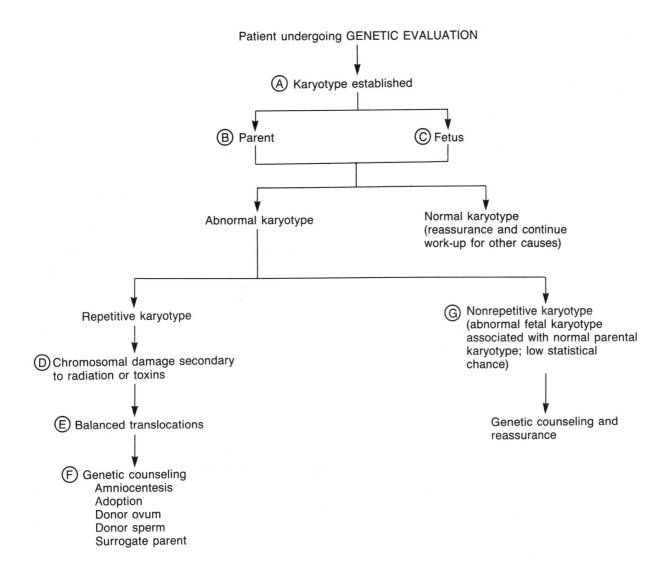

Patient undergoing GENETIC EVALUATION

(A) Karyotype established

(B) Parent   (C) Fetus

Abnormal karyotype

Normal karyotype
(reassurance and continue
work-up for other causes)

Repetitive karyotype

(G) Nonrepetitive karyotype
(abnormal fetal karyotype
associated with normal parental
karyotype; low statistical
chance)

(D) Chromosomal damage secondary
to radiation or toxins

(E) Balanced translocations

Genetic counseling and
reassurance

(F) Genetic counseling
Amniocentesis
Adoption
Donor ovum
Donor sperm
Surrogate parent

INFECTIOUS DISEASE EVALUATION

Robert A. Graebe, M.D.
Mary Lake Polan, M.D., Ph.D.

A. Acute systemic infections have been known for years to cause spontaneous miscarriage. The microorganisms and viruses include *Listeria, Vibrio, Salmonella*, and vaccinia. Although individual miscarriages may result from infections with these organisms, there are no controlled studies that clearly demonstrate that any of these agents causes habitual abortion.

B. One group of acute infections that may cause miscarriage and fetal abnormalities is known by the acronym TORCHES. Acute toxoplasmosis infection causes miscarriages, but a positive toxoplasmosis titer indicates that the woman has been exposed to the disease and has immunity. The same is true for rubella, and all nonimmune women should be vaccinated and postpone pregnancy for 3 months. Both cytomegalovirus and herpes are responsible for miscarriages during acute systemic infections. There is no therapy and no immunization is available. Active syphilis should be treated with appropriate antibiotics, since it may result in miscarriage early in pregnancy and in fetal abnormalities when acquired during the second or third trimester of pregnancy.

C. Although *Chlamydia* has been associated with miscarriage, it is more clearly associated with infertility and pelvic infection. Culture positive women and their husbands should be treated with tetracycline to eradicate infection. There are no controlled data that definitely link *Chlamydia* to habitual abortion.

D. Intrauterine bacterial infecton has also been implicated as a cause of habitual abortion. Cervical cultures are useless in this situation and uterine cultures must be obtained. If intrauterine aerobic or anaerobic organisms are encountered, the infections should be treated with appropriate antibiotics.

E. *Mycoplasma* and Ureaplasma have been implicated in the etiology of habitual abortion, and uncontrolled studies have shown an increased term pregnancy incidence after therapy with antibotics. The data are controversial, and many women who are culture positive for *Mycoplasma* carry pregnancies to term without difficulty.

F. If positive *Mycoplasma* cultures are found during early pregnancy in a patient with a history of miscarriages, therapy with erythromycin should be considered.

G. Prior to conception, patients with positive *Mycoplasma* cultures and their husbands should be treated with Vibramycin and, if miscarriage occurs again, should be treated during the next pregnancy with erythromycin.

References

Mead PB, Sweet RL. Looking for Chlamydia and finding it. Contemp Obstet Gynecol 1985; 25:50–55.

Quinn PA, Shewchuk AB, Shuber J, et al. Efficacy of antibiotic therapy in preventing spontaneous pregnancy loss among couples colonized with genital Mycoplasmas. Am J Obstet Gynecol 1983; 145:239–244.

Quinn PA, Shewchuk AB, Shuber J, et al. Serologic evidence of Ureaplasma urealyticum infection in women with spontaneous pregnancy loss. Am J Obstet Gynecol 1983; 145:245–250.

Rock JA, Zacur HA. The clinical management of repeated early pregnancy wastage. Fertil Steril 1983; 39:123–140.

Patient undergoing DISEASE EVALUATION

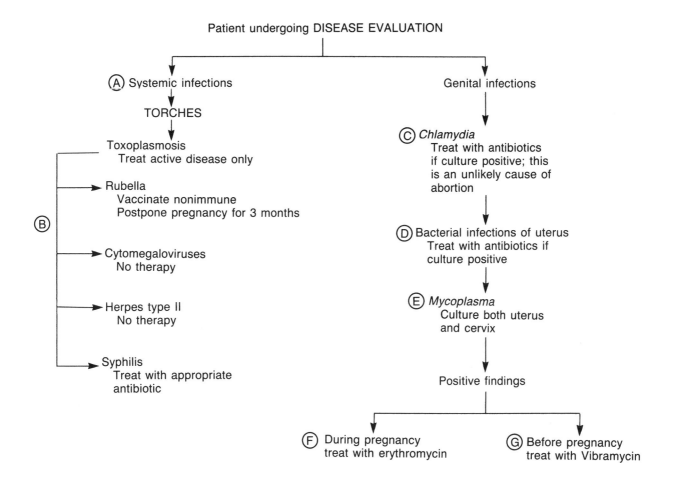

Ⓐ Systemic infections

TORCHES

Toxoplasmosis
Treat active disease only

Ⓑ

Rubella
Vaccinate nonimmune
Postpone pregnancy for 3 months

Cytomegaloviruses
No therapy

Herpes type II
No therapy

Syphilis
Treat with appropriate
antibiotic

Genital infections

Ⓒ *Chlamydia*
Treat with antibiotics
if culture positive; this
is an unlikely cause of
abortion

Ⓓ Bacterial infections of uterus
Treat with antibiotics if
culture positive

Ⓔ *Mycoplasma*
Culture both uterus
and cervix

Positive findings

Ⓕ During pregnancy
treat with erythromycin

Ⓖ Before pregnancy
treat with Vibramycin

IMMUNOLOGIC EVALUATION

Robert A. Graebe, M.D.
Mary Lake Polan, M.D., Ph.D.

A. The fetus appears to be protected from immunologic rejection by two factors—the immunosuppressive effects of progesterone and the presence of an IgG antibody, which acts to block fetal antigens and keep them from being recognized as foreign by the maternal immunologic system. In addition, early pregnancy factor appears within days after fertilization and has immunosuppressive properties that inhibit maternal lymphocyte activity. This activity exists well into the third trimester in normal pregnancies but is at a low level in women sustaining spontaneous abortions. The immunologic interaction between mother and fetus is poorly understood and controversial.

B. There appears to be greater sharing of the histocompatibility locus antigens (HLA) of the A and B loci in couples with a history of habitual abortion. This sharing of antigens may cause the failure of blocking antibody induction, allowing antibodies to be made against the fetus itself, resulting in fetal wastage. If many antigens are shared between mother and father, successful pregnancies have been achieved by maternal immunization with paternal leukocyte enriched plasma, eliciting the induction of blocking antibodies.

C. ABO blood group incompatibility does not appear to be a factor in habitual abortion. However, there have been reports of anti-PP1PK K antibodies against the blood's P system of antigens in a group of patients with otherwise idiopathic habitual abortion. Also there have been successful pregnancies in this group with maternal plasmaphoresis throughout pregnancy to remove antibodies and protect the fetus.

D. Women with collagen vascular disease, particularly lupus erythematosus, have been thought to have a higher incidence of pregnancy wastage as a result of poor vascularization of the uterus and decreased fetal blood flow. Recently a small percentage of women with lupus and a positive antinuclear antibody (ANA) screen have also been found to have an elevated circulating lupus anticoagulant level in association with repetitive fetal wastage.

E. Both full blown lupus erythematosus and the circulating lupus anticoagulant syndrome have been treated with high doses of steroids to decrease the maternal immune response. Up to 50 mg of prednisone a day has been used, resulting in successful term pregnancies. With circulating lupus anticoagulant and small microthrombi, additional therapy includes low doses of aspirin to retard platelet adhesiveness and reduce the formation of small thrombi.

F. Circulating lupus anticoagulant is a factor that impairs clotting, and its level is elevated in some women with positive antinuclear antibodies. It is measured in the partial thromboplastin (PT) assay in which it prolongs the partial thromboplastin time (PTT). In some studies as many as 10 to 20 percent of women with habitual abortion have been found to have elevated circulating lupus anticoagulant levels diagnosed with a PTT ratio of patient to control greater than 1.3. Paradoxically, although circulating lupus anticoagulant prolongs the PTT, it is associated pathologically with microthrombi in small vessels and seems to cause pregnancy wastage by a series of small thrombotic events impairing blood flow to the fetus.

References

Branch DW, et al. Obstetric complications associated with the lupus anticoagulant. N Engl J Med 1985; 313:1322–1326.

Menge AC, Beer AE. The significance of human leukocyte antigen profiles in human infertility, recurrent abortion, and pregnancy disorders. Fertil Steril 1985; 43:693–695.

Persitz E, Oksenberg JR, Margalioth EJ, et al. Histoincompatibility in couples with unexplained infertility. Fertil Steril 1985; 43:733–738.

Rock JA, Shirey RS, Braine HG, et al. Plasmaphoresis for the treatment of repetitive early pregnancy wastage associated with anti-P. Obstet Gynecol 1985; 66:575–578.

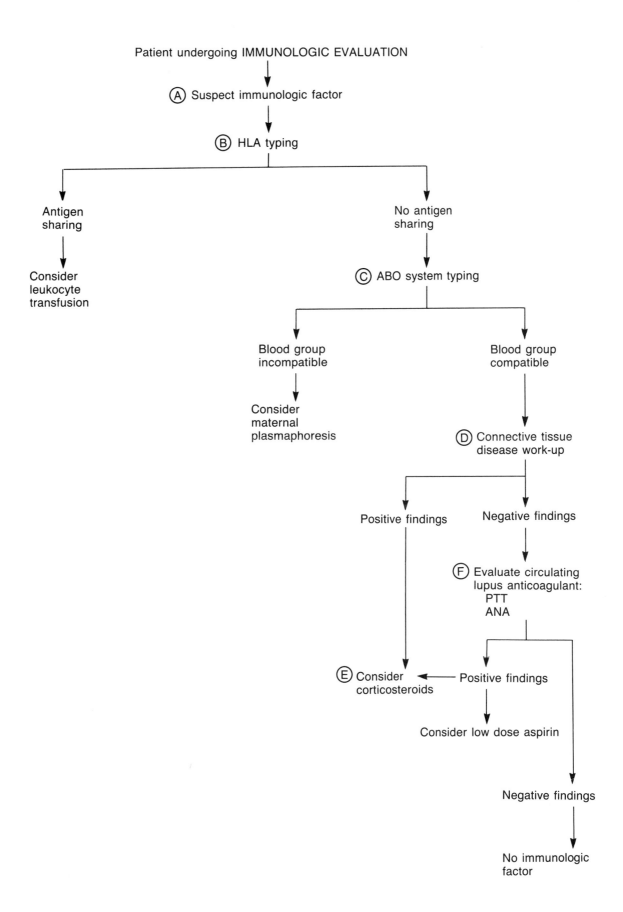

Patient undergoing IMMUNOLOGIC EVALUATION

Ⓐ Suspect immunologic factor

Ⓑ HLA typing

Antigen sharing

Consider leukocyte transfusion

No antigen sharing

Ⓒ ABO system typing

Blood group incompatible

Consider maternal plasmaphoresis

Blood group compatible

Ⓓ Connective tissue disease work-up

Positive findings

Negative findings

Ⓕ Evaluate circulating lupus anticoagulant:
PTT
ANA

Ⓔ Consider corticosteroids

Positive findings

Consider low dose aspirin

Negative findings

No immunologic factor

TUBAL SURGERY OVERVIEW I: HISTORY AND PHYSICAL EXAMINATION

James M. Wheeler, M.D.
Mary Lake Polan, M.D., Ph.D.

Assessment of fallopian tube function is a basic component in the evaluation of the infertile couple. Infertility caused by tubal disease has increased in the United States over the last decade, presumably because of the continuing epidemic of salpingitis. Infection of the tubes and ovaries is the leading cause of adnexal disease, accounting for about 15 percent of the cases of infertility. Surveys of infectious agents have implicated over 20 microorganisms, the most common being *Chlamydia trachomatis, Neisseria gonorrhoeae,* coliforms, and anaerobes. Typical clinical manifestations vary among the infecting organisms; chlamydial salpingitis is notorious as an indolent infection when compared with the typical acute salpingitis of gonorrhea. Further complicating the clinical course of these infections is the logarithmic increase in the incidence of infertility with repeated episodes of pelvic inflammatory disease (PID): 12 percent of patients are infertile with one episode, 23 percent with two episodes, and 54 percent with three or more episodes.

Most cases of PID are caused by ascending infection from the lower genital tract to the fallopian tubes. Infection can ascend within the genital tract to primarily infect the endosalpinx, or can extend via the lymphatics to involve the adnexa, the so-called exosalpingitis. The distinction between endo- and exosalpingitis is somewhat moot, since either can produce the two major sequelae that can cause infertility: intraluminal tubal damage and external tubal adhesions. Adhesions form when inflamed serosal surfaces agglutinate, sealed together by fibrin deposition and fibroblast proliferation. Adhesions may then impede ovum pick-up and transport. Intraluminal tubal damage is thought to represent more severe damage, and can reduce the usually ciliated endosalpingeal cells to a flattened cobblestone appearance. Once infected, tubes attempt to limit the spread of infection by closing both ends of the tube, perhaps initially because of cellular edema from inflammation. Typically, the larger the hydrosalpinx, the thinner the tubal mucosa and the more devastating the damage to ciliary and secretory cells.

A. Despite a careful history, half the women with pelvic adhesions do not have any history suggesting a possible etiology.

B. Postpartum endometritis and noninfectious complications of pregnancy, such as ruptured corpus luteum or ectopic pregnancy, may cause tubal damage. Septic abortion may be associated with damage to the proximal tube.

C. Inflammation from the infected tubes themselves often induces varying degrees of peritonitis. However, nongenital inflammation as seen with appendicitis or cholecystitis may also cause pelvic peritonitis and adhesions without severely affecting the intraluminal tubal mucosa. An increasingly frequent cause of tubal disease is a previous pelvic operation. All gynecologic surgeons must be cognizant that the *first* pelvic reconstructive procedure has the best chance for success.

D. Intrauterine devices (IUDs) are a known risk factor for PID, but their role in infertility in the asymptomatic woman is unknown (except when removal of the device is incomplete). Unusual organisms, including *Actinomyces* species, and unusual presentations such as unilateral salpingitis, are seen in IUD-associated PID.

E. A history of possible exposure to diethylstilbestrol (DES) should be elicited from couples. Changes in the female include anomalous development of the uterus, cervix, and tubes; changes in the male are less well defined.

F. Adnexal enlargement may represent tubo-ovarian complexes, isolated hydrosalpinges, endometrioma, or any other cause of pelvic mass. Adnexal tenderness in these patients may be due to resolving PID. Bimanual examination may reveal impeded adnexal mobility caused by restricting adhesions. Speculum examination may reveal DES-related changes of the exocervix. If a mass is palpated, further evaluation is necessary if any etiology other than PID is suspected; malignant tumors can be of any size, can be unilateral, and may occur in young women. Ultrasonography, computed tomography, and magnetic resonance imaging should be attempted prior to operative intervention.

G. If pelvic examination reveals persistent tenderness or a mass attributable to PID, a course of antibiotics is prescribed to allow inflammation to subside prior to hysterosalpingography (HSG). Typical antibiotic courses are doxycycline or Augmentin with metronidazole for 6 to 12 weeks. If there is no improvement after this time, HSG should *not* be performed owing to the risk of peritonitis; operative evaluation should be initiated.

H. Any person with a history or physical examination compatible with pelvic infection, and those women at risk of complications from bacteremia (e.g., mitral value prolapse) are treated with peri-HSG antibiotics. Typically, doxycycline, 24 hours before and 24 hours after HSG, is prescribed. According to these criteria, it can be expected that nearly half the patients will receive peri-HSG prophylaxis.

References

DeCherney AH. Infertility: General principles of evaluation. In: Kase NG, Weingold AB, eds. Principles and practice of clinical gynecology. New York: John Wiley, 1983:425.

Speroff L, Glass RH, Kase NG. Clinical gynecologic endocrinology and infertility. 3rd ed. Baltimore: Williams & Wilkins, 1983: 473.

Weström L. Incidence, prevalence, and trends of acute pelvic inflammatory disease and its consequences in industrialized countries. Am J Obstet Gynecol 1980; 138:880–892.

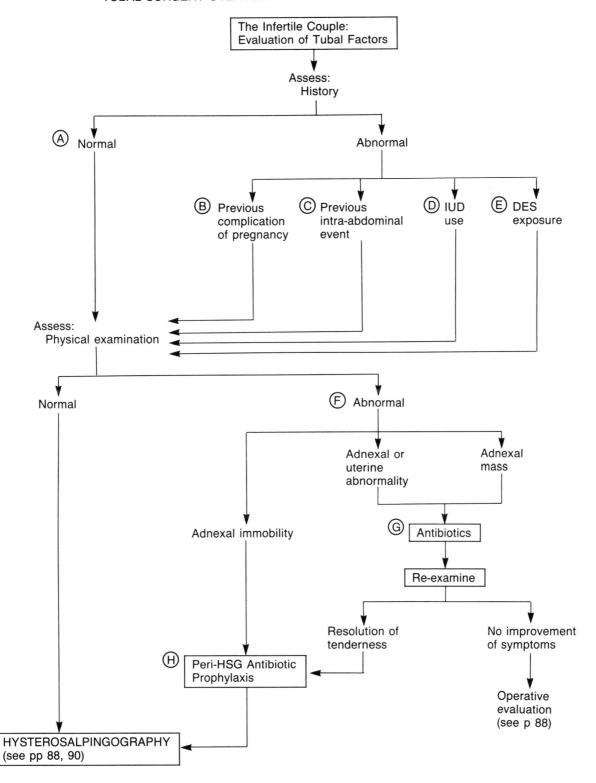

TUBAL SURGERY OVERVIEW II: HYSTEROSALPINGOGRAPHY AND LAPAROSCOPY

James M. Wheeler, M.D.
Mary Lake Polan, M.D., Ph.D.

The prehysterosalpingography (HSG) bimanual examination should demonstrate no adnexal tenderness; at least 6 months should elapse from an episode of acute pelvic inflammatory disease (PID) before an HSG is requested. HSG (see Fig. 1) is performed 3 to 6 days after cessation of menses; in patients with a history of PID, or other indication for antibiotic prophylaxis, doxycycline is ordered for 48 hours beginning the day before HSG. The risk of salpingitis following HSG may be as high as 3 percent within the first 24 hours. The best assessment of uterine contour and tubal architecture is obtained during the fluoroscopic examination. Three still radiographs are typically obtained: preinjection, spill from one or both tubes, and a delayed film showing distribution through the peritoneal cavity. Good technique assures minimal discomfort; minimal cervical dilation and manipulation are warranted.

A. Patency does not rule out pelvic adhesive disease involving the tube; HSG results are false negative in 20 percent of women with tubal disease diagnosed at laparoscopy.

B. Unilateral or bilateral proximal occlusion may be caused by spasm of the tubal muscular coat or faulty technique preventing adequate uterine filling.

C. Careful attention is paid to dilatation of the tube and the presence of tubal rugae representing mucosal folds. Undue filling pressure will not serve to open distal occlusion caused by significant disease.

D. Glucagon, 1 mg IV 10 minutes before HSG, helps diminish tubal spasm at HSG. If there is a compelling indication for laparoscopy regardless of HSG results, this stage may be omitted.

E. Ethiodol is injected if there is bilateral tubal patency. This oil-based medium is associated with a greater pregnancy incidence following HSG than water-based medium; complications, including lethal dye embolization, are rare with both media. If there is fluoroscopic evidence of intravasation during slow injection of Ethiodol, the HSG is stopped immediately, and the patient is observed closely.

F. Laparoscopy is the final diagnostic procedure of any infertility investigation because of its operative risks. It is the essential method of diagnosis of tuboperitoneal causes of infertility. If HSG is normal, laparoscopy may be delayed 6 months to allow any fertility-enhancing effect of the HSG to allow conception. If tubal disease warranting operation is discovered at HSG, the 6-month wait for laparoscopy is optional. The findings at laparoscopy agree with those of HSG in about two-thirds of patients. After complete infertility evaluation, at least half the patients undergoing laparoscopy have pelvic disease, usually endometriosis or pelvic adhesions. Laparoscopic examination should provide the following information: (1) the extent and severity of adhesions involving the adnexa and bowel; (2) the extent of other pathologic processes, e.g., endometriosis; (3) tubal patency via chromopertubation; (4) the status of the distal tubal segment, particularly in those patients requesting reversal of sterilization; and (5) some overall assessment of the prognosis for the proposed reconstructive operation.

G. Advising tubal surgery should only be done if the expected pregnancy incidence is greater than that offered by in vitro fertilization (IVF). At this time, severe tubal disease such as bipolar tubal occlusion is best treated by IVF rather than bilateral neosalpingostomy. A thorough, frank discussion with the infertile couple is mandatory prior to undertaking major tubal surgery. The surgeon should present contraindications, alternatives, complications, and success incidences of the proposed operative approach. Alternative approaches in many patients will be laparoscopic therapy of adhesions or in vitro fertilization. Complications are infrequent but are in proportion to the severity of abdominal adhesions present. In addition to complications, the clinician must inform all patients that there is significant risk (at least 10 percent) of ectopic pregnancy and possible recurrence of pelvic adhesions.

References

DeCherney AH, Kort H, Barner JB, DeVore GR. Increased pregnancy rate with oil-soluble hysterosalpingography dye. Fertil Steril 1980; 33:407–410.

Gillespie HW. The therapeutic aspect of hysterosalpingography. Br J Radiol 1965; 38:301–302.

Soules MR. Infertility surgery. In: DeCherney AH, ed. Reproductive failure. New York: Churchill Livingstone, 1986:117.

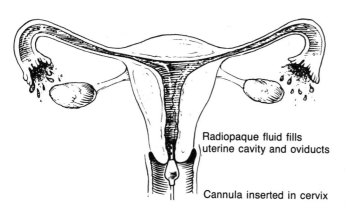

Radiopaque fluid fills uterine cavity and oviducts

Cannula inserted in cervix

Figure 1 Hysterosalpingography.

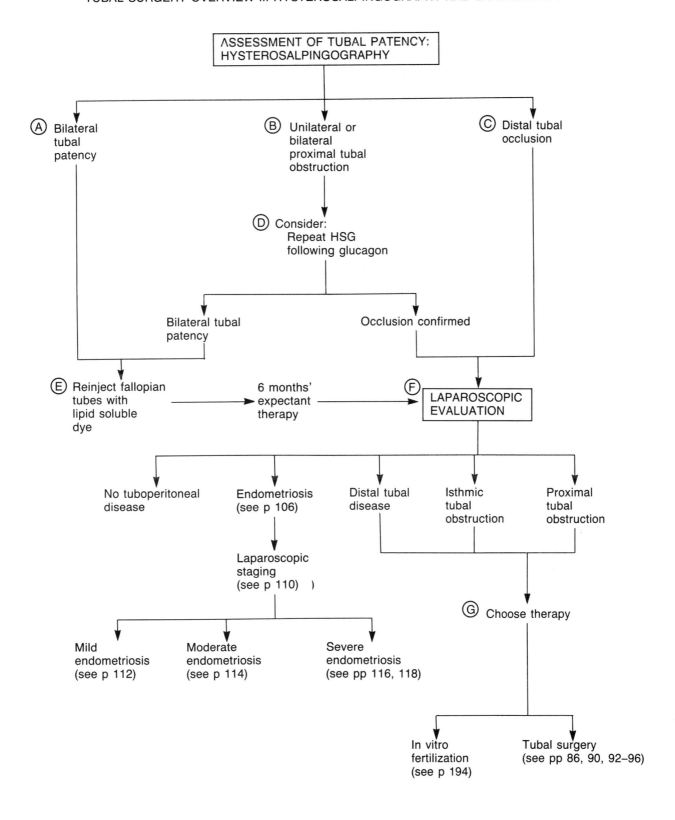

HYSTEROSALPINGOGRAPHY

Michael P. Diamond, M.D.
Mary Lake Polan, M.D., Ph.D.

A. Hysterosalpingography is usually performed as a diagnostic procedure; however, at times it may also be used therapeutically.

B. The hysterosalpingogram can be used to assess the anatomic shape of the uterine cavity as well as fallopian tube patency, length, and caliber. Depending on the technique utilized for injection of the dye, it is sometimes possible to visualize the cervical canal.

C. Hysterosalpingography can yield information about the uterine cavity, e.g., a normal cavity, uterine synechiae (adhesions) as in Asherman's syndrome, polyps or myomas, a uterine septum, products of conception, or a T shaped uterus suggesting diethylstilbestrol (DES) exposure.

D. Hysterosalpingography can also yield information regarding the status of the fallopian tubes, both simple patency and other subtler details that bear on fertility.

E. Tubal patency can be evaluated by observation of the passage of dye into the peritoneal cavity. However, pelvic adhesions, which could prevent passage of an egg from the ovary to the tube, are difficult to identify by this means.

F. Tubal blockage can be identified in the proximal, middle, and distal portions of the fallopian tube. Complete blockage is identified with more certainty than partial occlusion, which can be difficult to detect. However, tubal spasm cannot be ruled out, particularly when there is a proximal block. In occluded tubes the extent of damage can be partially determined by the size of a hydrosalpinx and the presence or absence of rugae.

G. Salpingitis isthmica nodosa can be identified by the presence of multiple channels in the isthmic portion of the fallopian tubes.

H. DES exposure can also be manifested in the fallopian tubes by shortening, but this is more difficult to identify than the uterine findings following DES exposure.

I. Tubal ectopic pregnancies often can be identified by hysterosalpingography.

J. Hysterosalpingography can be performed using either water base or oil base dyes. Several studies suggest that the use of oil base dye is associated with an increase in the pregnancy incidence in the successive three to four cycles. The mechanism by which this occurs is unclear. Potential complications of the use of oil dye are extravasation with resultant embolus or granuloma production in the fallopian tubes. We perform hysterosalpingography using a water soluble dye. If the tubes appear normal and the patient has no history of peritoneal disease, 3 cc of Ethiodol is then placed into the uterine cavity.

References

DeCherney AH, Kort H, Barney JB, DeVore GR. Increased pregnancy rate with oil-soluble hysterosalpingography dye. Fertil Steril 1980; 33:407–410.

Schwartz PE, et al. Routine use of hysterography in endometrial carcinoma and postmenopausal bleeding. Obstet Gynecol 1975; 45:378–384.

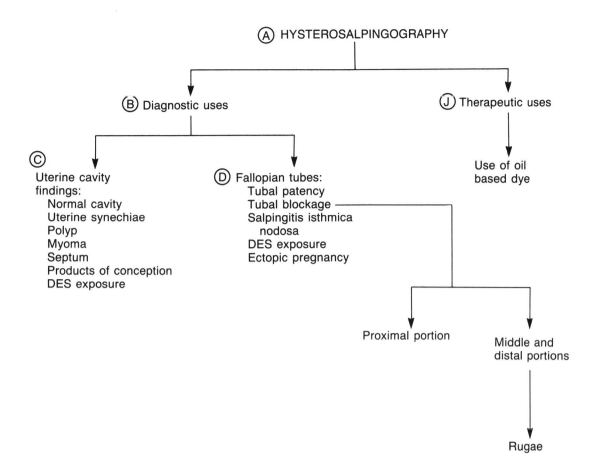

Ⓐ HYSTEROSALPINGOGRAPHY

Ⓑ Diagnostic uses

Ⓙ Therapeutic uses

Use of oil
based dye

Ⓒ
Uterine cavity
findings:
    Normal cavity
    Uterine synechiae
    Polyp
    Myoma
    Septum
    Products of conception
    DES exposure

Ⓓ Fallopian tubes:
    Tubal patency
    Tubal blockage
    Salpingitis isthmica
        nodosa
    DES exposure
    Ectopic pregnancy

Proximal portion

Middle and
distal portions

Rugae

PREVENTION OF POSTOPERATIVE ADHESION DEVELOPMENT

Michael P. Diamond, M.D.
Mary Lake Polan, M.D., Ph.D.

A. The postoperative development of pelvic adhesions is a major problem for the surgeon. They occcur in the majority of women who undergo operative procedures to restore fertility. Such adhesions reduce the likelihood that these women will conceive.

B. The etiology of the development of adhesions is not well established. In large part it is related to tissue ischemia and resultant reductions in plasminogen activator activity. Tissue ischemia, including devascularization, results from trauma to tissues during an operative procedure. The introduction of foreign bodies into the abdominal cavity, whether glove talc, suture material, or other sources, is considered to be a potentiating factor. The presence of continued oozing at the completion of a procedure is also thought to be associated with adhesion development; the role of blood or preformed clots is less well established.

C. A wide variety of surgical approaches and surgical adjuvants have been utilized in attempts to reduce postoperative adhesion development. To date these attempts have not been completely successful, as evidenced by the large number of women who have pelvic adhesions at the time of "second look" laparoscopy.

D. The use of microsurgical techniques is thought to reduce postoperative adhesion development. These tenets include the use of magnification, achievement and maintenance of meticulous hemostasis, precise reapproximation of tissue planes, copious tissue irrigation, and avoidance of introduction of foreign material into the operative field. It had been thought that the use of lasers would reduce postoperative adhesion development, but this has not been observed in either animal or human studies to date. It has also been suggested that the use of operative laparoscopy as opposed to laparotomy would reduce postoperative adhesion development; this issue has not as yet been thoroughly evaluated.

E. A wide variety of adjuvants have been utilized in attempts to reduce postoperative adhesion development. These are often administered in various regimens, including preoperative, intraoperative, and postoperative administration. Drugs utilized in this fashion include antibiotics, particularly Vibramycin and the cephalosporins. A wide variety of anti-inflammatory drugs have been utilized, including corticosteroids and antiprostaglandins. Heparin is utilized by many surgeons in the irrigation fluid. Before closing, 32 percent Dextran 70 is frequently placed intra-abdominally; its efficacy, however, is debated. The mechanisms by which it may work include its hydrofloatation, siliconizing, and anticoagulant effects. To prevent development of adhesions between adjoining structures, a variety of barriers have been utilized. These include biologic tissues, such as preperitoneal or omentum grafts and amnion, and synthetic materials. The latter include materials that require removal at a subsequent operative procedure as well as those that subsequently are reabsorbed.

References

Diamond MP, Daniell JF, Feste J, et al. Adhesion reformation and de novo adhesion formation following reproductive pelvic surgery. Fertil Steril 1987; 47:864–866.

Diamond MP, DeCherney AH. Pathogenesis of adhesion formation/reformation; application to reproductive surgery. Mirosurgery (in press).

Di Zerega GS. The causes and prevention of postsurgical adhesions. Bethesda: Pregnancy Research Branch, National Institutes of Health and Human Development, 1980.

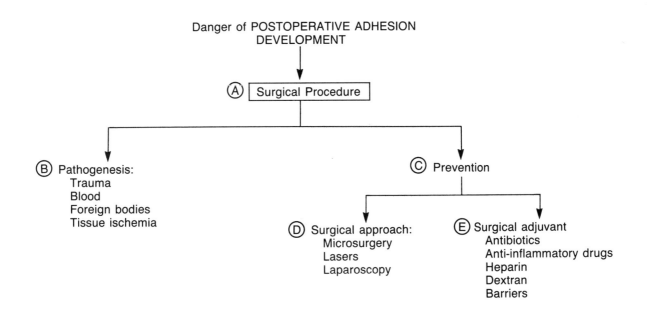

Danger of POSTOPERATIVE ADHESION
DEVELOPMENT

(A) Surgical Procedure

(B) Pathogenesis:
Trauma
Blood
Foreign bodies
Tissue ischemia

(C) Prevention

(D) Surgical approach:
Microsurgery
Lasers
Laparoscopy

(E) Surgical adjuvant
Antibiotics
Anti-inflammatory drugs
Heparin
Dextran
Barriers

PROXIMAL TUBAL DISEASE

James M. Wheeler, M.D.
Mary Lake Polan, M.D., Ph.D.

Proximal tubal disease is usually caused by salpingitis isthmica nodosa or pelvic inflammatory disease (PID). Less common causes are endometriosis, leiomyomas, congenital atresia, polyps, and sequelae of previous surgery (e.g., tubal sterilization).

A. The differential diagnosis of bilateral proximal occlusion on hysterosalpingography (HSG) includes tubal spasm, artifactual occlusion by air bubbles, or pathologic occlusion of the tubes. If HSG demonstrates bilateral proximal occlusion, a repeat HSG may be performed, but most clinicians proceed to chromotubation under laparoscopy for confirmation. Whereas most experts first perform HSG as the current standard in evaluating the uterine cavity and tubal isthmus, some perform hysteroscopy at the time of laparoscopy. Following assessment of tubal patency at transcervical chromotubation, the pelvis is surveyed for concomitant disease. Corrective surgery for proximal occlusion is contraindicated in the presence of acute or subacute infection, concomitant distal occlusion, a frozen pelvis, tuberculosis, or an anticipated post-repair tubal length of less than 3 cm.

B. At this time, the incidence of success through in vitro fertilization is better than that with surgical correction of bipolar tubal disease.

C. Surgery is scheduled during the proliferative phase. An intrauterine pediatric Foley catheter attached to a syringe filled with dilute indigocarmine dye is placed. The cornu may be circumferentially injected with dilute Pitressin.

The initial incision is made with the Gomel knife 1 cm from the apparent cornu-tubal junction; subsequent cuts are made proximally until dye flows freely from the new opening. If sufficient uterine myometrium remains to permit tubocorneal anastomosis, the procedure continues; if the serial cuts extend all the way to the uterine cavity, most surgeons proceed with an implantation procedure (see F). Careful bipolar cautery is used to achieve hemostasis.

D. For tubocornual anastomosis (Fig. 1), a bulb syringe with dilute indigocarmine dye is used to flush the distal tube via the fimbria; serial sharp cuts are made until dye is seen to be flowing freely from the new proximal opening of the distal tubal segment. Absorbable muscularis 7–0 sutures are placed at the 6-, 3-, 9- and 12-o'clock positions in order; they are tied in the same order. The serosa is closed with interrupted 6–0 absorbable sutures. The mesosalpinx can be anchored to the uterine serosa with a 5–0 suture. A successful anastomosis reestablishes patency of tubes with undamaged mucosa, a preserved blood supply, and a minimal length of 5 cm.

E. Tubal implantation (Fig. 2) traditionally involves remov-

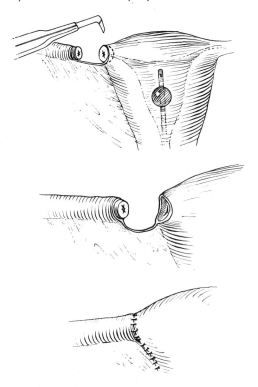

Figure 1 Tubocornual anastomosis.

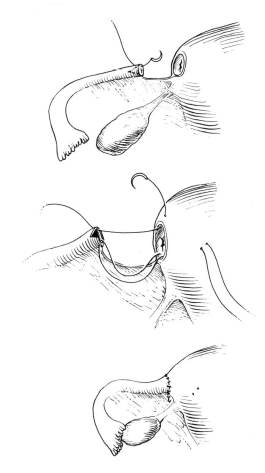

Figure 2 Tubouterine implantation.

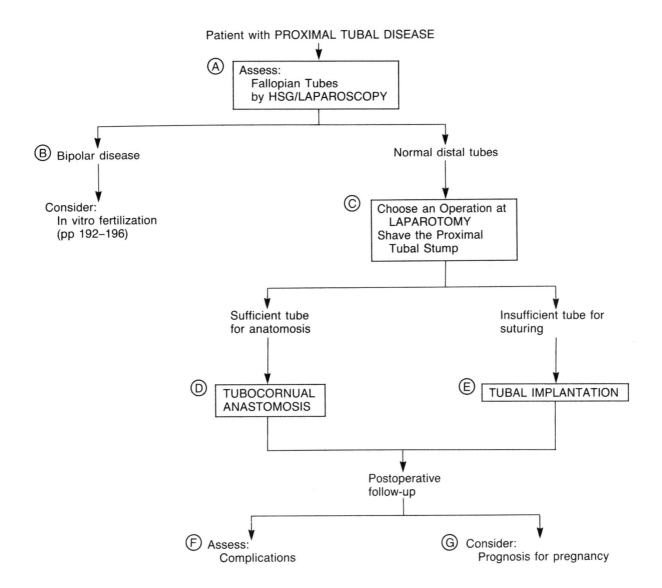

Patient with PROXIMAL TUBAL DISEASE

(A) Assess:
Fallopian Tubes
by HSG/LAPAROSCOPY

(B) Bipolar disease

Normal distal tubes

Consider:
In vitro fertilization
(pp 192–196)

(C) Choose an Operation at
LAPAROTOMY
Shave the Proximal
Tubal Stump

Sufficient tube
for anatomosis

Insufficient tube for
suturing

(D) TUBOCORNUAL
ANASTOMOSIS

(E) TUBAL IMPLANTATION

Postoperative
follow-up

(F) Assess:
Complications

(G) Consider:
Prognosis for pregnancy

ing the interstitial portion of the tube by using a sharp cork borer or a no. 11 scalpel blade. The distal tube is prepared as for tubocornual anastomosis, except that the proximal end is incised perpendicular to the axis of the mesosalpinx for about 1.5 cm (so-called "fish-mouthing"). The first layer of sutures attaches tubal muscularis to uterine myometrium; 6–0 absorbable suture is used. The serosa is closed with interrupted 5–0 absorbable suture. Implantation may also be performed via a transverse incision in the posterior wall of the uterus. The tubes are implanted into the corners of the incision with 4–0 sutures, and the uterine wall is then closed with 4–0 suture. Posterior implantation using the cork borers is another option.

F. Bleeding is easily controlled with Pitressin and bipolar cautery. Infection is possible but uncommon. A failed anastomosis or implantation may be related to technical errors, including separation of the tube from the uterus due to excess tension, poor healing due to poor suturing technique, and local hemorrhage due to poor preparation of the cornua. The ectopic pregnancy incidence is 2 to 5 per 100 live births, compared to the general population risk of about 1 per 100 live births. Proximal occlusion caused by PID is associated with an even

higher incidence of ectopic pregnancy. In the case of intrauterine pregnancy, cesarean section is indicated with all tubal implantation procedures, but not for tubocornual anastomoses. Uterine rupture and silent dehiscence have been reported at the site of a posterior wall incision; rupture is reportedly rarer if cork borers are used.

G. Live pregnancy incidences of up to 60 percent following cornual-isthmic anastomosis are reported, compared to about 50 percent after cornual-ampullary anastomosis. Posterior wall implantation procedures are generally less successful than anastomoses, but some series report up to 68 percent success in selected cases; an "average" incidence after implantation would be 40 percent.

References

Gomel V. Microsurgery in female infertility. Boston: Little, Brown, 1983.
Peterson EP, Musich JR, Behrman SJ. Uterotubal implantation and obstetric outcome after previous sterilization. Am J Obstet Gynecol 1977; 128:662–667.

DISTAL TUBAL DISEASE

James M. Wheeler, M.D.
Mary Lake Polan, M.D., Ph.D.

A. The most common etiology for postinflammatory distal tubal disease is bacterial infection, exemplified by the endosalpingitis associated with gonorrhea and *Chlamydia*. Pelvic inflammatory disease (PID) associated tubal damage is the most common cause of infertility in women 25 years of age and younger. Of note, it is estimated that use of low-dose oral contraceptives decreases an individual woman's chance of PID and thus perhaps its sequelae of tubal disease by 50 percent. Less common causes of distal tubal disease are iatrogenic (postfimbriectomy) and congenital (atresia or deformity sometimes associated with intrauterine diethylstilbestrol [DES] exposure). The hysterosalpingographic (HSG) appearance of postinflammatory distal tubal disease may involve tubal closure, as seen with hydrosalpinx or distortion and sacculation due to adhesions, which distort the tube (Fig. 1). If a hydrosalpinx is identified, demonstration of tubal rugae is a favorable prognostic sign. Laparoscopy follows HSG in the evaluation of tubal disease. Asymmetry in tubal disease is noted, and each tube is assessed for its dilation, thickness of wall, and condition of fimbria and ovary. Upon chromopertubation, if dye fails to reach the distal tube because of proximal hindrance or if the tube appears thin and attentuated, the prognosis following repair is poor. Hydrosalpinges more than 2 cm in diameter have less than half the success rate of lesser degrees of dilation.

B. Laparoscopic lysis of adhesions is a standard technique, whereas laparoscopic fimbrioplasty is not. In patients with severe disease, e.g., bilateral dilated hydrosalpinges, laparoscopic neosalpingostomy would probably produce the same dismal results as the operation performed at laparotomy with less risk and discomfort to the patient.

C. Salpingostomy is surgical correction of the fallopian tube that is completely occluded with no recognizable fimbria on inspection prior to opening the tube. A central dimple is often identified and represents the best point of puncturing the hydrosalpinx. A titanium rod is inserted into the opening, and three or four radial incisions are made with minimal trauma using finepoint laser or cautery. Should bleeding be encountered, careful bipolar electrocautery is used. The edges of the neosalpingostomy are everted by using the defocused laser beam on the tubal serosa or sparing placement of 8-0 or finer nylon sutures.

D. Fimbrioplasty is surgical correction of the distal fallopian tube in the presence of definite fimbrial tissue. The fimbria is more diseased than seen at salpingo-ovariolysis, yet is visible in comparison to the denuded tube seen with hydrosalpinx. The tube may be completely or partially occluded at its opening. Magnification and microsurgical technique are absolute prerequisites for fimbrioplasty. "Phimosis" of the tube by a collar of adhesions constricting the lumen of the ampulla is corrected by lysis at the antimesenteric aspect of the tube. Fimbrial agglutination involves usually fine adhesions over the surface of the fimbria. If the edges of the fimbria are inverted, serial incisions along avascular planes of the tubal serosa are made, and the edges are everted using either the defocused CO_2 laser, or a few 8-0 or finer permanent sutures.

E. Salpingo-ovariolysis offers the best prognosis of any surgery involving the distal tube since the fimbria is preserved in a normal state but distorted in its normal relationship to the ovary because of external adhesions. Adhesions are serially lysed, from opening the peritoneal cavity, down to the pelvis to free omentum and bowel, and finally detailed lysis of adnexal adhesions.

F. Operative complications of bleeding and infection are rare. The most common and serious complication resulting from distal tubal surgery is tubal ectopic pregnancy. The reported range of ectopic pregnancy is from 4 percent to 20 percent; the incidence seems to be directly related to the degree of intraluminal disease present at surgical correction. Macro- versus microsurgical and laser versus cautery technique seem not to be associated with a change in the incidence of ectopic presurgery.

G. Success is directly related to the degree of disease discovered in the tubes. Salpingo-ovariolysis is associated with a 60 percent incidence of success because of the normalcy of the fimbria and ampulla; pregnancy inci-

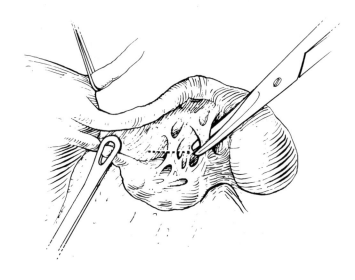

Figure 1 Lysis of peritubal and periovarian adhesions.

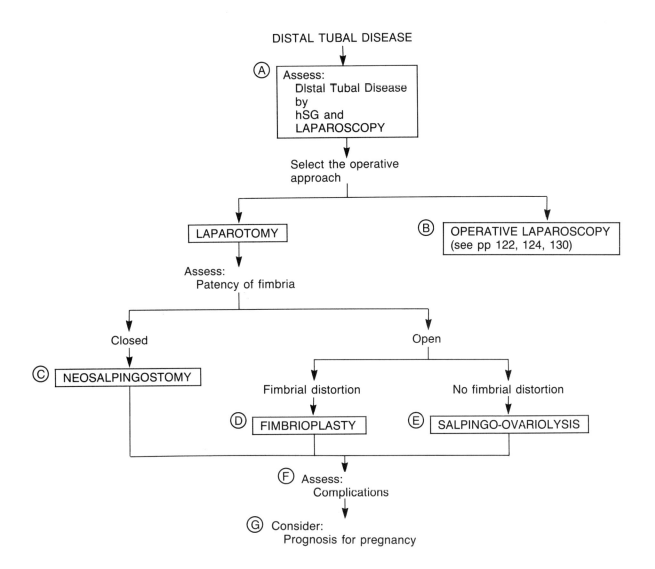

DISTAL TUBAL DISEASE

Ⓐ Assess:
Distal Tubal Disease
by
hSG and
LAPAROSCOPY

Select the operative
approach

LAPAROTOMY

Ⓑ OPERATIVE LAPAROSCOPY
(see pp 122, 124, 130)

Assess:
Patency of fimbria

Closed

Open

Ⓒ NEOSALPINGOSTOMY

Fimbrial distortion

No fimbrial distortion

Ⓓ FIMBRIOPLASTY

Ⓔ SALPINGO-OVARIOLYSIS

Ⓕ Assess:
Complications

Ⓖ Consider:
Prognosis for pregnancy

dences after fimbrioplasty are as high as 50 percent. Salpingostomy results are strongly correlated with the native disease; if fimbria is discovered within the hydrosalpinx and rugal folds are present, pregnancy incidences can approach 30 percent. In the presence of bilaterally thinned-out, adhesed tubes dilated more than 2 cm, lacking any identifiable fimbria or proximal tubal opening, pregnancy results in 5 percent or less of cases; therefore, in vitro fertilization would likely be more successful.

References

Gomel V. Salpingo-ovariolysis by laparoscopy in infertility. Fertil Steril 1983; 40:607–611.

Gomel V, Swolin K. Salpingostomy: microsurgical technique and results. Clin Obstet Gynecol 1980; 23:1243–1258.

Mage G, Bruhat M-A. Pregnancy following salpingostomy; comparison between CO_2 laser and electrosurgery procedures. Fertil Steril 1983; 40:472–475.

TUBAL ANASTOMOSIS

James M. Wheeler, M.D.
Mary Lake Polan, M.D., Ph.D.

A. Occlusion of the tubal isthmus involves a variable length of the tube depending on the underlying cause. Laparoscopic unipolar coagulation for sterilization is associated with the most widespread destruction of the isthmus, and histologic damage may extend to the intramural and ampullary aspects of the tube. Bipolar burns are usually less widespread than unipolar burns; however, many surgeons apply a bipolar burn to three distinct points on the isthmus during sterilization. The Falope ring usually destroys 1 to 2 cm of tube, and the Hulka clip about 0.5 cm of isthmus. Records of previous sterilization should be reviewed. As disparity between dictated operative records and subsequent laparoscopic evaluation is not uncommon, care must be exercised in refusing to further evaluate a patient for anastomosis solely on the basis of an operative report.

B. Hysterosalpingography (HSG) remains the best way to measure the length of proximal tube remaining after the sterilization. As prognosis for pregnancy is directly and positively correlated with the length of the repaired tube, at least 2 cm of proximal tube is important for successful anastomosis.

C. The most important finding at laparoscopy is the presence or absence of an intact fimbria; if the patient has had a previous fimbriectomy, anastomosis is not possible.

D. The patient is advised that anastomosis is contraindicated if the total tubal length is less than 3 cm. For a total length of 4 cm or more, the prognosis for pregnancy is 50 percent, and for 6 cm or more it approaches 70 percent.

E. Although research is under way to perfect the technique for laparoscopic anastomosis of ligated fallopian tubes, the current standard requires laparotomy. A low transverse incision is usually used. Careful microsurgical technique and magnification are prerequisites to a successful anastomosis.

F. An intrauterine pediatric Foley catheter or Harrison uterine manipulating injector (HUMI) is connected to a 30 cc syringe filled with a dilute indigocarmine dye solution. The proximal tube is serially sectioned using a sharp knife until a nipple of tubal mucosa that freely expresses dye is uncovered. The tubal mucosa should appear normal under magnification. Hemostasis is achieved by careful bipolar electrocauterization. Ideally, the serosa is 3 to 4 mm shorter than the mucosa and muscularis of the tube to facilitate suturing. If either proximal tubal segment is not suitable for anastomosis, transposition of contralateral segments is possible. Transposition and anastomosis of tubal segments have been accomplished in a few patients, and an occasional conception has occurred. The first successful "transplantation," involved transposing a left fimbrial segment and its vasculature to the proximal right tubal segment, anastomosing the tubal vessels, and allowed the patient to conceive and carry to term.

G. The distal tubal segment is flushed with an eyedrop syringe filled with dilute indigocarmine dye. The occluded end is serially cut with a knife until the lumen appears normal under magnification and dye flows freely. A no. 1 nylon stent is threaded through the fimbria into the new opening in the proximal tubal segment (Fig. 1). The stent should *not* be threaded into the intramural portion of the tube owing to the risk of developing a false passage. The mesosalpinx is approximated with interrupted 6–0 absorbable suture to take tension off the anastomosis sutures. The mucosa of the tubal segments is not traversed by the needles or manipulated by forceps. The muscularis is approximated with interrupted 8–0 absorbable sutures at 6, 3, 9, and 12 o'clock positions in order; these sutures are then tied snugly but not tightly in the same order. The knots are directed away from the mucosa. The serosa is approximated with four 6–0 absorbable sutures. Chromopertubation should demonstrate tubal patency without leakage at the anastomotic site.

H. Serious complications of bleeding and infection are rare. Ectopic pregnancy occurs in about 5 percent of patients; microsurgical technique and magnification are thought to decrease the risk for tubal ectopic pregnancy.

I. The prognosis for pregnancy depends on several factors, including the site of anastomosis. The highest incidence of pregnancy occurs with isthmic-isthmic (63 percent) and isthmic-cornual (60 percent) anastomoses and the lowest with ampullary-ampullary (50 percent) anastomosis and ampullary-cornual (40 percent) anastomosis.

References

Gomel V. Tubal reanastomosis by microsurgery. Fertil Steril 1977; 28:59–65.

Haney AF. Utilization of contralateral fallopian tube segments in tubal reanastomosis. Fertil Steril 1982; 37:701–703.

Siegler AM, Koutopoulos V. An analysis of macrosurgical and microsurgical techniques in the management of the tuboperitoneal factor in infertility. Fertil Steril 1979; 32:377–383.

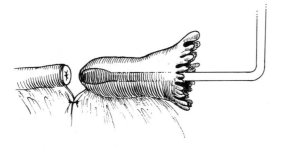

Figure 1 Isthmic-ampullary anastomosis. Preparation of the ampullary segment.

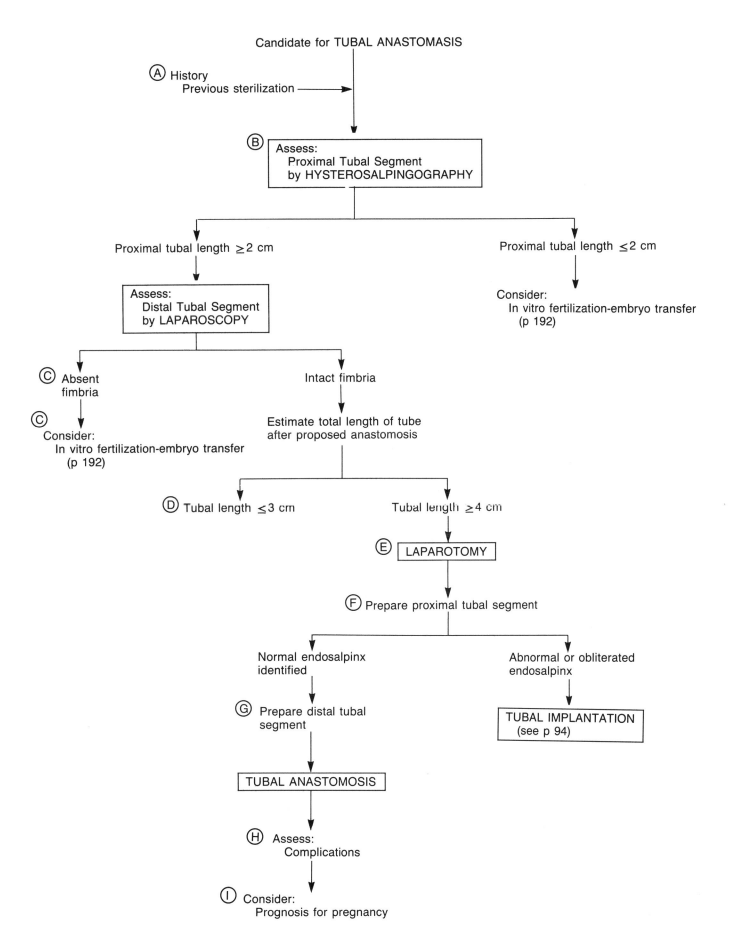

Candidate for TUBAL ANASTOMASIS

(A) History
Previous sterilization ⟶

(B) Assess:
Proximal Tubal Segment
by HYSTEROSALPINGOGRAPHY

Proximal tubal length ≥2 cm

Proximal tubal length ≤2 cm

Assess:
Distal Tubal Segment
by LAPAROSCOPY

Consider:
In vitro fertilization-embryo transfer
(p 192)

(C) Absent
fimbria

Intact fimbria

(C) Consider:
In vitro fertilization-embryo transfer
(p 192)

Estimate total length of tube
after proposed anastomosis

(D) Tubal length ≤3 cm

Tubal length ≥4 cm

(E) LAPAROTOMY

(F) Prepare proximal tubal segment

Normal endosalpinx
identified

Abnormal or obliterated
endosalpinx

(G) Prepare distal tubal
segment

TUBAL IMPLANTATION
(see p 94)

TUBAL ANASTOMOSIS

(H) Assess:
Complications

(I) Consider:
Prognosis for pregnancy

99

INFERTILITY OPERATIONS ON THE OVARY

James M. Wheeler, M.D.,
Mary Lake Polan, M.D., Ph.D.

A. The goal of the infertility surgeon is to maximize the individual patient's chances for pregnancy. This may require removal of an ovary in the presence of severe disease. Although a single ovary is adequate for steroid secretion and consistent ovulation, it remains functional only if its blood supply is preserved.

B. If the substance of the ovary is destroyed by endometriosis or if any ovary's blood supply is irreparably compromised by disease or attempted surgical repair, oophorectomy, especially in the presence of a normal contralateral adnexa, is the preferred operation.

C. In addition to preserving ovaries, the proper association of the salvaged ovary to its fallopian tube must be assured. Efficient ovum pickup does not occur if the ovary is trapped by pelvic adhesions or if the fimbria is restricted by adhesions. Entrapped ovaries are more likely to cause pain and form cysts. The ovarian capsule is not as amenable to suturing as peritoneum and serosal surfaces and should not be incised unless tissue within the ovary must be removed. Following ovarian repair, additional steps to prevent re-formation of adhesions to the ovary is indicated, e.g., ovarian suspension and intraperitoneal dextran solution.

D. Tumors within the ovary may vary from a barely appreciable 5 mm to many centimeters, seemingly displacing the ovary. An ovarian tumor should be removed if it is large, likely to grow, of unknown pathologic nature, or represents a condition deleterious to fertility, e.g., endometriosis. The capsule is incised along the antimesenteric edge over the tumor in such a way as to avoid the hilum. Sharp incision with the knife or laser should cleanly incise the capsule only, avoiding the underlying ovarian stroma. The tumor is removed intact using sharp dissection with scissors, preserving as much ovarian stroma and capsule as possible. Suture closure is accomplished using 3–0 to 5–0 absorbable sutures to effect hemostasis in the stroma. The goal of ovarian closure is maintenance of the ovarian blood supply while minimizing risk of adhesions. A running subcapsular 5–0 absorbable suture is brought out at the apex of the ovarian incision and then used to close the cortex in a smooth manner. Care should be taken not to tear the capsule or imbricate cortex, either of which could produce cysts. Even with large tumors, some ovarian tissue can often be preserved. Following repair, careful attention must be paid to the contralateral ovary owing to the varying incidence of bilateral disease. Frozen section of the excised tumor often aids the surgeon in determining the need for further surgery. Cosmetic results from plastic closure of the ovary are good, although adhesions form in up to 40 percent of the cases. Ovarian steroid production is more difficult to compromise than ovulation and ovum pick-up; pregnancy incidences depend on the underlying disease and proportionate mass of ovary remaining.

E. Wedge resection is the last option for women with polycystic ovarian disease (PCOD) who fail to ovulate despite optimum medical therapy. Sharp elliptical incision of the capsule is followed by excision of a wedge of stromal tissue deep into the ovary. Closure is the same as described above for ovarian cystectomy. Ovulation will follow in reportedly 6 to 95 percent of cases for a variable period of time. Pelvic adhesions occur in over one-fourth of wedge-resected patients. If pregnancy does not ensue, the hormonal milieu returns to its preoperative state with time, and ovulation is again inhibited by high tonic levels of luteinizing hormone.

F. Ovarian suspension may increase the distance between the ovary and the fimbria and therefore probably does not promote endogenous fertility. However, ovarian suspensions are used when the posterior cul de sac is severely diseased, and the ovary is lifted up from the cul de sac by shortening the utero-ovarian ligament.

G. As transvaginal ultrasound-guided oocyte aspiration becomes the dominant form of oocyte harvesting, there is less reason to suspend the ovaries superiorly, since lower ovaries are more amenable to the ultrasonographic retrieval technique.

References

Buttram VC, Vaquero C. Post-ovarian wedge resection adhesive disease. Fertil Steril 1975; 26:874–876.

Judd HL, Rigg LA, Anderson DC, Yen SSC. Effects of ovarian wedge resection on gonadotropin and steroid levels in polycystic ovary syndrome. J Clin Endocrinol Metab 1976; 43:347–355.

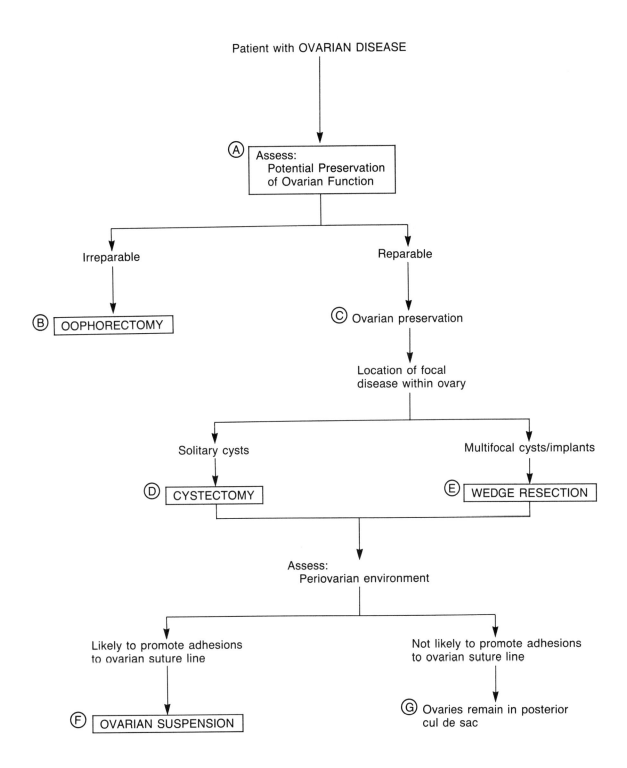

Patient with OVARIAN DISEASE

(A) Assess:
　Potential Preservation
　of Ovarian Function

Irreparable

(B) OOPHORECTOMY

Reparable

(C) Ovarian preservation

Location of focal
disease within ovary

Solitary cysts

(D) CYSTECTOMY

Multifocal cysts/implants

(E) WEDGE RESECTION

Assess:
Periovarian environment

Likely to promote adhesions
to ovarian suture line

(F) OVARIAN SUSPENSION

Not likely to promote adhesions
to ovarian suture line

(G) Ovaries remain in posterior
cul de sac

ECTOPIC PREGNANCY: DIAGNOSIS

James M. Wheeler, M.D.
Mary Lake Polan, M.D., Ph.D.

A pregnancy developing outside the endometrial cavity is ectopic. A primary ectopic pregnancy develops at the point of nidation; a secondary ectopic pregnancy results from implantation following tubal abortion or rupture. Tubal pregnancy is found in 99 percent of ectopic pregnancies. Following tubal abortion or rupture, a tubal ectopic pregnancy can implant as a secondary abdominal pregnancy (0.03 percent of ectopics). Heterotopic pregnancy is defined as the simultaneous existence of an intrauterine and extrauterine pregnancy; the incidence is classically given as 1 in 30,000 births, but some authorities feel the incidence approaches 1 in 5,000 live births.

In women of reproductive age in the United States, the incidence of ectopic pregnancy has been variously estimated at 49 to 84 per 100,000 live births. Pathologic evidence of tubal damage caused by tubal infection occurs in about 45 percent of patients. Intramural polyps and tubal diverticula may alter migration of spermatozoa or fertilized ova. Tubal infertility surgery is associated with an average 10 percent incidence of ectopic pregnancies; terminal neosalpingostomy may be associated with a 40 percent incidence. Although pregnancy follows only 0.5 percent of tubal sterilizations, half the pregnancies are ectopic. Intrauterine devices (IUDs) reduce the risk of intrauterine pregnancy by 99.5 percent, but tubal pregnancy by only 95 percent, with no reduction in the incidence of ovarian pregnancy; a greater proportion of pregnancies associated with IUD use are therefore ectopic. The same phenomenon has been described in failures of combined therapy with oral contraceptives or progestins.

A. The classic triad of pain, uterine bleeding, and adnexal mass occurs in 75 percent of ruptured ectopic pregnancies. Orthostatic symptoms or signs may be elicited; evidence of hypovolemia signals massive intraperitoneal blood loss.

B. Symptoms and signs of an early ectopic gestation are nonspecific and difficult to differentiate from complaints of early intrauterine pregnancy. Patients with a history of any of the etiologic factors listed above are suspect. The strongest risk factors are those of previous tubal surgery or pelvic inflammatory disease (PID). Patients' complaints range from a vague sense of discomfort in the lower abdomen to a sharp localized pain. Abnormal uterine bleeding is common. The uterus may be small or slightly softened; adnexal tenderness is usually present but can be absent. In one series, 68 percent of patients operated upon for ectopic pregnancies had been seen earlier by a physician an average of 2.5 times before the diagnosis was made.

C. Urine pregnancy tests may be negative in up to one-half of ectopic pregnancies depending on test sensitivity. Serum testing has a 1 percent false-negative incidence. The sensitivity of the urine or serum pregnancy test *must* be known by practitioners caring for women; appropriately sensitive tests reliably detect 25 to 50 mIU of β-human chorionic gonadotropin (hCG) per milliliter of serum.

D. In the event of a negative sensitive pregnancy test in this serious clinical scenario, immediate consultation is warranted for possible appendicitis, cholecystitis, or other abdominal complications.

E. Culdocentesis is positive (i.e., retrieves more than 3 ml of nonclotting blood) in 85 percent of ruptured ectopic pregnancies. Culdocentesis facilitates proper triage of patients: positive results warrant surgery and negative or inconclusive results merit further observation.

F. The patient should be observed and evaluated for other disease. There is a 1 to 2 percent false-negative incidence for sensitive pregnancy tests; a second test is warranted by a strong clinical suspicion of ectopic pregnancy.

G. Ultrasonography can detect an intrauterine gestation between 6 and 8 weeks of pregnancy, and except for heterotopic pregnancy, excludes the possibility of ectopic gestation. If an intrauterine pregnancy is not seen, a quantitative β-hCG determination is done. Lack of an ultrasonographically diagnosed gestational sac when the hCG reaches 6,500 IU per L is associated with a 93.5 percent probability of ectopic pregnancy. If the quantitative hCG is less than 6,000, further testing of the patient is warranted.

H. Serum β-hCG doubles every 2.2 days; failure of the titer to increase by 66 percent every 2 days suggests an abnormal pregnancy. Thus, if hCG levels fall, plateau, or fail to rise normally, curettage is performed, and if no intrauterine villi are retrieved, laparoscopy is indicated to search for an ectopic pregnancy.

I. The combined use of serum hCG and ultrasonography should not delay laparoscopy and treatment to the point of tubal rupture. Laparoscopy remains the mainstay of diagnosis, and its use in diagnosing ectopic pregnancies is contraindicated only in the presence of shock.

References

DeCherney AH. Ectopic pregnancy. Rockville, MD: Aspen Publications, 1986.

DeCherney AH, Kase N. The conservative surgical management of unruptured ectopic pregnancy. Obstet Gynecol 1979; 54:451–455.

DeCherney AH, Maheux R. Modern management of tubal pregnancy. Curr Probl Obstet Gynecol 1983; 9:15.

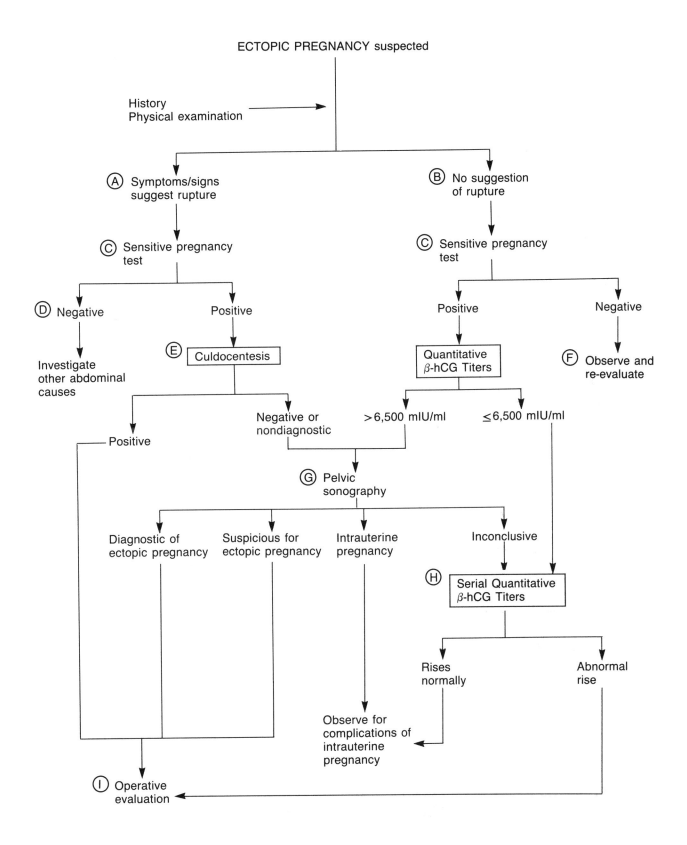

ECTOPIC PREGNANCY suspected

History
Physical examination

(A) Symptoms/signs
suggest rupture

(B) No suggestion
of rupture

(C) Sensitive pregnancy
test

(C) Sensitive pregnancy
test

(D) Negative   Positive

Positive   Negative

Investigate
other abdominal
causes

(E) Culdocentesis

(F) Observe and
re-evaluate

Quantitative
β-hCG Titers

Positive   Negative or
nondiagnostic   >6,500 mIU/ml   ≤6,500 mIU/ml

(G) Pelvic
sonography

Diagnostic of
ectopic pregnancy   Suspicious for
ectopic pregnancy   Intrauterine
pregnancy   Inconclusive

(H) Serial Quantitative
β-hCG Titers

Rises
normally   Abnormal
rise

Observe for
complications of
intrauterine
pregnancy

(I) Operative
evaluation

ECTOPIC PREGNANCY: TREATMENT

James M. Wheeler, M.D.,
Mary Lake Polan, M.D., Ph.D.

A. Laparoscopy is warranted in the patient with stable vital signs for diagnosis and evaluation of suspected ectopic pregnancy.

B. During laparoscopy, blood may be aspirated, revealing a bleeding corpus luteum amenable to laparoscopic electrocoagulation. Similarly, a tubal abortion is occasionally complete, indicating no further surgery.

C. Salpingostomy can be successfully completed via laparoscopy. In cases with tubal swelling less than 3 cm in diameter, the experienced operative laparoscopist can attempt salpingostomy. A 1-cm incision is made over the ectopic pregnancy on the antimesenteric side of the tube. The products of conception are removed by forceps and retrieved for histologic examination. Laser beam cautery stops pinpoint bleeding. Manipulation of the endosalpinx is minimized; the peritoneal cavity is lavaged. Hysterosalpingography (HSG) 6 to 8 weeks after salpingostomy will dictate further attempts at achieving pregnancy.

D. Crystalloid is begun immediately in a large bore intravenous catheter. Urine output is followed closely. A clot is sent to the blood bank for pretransfusion studies. Immediate consultation with the anesthesia service is arranged in anticipation of emergency laparotomy.

E. At laparotomy blood is aspirated, and bleeding stopped immediately by finger pressure across the mesosalpinx. The site of the ectopic is inspected for condition of the involved tube.

F. The available surgical options depend on the site of the tube involved and its potential necessity.

G. The ampulla is involved in 80 percent or more of tubal pregnancies.

H. In women who desire preservation of their fertility potential, there are several options available. In the 1950s salpingotomy—the opening of the tube, removal of the pregnancy, and primary closure—was the first conservative operation advocated. This has been replaced by a salpingostomy that differs by leaving the tube open to close by secondary intention. Most experts now prefer salpingostomy since there appears to be no advantage in time taken to close the tubal incision; salpingostomy incisions are uniformly healed and closed within 4 months of surgery. Surgeons may elect maneuvers in addition to salpingostomy in the treatment of ectopic pregnancy. Most experts recommend not milking the products from the open end of the tube because of increased tissue damage and the chance for incomplete removal of products. The Gepfert procedure can be used if nidation has occurred in the distal end of the tube. The linear incision is extended to the implantation site and products extracted. The mucosa is everted using a defocused laser beam or fine sutures. This procedure is associated with a lower pregnancy incidence than salpingostomy, presumably owing to disruption of the fimbrial mechanism.

I. If the woman has completed childbearing, salpingectomy is the best procedure to correct the problem and prevent its recurrence. The ipsilateral ovary should be preserved if it is anatomically normal.

J. If the patient's childbearing is completed, salpingectomy is performed. If fertility is desired, and the contralateral tube and ovary are normal, salpingectomy may again be indicated. If the contralateral tube is diseased, partial salpingectomy is indicated, removing as short a portion of tube as possible. Although anastomosis at the time of segmental salpingectomy has been reportedly successful, an improved chance for pregnancy is obtained if anastomosis is delayed until the vascular changes of pregnancy have resolved 6 to 8 weeks after treatment of the ectopic pregnancy. Although laparoscopic partial salpingectomy has been performed, complications with bleeding dictate that this procedure is one still best treated at laparotomy. Linear salpingostomy of isthmic ectopic pregnancies have been uniformly associated with occluded tubes at postoperative HSG.

K. Patients with interstitial ectopic pregnancies are notorious for late presentation often at 16 to 18 weeks of gestation. Frequently, hysterectomy is necessary because of the destruction of the cornu and associated bleeding. Excision of an interstitial pregnancy and tubouterine implantation into the cornu have been abandoned. Patients with cervical ectopic pregnancies are notorious for excessive bleeding and are almost invariably treated by hysterectomy. Abdominal pregnancies are debrided more than excised; placental tissue invading vascular tissues is not removed as life-threatening bleeding may ensue. Ovarian pregnancies are treated by conservative excision of the pregnancy; oophorectomy is warranted only if the ovary is destroyed by the pregnancy.

References

Bruhat MA, Manhes H, Mage G, Pouly JL. Treatment of ectopic pregnancy by means of laparoscopy. Fertil Steril 1980; 33:411–414.

DeCherney AH, Maheux R. Modern management of tubal pregnancy. Curr Probl Obstet Gynecol 1983; 9:15.

Weinstein L, Morris MB, Dotters D, Christian CD. Ectopic pregnancy: a new surgical epidemic. Obstet Gynecol 1983; 61:698–701.

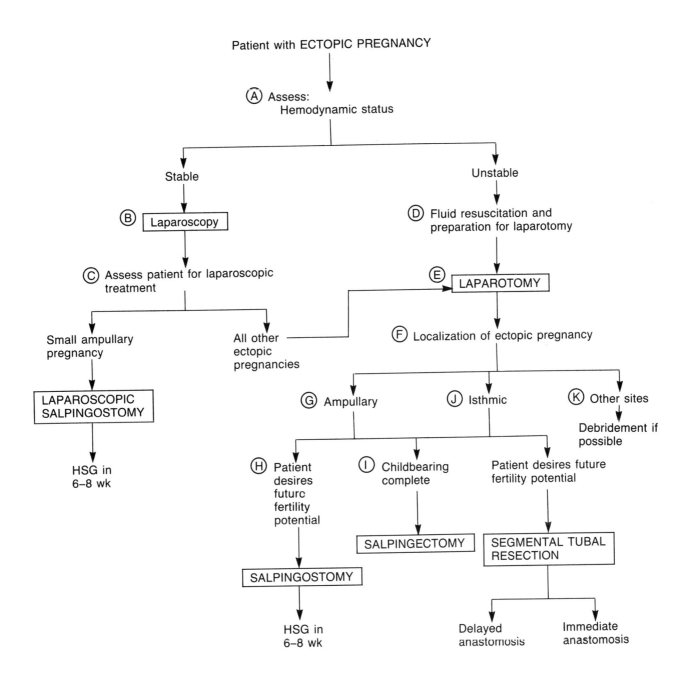

Patient with ECTOPIC PREGNANCY

(A) Assess:
Hemodynamic status

Stable

(B) Laparoscopy

(C) Assess patient for laparoscopic treatment

Small ampullary pregnancy

All other ectopic pregnancies

LAPAROSCOPIC SALPINGOSTOMY

HSG in 6–8 wk

Unstable

(D) Fluid resuscitation and preparation for laparotomy

(E) LAPAROTOMY

(F) Localization of ectopic pregnancy

(G) Ampullary

(J) Isthmic

(K) Other sites

Debridement if possible

(H) Patient desires future fertility potential

(I) Childbearing complete

Patient desires future fertility potential

SALPINGOSTOMY

SALPINGECTOMY

SEGMENTAL TUBAL RESECTION

HSG in 6–8 wk

Delayed anastomosis

Immediate anastomosis

ENDOMETRIOSIS

Mary Lake Polan, M.D., Ph.D.

A. Pelvic endometriosis is thought to be due to retrograde menstruation of viable endometrium, which implants on peritoneal surfaces. Although more frequently found in older nulliparous women, active endometriosis has been described in teenagers as well. Endometriotic lesions frequently occur on the uterosacral ligaments, leading to uterine retroversion and painful nodules palpable on vaginal examination. These nodules are frequently accompanied by pain on intercourse and severe dysmenorrhea. The finding of an adnexal mass in an asymptomatic patient must also lead to a suspicion of endometriosis, since the degree of pain or lack of it often does not correlate with palpable evidence of the disease. Finally, as many as 30 to 40 percent of the patients with endometriosis have associated infertility as a presenting complaint.

B. If infertility is a presenting complaint, laparoscopy should be performed at the end of a thorough infertility workup including semen analysis, a postcoital test, documentation of ovulation, and hysterosalpingography. If pain is the only presenting complaint, hysterosalpingography is still indicated prior to laparoscopy. At the time of laparoscopy, tubes should be lavaged with indigo carmine dye to assess patency and the pelvis examined systematically in a clockwise fashion. All areas of active endometriosis, scarring, and evidence of ovarian endometriosis should be documented using the American Fertility Society criteria. If the laparoscopy is done during the luteal phase, an endometrial biopsy may be performed simultaneously.

C. Since the incidence of pregnancy in patients with mild disease is similar regardless of whether management is expectant, medical, or surgical, the choice of therapy depends on other factors, such as age and the extent of pain. It must be remembered that the incidence of miscarriage in untreated and mild cases of endometriosis may range as high as 50 percent and is decreased after danazol or surgical therapy. By using the new technology of carbon dioxide and argon lasers, small endometriotic lesions often can be adequately treated and vaporized at the time of diagnostic laparoscopy.

D. Patients with moderate endometriosis at the time of laparoscopy who desire pain relief may be given medical therapy with danazol or a luteinizing hormone releasing factor (LRF) analogue. Although cessation of medical therapy often results in a recurrence of symptoms within 6 months to 1 year, another course of treatment is possible. Women desiring pregnancy can be treated with either medical therapy or conservative surgery, both of which are associated with a 50 to 60 percent incidence of pregnancy.

E. Women with severe disease can be treated with medical therapy for pain relief, and 85 to 90 percent experience a cessation of symptoms. Those who desire pregnancy should undergo conservative surgery, which is associated with a 30 to 40 percent incidence of pregnancy.

F. At the time of conservative surgery for endometriosis, several other adjunctive procedures may be considered. Uterine suspension and uterosacral plication have frequently been performed to antevert the uterus and, in the case of the latter procedure, to provide a shelf on which the ovaries may rest. Presacral neurectomy has frequently been performed in cases of severe pain and dysmenorrhea and relieves symptoms in 75 percent of the cases. All other areas of endometriosis that can be safely resected should be removed; however, appendectomy should be performed only when the appendix is involved with endometriosis.

G. Failure of both conservative surgical and medical therapy to reduce pain or result in pregnancy leaves the patient with few alternatives. When fertility is not a consideration, extirpative surgery with removal of the uterus and both ovaries is a reasonable alternative. In such situations estrogen replacement therapy should be instituted, because complications with residual endometriosis are rare when exogenous estrogen is used. Women who continue to hope for fertility may undergo repeat conservative surgery, which promises only an 8 to 12 percent pregnancy incidence. Recently the introduction of in vitro fertilization (IVF) programs across the country has given a third alternative to women who do not conceive after conservative surgery.

References

Batt RE, Naples JD. Conservative surgery for endometriosis in the infertile couple. Curr Probl Obstet Gynecol 1982; 6(1).

Buttram VC Jr, Belue JB, Reiter R. Interim report of a study of danazol for the treatment of endometriosis. Fertil Steril 1982; 37:478–483.

Polan ML. Endometriosis. Semin Reprod Endocrinol 1984; 2:186–196.

Rock JA, Guzick DS, Sengos C, et al. The conservative surgical treatment of endometriosis: evaluation of pregnancy success with respect to the extent of disease as categorized using comtemporary classification systems. Fertil Steril 1981; 35:131–137.

Wheeler JM, Johnston BM, Malinak LR. The relationship of endometriosis to spontaneous abortion. Fertil Steril 1983; 39:656–700.

ENDOMETRIOSIS suspected

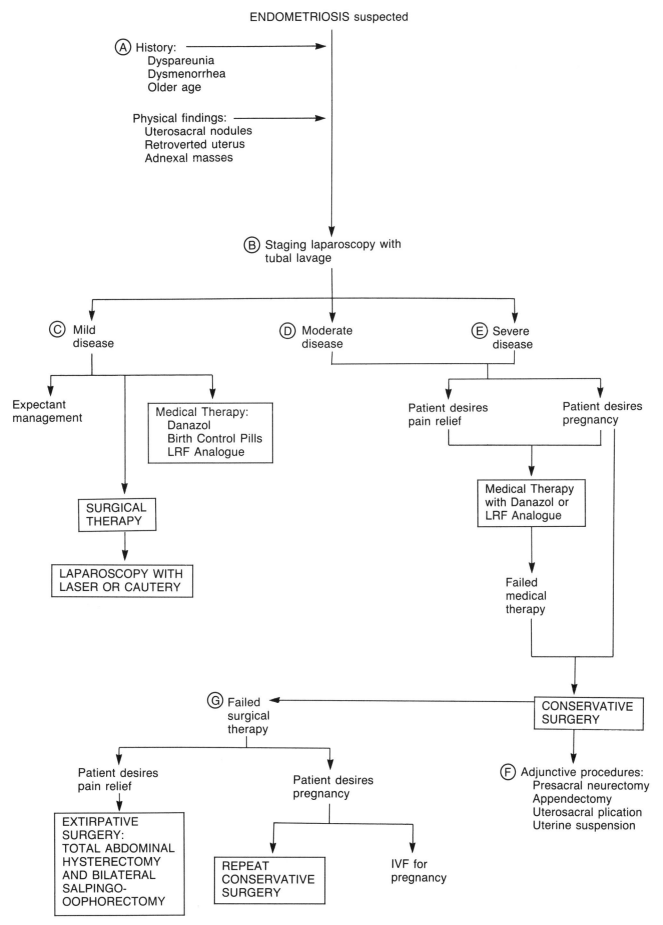

ENDOMETRIOSIS: DIAGNOSIS

Gad Lavy, M.D.
Mary Lake Polan, M.D., Ph.D.

A. Endometriosis is traditionally described in older white professional women. It is important to emphasize that it can be found in any woman regardless of age, race, or socioeconomic status.

B. A familial tendency to develop endometriosis has been described. In a study of patients with endometriosis, 5.8 percent of the sisters and 8.1 percent of the mothers were also found to be affected. The severity of the disease in the familial group seemed to be increased; severe disease was found in 64 percent of the familial group as compared with 24 percent of the nonfamilial group.

C. Endometriosis is defined as the presence of ectopic tissue that possesses the histologic structure and function of uterine mucosa. It is thought to be due to retrograde menstruation of viable endometrium, which implants on peritoneal surfaces. The symptoms tend to reflect the location of the disease process. The common symptoms—dyspareunia and dysmenorrhea—arise from involvement of the uterus and the cul de sac. Involvement of unusual locations (cervix, perineum, umbilicus, lung, brain) can give rise to atypical symptoms. Frequently the symptoms do not correlate with the extent of organ involvement. Women with mild disease can present with severe pain, while those with the severe forms may have minimal or no symptoms.

D. The common involvement of the uterosacral ligaments in the disease process gives rise to the typical finding of endometriosis, i.e., indurated and nodular uterosacral ligaments. The uterus is often retroverted owing to adhesions in the cul de sac. The finding of an enlarged ovary even in an asymptomatic young woman should raise the suspicion of endometriosis.

E. Approximately 30 to 40 percent of the patients with endometriosis have associated infertility as a presenting symptom. Possible causes of infertility in these patients include one or more of the following: tubal or ovarian adhesions, excess prostaglandin production interfering with tubal motility, and possibly the "luteinized unruptured follicle" syndrome. When infertility is the presenting symptom or when pregnancy is desired, a thorough infertility evaluation is mandatory in order to exclude other potential causes of infertility. The incidence of spontaneous abortion is increased in patients with endometriosis. The spontaneous abortion incidence in mild cases is higher (47 percent) than in moderate or severe cases (25 percent). The high incidence is reduced following surgery or medical therapy.

F. Endometriosis can be found outside the peritoneal cavity. Involvement of surgical scars, cervix, vagina, perineum, umbilicus, lung, and brain is occasionally seen. Its presence in strategic areas can give rise to life threatening conditions (e.g., pneumothorax when the lung is involved).

References

Chatman DL. Endometriosis in the black woman. J Reprod Med 1976; 16:303–306.

Melinak LR, Buttram VC Jr, Elias S, Simpson JL. Heritable aspects of endometriosis. Clinical characteristics of familial endometriosis. Am J Obstet Gynecol 1980; 137:332–337.

Paull T, Tedeschi LG. Perineal endometriosis at the site of episiotomy scar. Obstet Gynecol 1972; 40:28–34.

Schifrin BS, Erez S, Moore JG. Teenage endometriosis. Am J Obstet Gynecol 1973; 116:973–980.

Schoenfeld A, Ziv E, Zeelel Y, Ovadia J. Catamenial pneumothorax—a literature review and report of an unusual case. Obstet Gynecol Surv 1986; 41:20–24.

DIAGNOSIS AND EVALUATION IN ENDOMETRIOSIS

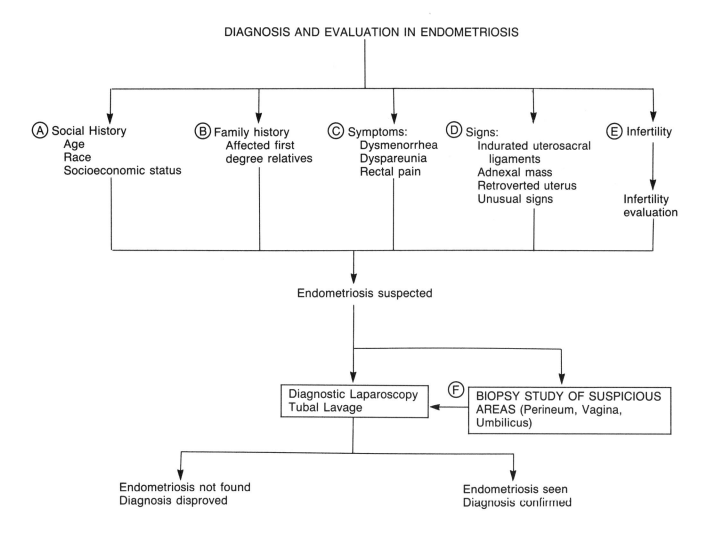

Ⓐ Social History
Age
Race
Socioeconomic status

Ⓑ Family history
Affected first
degree relatives

Ⓒ Symptoms:
Dysmenorrhea
Dyspareunia
Rectal pain

Ⓓ Signs:
Indurated uterosacral
ligaments
Adnexal mass
Retroverted uterus
Unusual signs

Ⓔ Infertility

Infertility
evaluation

Endometriosis suspected

Diagnostic Laparoscopy
Tubal Lavage

Ⓕ BIOPSY STUDY OF SUSPICIOUS
AREAS (Perineum, Vagina,
Umbilicus)

Endometriosis not found
Diagnosis disproved

Endometriosis seen
Diagnosis confirmed

ENDOMETRIOSIS: STAGING LAPAROSCOPY

Gad Lavy, M.D.
Mary Lake Polan, M.D., Ph.D.

A. The diagnosis of endometriosis should always be confirmed by laparoscopy, and treatment should never be started without a laparoscopic diagnosis. When laparoscopy is done during the follicular phase, the preovulatory follicle can be evaluated. In the luteal phase, laparoscopy can be combined with an endometrial biopsy to assess the adequacy of the luteal phase. The endometriotic lesions tend to become more vascular and friable during the luteal phase, and if possible the laparoscopy should therefore be performed during the follicular phase of the cycle. At laparoscopy the pelvis is inspected in a clockwise or counterclockwise fashion. The endometriotic lesions should be carefully documented.

B. The involvement of peritoneal surfaces and the extent and severity of adhesion formation should be carefully evaluated and recorded. Special attention should be directed to the sites that tend to be involved most frequently—bladder, peritoneum, pelvic sidewall, veriform appendix, and rectosigmoid. For staging purposes the surface of the uterus is considered to be a peritoneal surface.

C. The uterosacral ligaments and cul de sac are the most common sites for endometriotic implants. These areas should be carefully exposed and investigated. Common findings in this area include endometriotic implants, shortening and scarring of the uterosacral ligaments, and obliteration of the cul de sac by adhesions.

D. The extent of ovarian involvement is critical in determining the prognosis for future fertility. Implants of endometriosis, endometriomas, and periovarian adhesions are the common findings.

E. Endometriosis frequently involves the fallopian tubes and leads to infertility by compromising tubal motility or patency. The fallopian tubes are evaluated for endometriotic implants and adhesions, and tubal patency is assessed by tubal lavage at the time of laparoscopy.

F. A standard approach to the diagnosis and treatment of endometriosis is important if any meaningful conclusions are to be drawn. The American Fertility Society has devised a point-based staging system for endometriosis that places patients into minimal, mild, moderate, and severe categories on the basis of the extent of involvement, the size of the lesions, depth of penetration, and adhesion formation. This classification is designed to be used in infertile patients, as the prognosis for pregnancy is clearly related to the extent of the disease.

G. Laparoscopic lysis of adhesion and fulguration of the endometriotic implants at the time of the initial laparoscopy can make the procedure therapeutic as well as diagnostic. Fulguration can be accomplished by the use of electrocautery or laser. The procedure should be performed only by an experienced laparoscopist.

References

Acosta AA, Buttram VC Jr, Besch PK, et al. A proposed classification of pelvic endometriosis. Obstet Gynecol 1973; 42:19–25.

American Fertility Society. Revised American Fertility Society classification of endometriosis 1985. Fertil Steril 1985; 43:351–352.

Buttram VC Jr. Evolution and the revised American Fertility Society classification of endometriosis. Fertil Steril 1985; 43:347–350.

Hasson HM. Electrocoagulation of pelvic endometriotic lesions with laparoscopic control. Am J Obstet Gynecol 1979; 135:115–121.

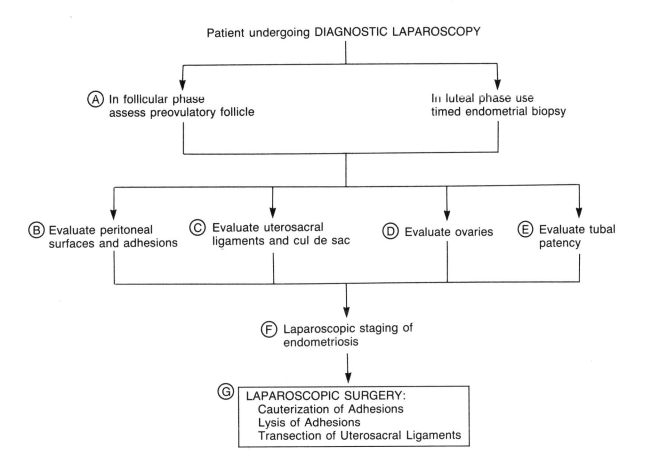

Patient undergoing DIAGNOSTIC LAPAROSCOPY

(A) In follicular phase
assess preovulatory follicle

In luteal phase use
timed endometrial biopsy

(B) Evaluate peritoneal
surfaces and adhesions

(C) Evaluate uterosacral
ligaments and cul de sac

(D) Evaluate ovaries

(E) Evaluate tubal
patency

(F) Laparoscopic staging of
endometriosis

(G) LAPAROSCOPIC SURGERY:
Cauterization of Adhesions
Lysis of Adhesions
Transection of Uterosacral Ligaments

MILD ENDOMETRIOSIS

Gad Lavy, M.D.
Mary Lake Polan, M.D., Ph.D.

A. In minimal and mild endometriosis the extent of involvement is limited. According to the American Fertility Society (AFS) classification, endometriosis is considered mild when the ovarian implants, if present, are superficial and periovarian or peritubal adhesions, if present, are filmy or do not enclose the entire ovary or tube. According to the point-based classification system, minimal endometriosis is given 1 to 5 points and mild endometriosis, 6 to 15 points (Fig. 1).

B. The drawback of fulgurating endometriosis by electrocautery, namely, organ damage by deeply penetrating electrical current, may be avoided by using the new argon lasers. With a wavelength of 488 to 514 μm, the energy is selectively absorbed by red objects, such as endometrial implants. In addition, the amount of energy needed for destruction of the implants is low enough to avoid deep penetration and minimize potential organ damage.

C. Operative laparoscopy can be used for pain relief in patients with endometriosis. Endometrial implants and adhesions, which are often the source of pain, can be lysed. In cases of chronic pelvic pain, interruption of the sensory nerve supply of the uterus traveling through the uterosacral ligaments can be accomplished by fulgurating these structures, with a high incidence of pain relief.

D. Following extirpative surgery in young women, estrogen replacement should be given unless a contraindication exists. The main objective of estrogen replacement is the prevention of osteoporosis. In addition, menopausal hot flashes and vaginal atrophy are avoided.

E. When pain persists after laparoscopic surgery and when medical therapy has failed to provide relief of pain, a laparotomy should be considered. In young patients and in those who wish to preserve their reproductive potential, conservative surgery is the procedure of choice. Lesions that are too large to be managed laparoscopically can be removed at laparotomy and a more complete lysis of adhesions performed.

F. Several investigators have recently demonstrated high conception incidences of up to 70 percent in infertile patients with mild endometriosis treated with expectant management. These figures compare favorably with the results of either medical therapy or conservative surgery. However, expectant management does not mean no therapy. During this observation period, all other identifiable causes of infertility are corrected.

G. The medical treatment of endometriosis is suppressive in nature. The various drugs used for therapy render the active lesions atrophic and prevent the appearance of new lesions during the treatment period. The cessation of therapy can lead to reactivation of the lesions. In addition chronic lesions, which consist mostly of scar tissue, are not affected by drugs. The major groups of drugs include those that induce a pseudopregnancy state (i.e., orally administered contraceptives) and those that induce pseudomenopause (i.e., danazol and gonadotropin releasing hormone analogues).

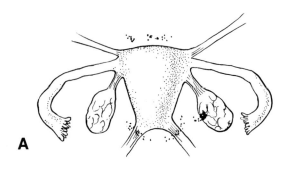

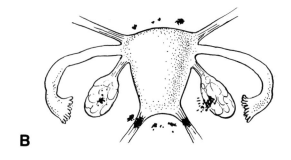

Figure 1 Mild endometriosis: *A*, stage I (minimal); *B*, stage II (mild).

References

Naples ND, Batt RE, Sadigh H. Spontaneous abortion rate in patients with endometriosis. Obstet Gynecol 1981; 57:509–512.

Schenken RS, Malinak LR. Conservative surgery versus expectant management for infertile patient with mild endometriosis. Fertil Steril 1983; 37:183–186.

Wheeler JM, Johnson BM, Malinak LR. The relationship of endometriosis to spontaneous abortion. Fertil Steril 1983; 39:656–660.

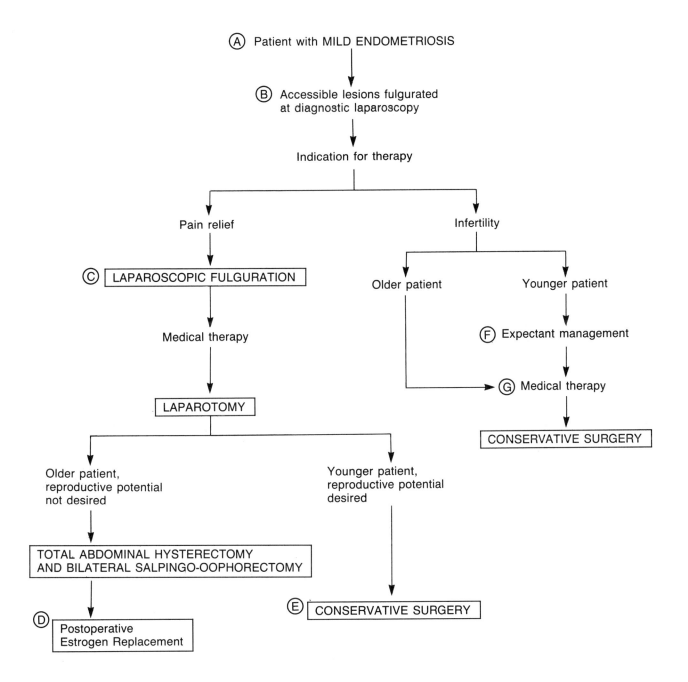

(A) Patient with MILD ENDOMETRIOSIS

(B) Accessible lesions fulgurated
at diagnostic laparoscopy

Indication for therapy

Pain relief

Infertility

(C) LAPAROSCOPIC FULGURATION

Older patient

Younger patient

Medical therapy

(F) Expectant management

LAPAROTOMY

(G) Medical therapy

Older patient,
reproductive potential
not desired

Younger patient,
reproductive potential
desired

CONSERVATIVE SURGERY

TOTAL ABDOMINAL HYSTERECTOMY
AND BILATERAL SALPINGO-OOPHORECTOMY

(D) Postoperative
Estrogen Replacement

(E) CONSERVATIVE SURGERY

MODERATE ENDOMETRIOSIS

Gad Lavy, M.D.
Mary Lake Polan, M.D., Ph.D.

A. According to the American Fertility Society (AFS) classification, moderate endometriosis implies the presence of a more extensive disease process than the mild form. Dense or filmy tubal and ovarian adhesions and superficial and deep ovarian and peritoneal implants that yield 16 to 40 points on the weighted system are compatible with moderate endometriosis. Dense adhesions and large implants that are present only unilaterally are still compatible with moderate endometriosis (Fig. 1).

B. Of the various drugs available for the treatment of endometriosis, orally administered contraceptives should be used for younger women who desire pain relief and are not interested in pregnancy in the immediate future. Oral doses of contraceptives are given continually and result in atrophy of the lesions. Danazol, by its androgenic effects, and the more recent gonadotropin releasing hormone (GnRH) agonist create a temporary menopause. The androgenic side effects of danazol are often disturbing and may limit its use; however, pregnancy incidences in patients with moderate endometriosis treated with danazol are 50 to 60 percent and are similar to those with conservative surgery. The side effects of the GnRH agonist are mainly those of a temporary menopause.

C. At the time of laparotomy, in addition to removing endometriotic implants and adhesions, procedures for pain relief may be performed. A presacral neurectomy, which disrupts the sensory output from the uterus, results in pain relief in a large proportion of patients. Uterine suspension can be performed when a retroverted uterus is a cause of dyspareunia.

D. When the indication for therapy is infertility, a complete infertility evaluation should precede therapy directed at endometriosis. Only after all other factors have been corrected and pregnancy still fails to occur should endometriosis be blamed for the infertility.

E. Pregnancy incidences of 50 to 60 percent are achieved with either medical or surgical therapy in patients with moderate endometriosis. The decision about the treatment modality depends on such factors as the patient's age and coexisting symptoms.

F. The incidence of recurrence after surgery is estimated to be 20 to 40 percent. In these patients the incidence of pregnancy following reoperation is low (9 to 12 percent). In addition, an equivalent number of patients require a third extirpative procedure. Repeat surgery after a failed conservative procedure requires careful consideration and counseling and is generally not recommended.

G. The failure to achieve a pregnancy following medical therapy or conservative surgery leaves the patient with few alternatives. If the symptoms are not severe enough to warrant extirpative surgery, in vitro fertilization and embryo transfer are the only remaining options prior to adoption.

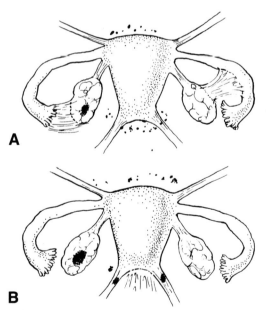

Figure 1 Moderate endometriosis. *A*, stage III (moderate). Note the filmy adhesions between the right ovary and the right fallopian tube, the deep left ovarian implants, and dense adhesions between the left tube and left ovary. *B*, stage III (moderate). Note the deep left ovarian implants and peritoneal adhesions.

References

Dmowski WP, Cohen MR. Antigonadotropin (danazol) in the treatment of endometriosis: evaluation of posttreatment: fertility and three-year follow-up data. Am J Obstet Gynecol 1978; 130:41–48.

Lemay A, Quesnel G. Potential new treatment of endometriosis: reversible inhibition of pituitary-ovarian function by chronic intranasal administration of a luteinizing hormone-releasing hormone (LH-RH) agonist. Fertil Steril 1982; 38:376–379.

Puleo JG, Hammond CB. Conservative treatment of endometriosis externa: the effects of danazol therapy. Fertil Steril 1983; 40:164–169.

Schenken RS, Malinak LR. Reoperation after initial treatment of endometriosis with conservative surgery. Am J Obstet Gynecol 1978; 131:416–424.

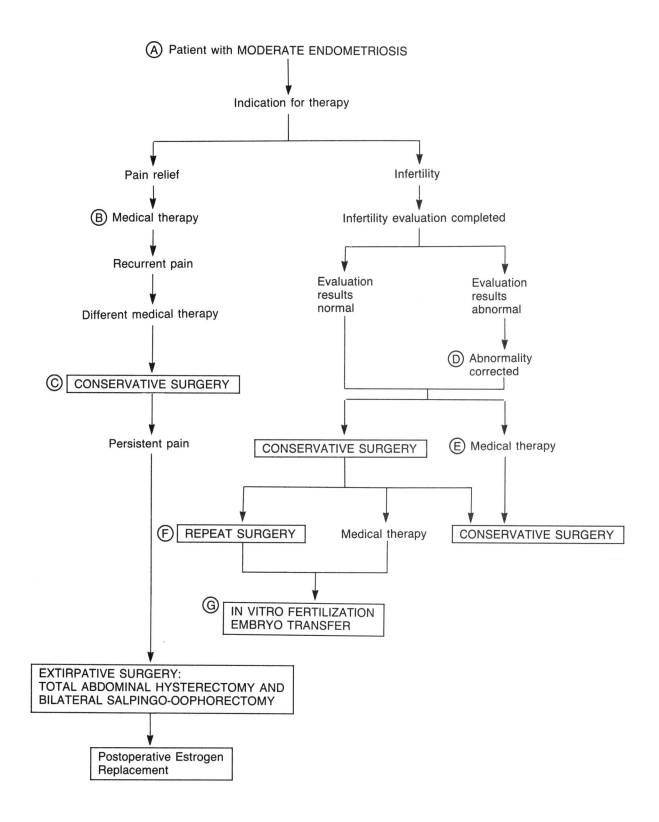

SEVERE ENDOMETRIOSIS

Gad Lavy, M.D.
Mary Lake Polan, M.D., Ph.D.

A. Severe endometriosis implies extensive involvement of the pelvic organs. On the point weighed staging system, 40 points or more are compatible with severe endometriosis. Bilateral large (more than 3 cm) ovarian endometriomas, dense ovarian adhesions enclosing more than two-thirds of the ovarian surface, complete obliteration of the cul de sac, or any combination of swollen lesions that gives a total of 40 points or more places the patient in the "severe" category (Fig. 1).

B. Patients with severe endometriosis treated with medical therapy experience relief of symptoms 85 to 90 percent of the time. The symptoms often recur within 6 to 12 months after cessation of therapy. When the pain recurs, an additional course of therapy is possible, but surgery offers a more permanent solution. The choice of conservative surgery or extirpative surgery depends on the patient's desire to preserve her child-bearing potential.

C. The benefits of estrogen replacement in young women after oophorectomy far outweigh the risks. The reactivation of the residual endometriotic implants with the hormonal therapy is only theoretical, for its occurrence is unusual in these patients.

D. The use of danazol prior to conservative surgery has the theoretical advantage of reducing the size of the implants and therefore facilitating the surgical procedure. In contrast with progesterone, danazol does not soften endometriomas and does not make them more likely to rupture at the time of surgery. On the other hand the administration of danazol preoperatively may mask small endometriotic implants that otherwise could have been removed. No definitive data exist to support or discourage the preoperative administration of danazol.

E. Areas of endometriosis that cannot be removed at surgery because of proximity to vital structures can be a source of postoperative pain and adhesion formation.

F. When a large amount of residual disease is left behind at the time of conservative surgery, a course of danazol given postoperatively can increase the chances for pregnancy. The incidence of pregnancy following surgery alone is 30 percent. A postoperative course of danazol has been shown to increase the pregnancy incidence to 79 percent.

G. After failure of conservative surgery, an attempt at medical therapy is recommended. The incidence of pregnancy when reoperation is attempted is low and in the range of that with in vitro fertilization and embryo transfer. Some of these patients eventually need an extirpative procedure after reoperation.

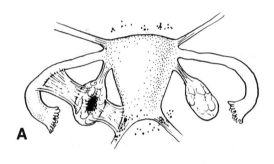

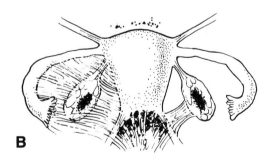

Figure 1 Severe endometriosis. Stage IV: *A*, dense adhesions and deep ovarian implant; *B*, complete obliteration of the cul de sac, dense ovarian adhesion, and bilateral large ovarian endometriomas.

References

Buttram VC Jr, Belue JB, Reiter R. Interim report of a study of danazol for the treatment of endometriosis. Fertil Steril 1982; 37:478–483.

Schenken RS, Malinak LR. Reoperation after initial treatment of endometriosis with conservative surgery. Am J Obstet Gynecol 1978; 131:416–424.

Wheeler JM, Malinak LR. Postoperative danazol therapy in infertility patients with severe endometriosis. Fertil Steril 1981; 36:460–463.

Patient with SEVERE ENDOMETRIOSIS

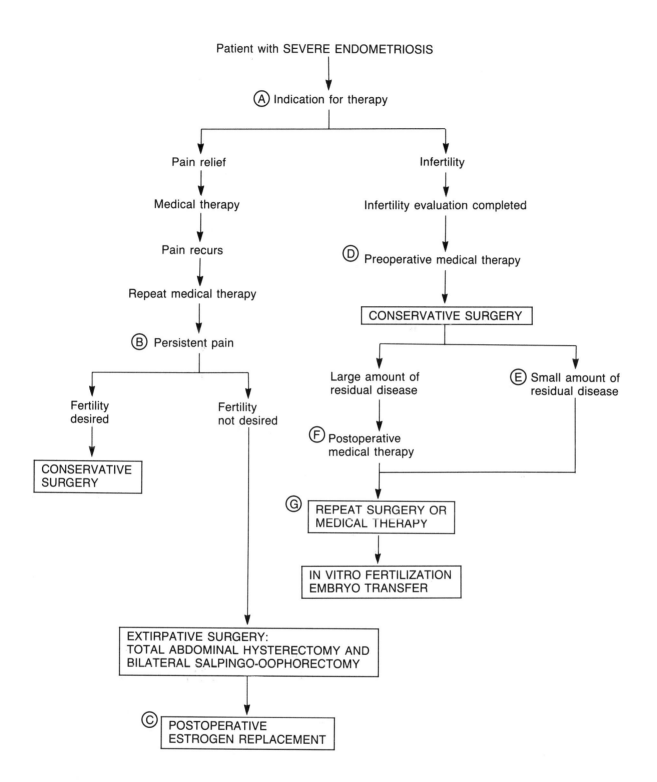

EXTIRPATIVE SURGERY:
TOTAL ABDOMINAL HYSTERECTOMY AND
BILATERAL SALPINGO-OOPHORECTOMY

CONSERVATIVE SURGERY FOR ENDOMETRIOSIS

Gad Lavy, M.D.
Mary Lake Polan, M.D., Ph.D.

A. Microsurgical technique should be employed in any woman in the reproductive age group undergoing abdominal or pelvic surgery. Microsurgical technique implies gentle handling of tissues, meticulous hemostasis, constant irrigation to prevent drying of tissue, avoidance of tissue ischemia, and the occasional use of magnification when needed.

B. One of the major obstacles to the success of surgical therapy is the recurrence of adhesions or the formation of new adhesions postoperatively. Various drugs are used to minimize this problem, although their effectiveness is still not proven. We currently employ the intravenous administration of Vibramycin, dexamethasone, and Phenergan perioperatively with high molecular weight dextran (Hyskon) instilled into the peritoneal cavity prior to closure.

C. Raw peritoneal surfaces can be a source of postoperative adhesion formation. The surgical removal of endometrial implants and lysis of adhesions can often create large raw surfaces. These surfaces can be covered with peritoneal or omental grafts. The use of relatively inert synthetic materials (polyglycolic acid polymers) has yielded disappointing results.

D. During surgery, an attempt should be made to meticulously remove all visible endometriotic implants. Ovarian endometriomas should be removed using microsurgical technique. Removal of an endometrioma is illustrated in Figure 1.

E. The appendix, owing to its close proximity to the pelvic organs, is frequently involved in the endometriotic process. Appendectomy should be performed only when involvement of the organ is demonstrated or when a fecolith is dislodged.

F. Frequently the uterus is retroverted because of adhesions in the cul de sac. Uterine suspension at the time of laparotomy at least temporarily keeps the uterus out of the cul de sac during the healing process. The uterus tends to return to its retroverted position some months following surgery when the round ligaments used for the suspension elongate. The uterosacral plication involves approximation of the uterosacral ligaments, thus obliterating the cul de sac and preventing adhesion formation in that area.

G. Presacral neurectomy is performed when significant central pelvic pain and dysmenorrhea exist. The procedure relieves these symptoms in up to 75 percent of the patients. The procedure disrupts the efferent nerve supply from the uterus. Women conceiving after this procedure may experience reduced pain sensation in labor.

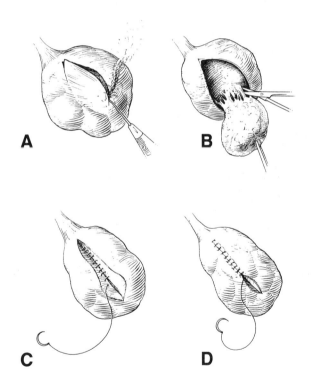

Figure 1 Excision of an endometrioma. *A*, an elliptical incision is made using the electrode. *B*, the endometrioma is excised. *C*, ovarian reconstruction is accomplished in two layers. *D*, the ovarian capsule is closed.

References

Adhesion Study Group. Reduction of postoperative pelvic adhesions with intraperitoneal 32% dextran 70: a prospective randomized clinical trial. Fertil Steril 1983; 40:612–619.

Buckman RF, Woods M, Sargent L, Gervin AS. A unifying pathologic mechanism in the etiology of intraperitonial adhesions. J Surg Res 1976; 20:1–5.

Collins DC. Endometriosis of the vermiform appendix. AMA Arch Surg 1951; 63:617–622.

Polan ML, DeCherney AH. Presacral neurectomy for pelvic pain in infertility. Fertil Steril 1980; 34:557–560.

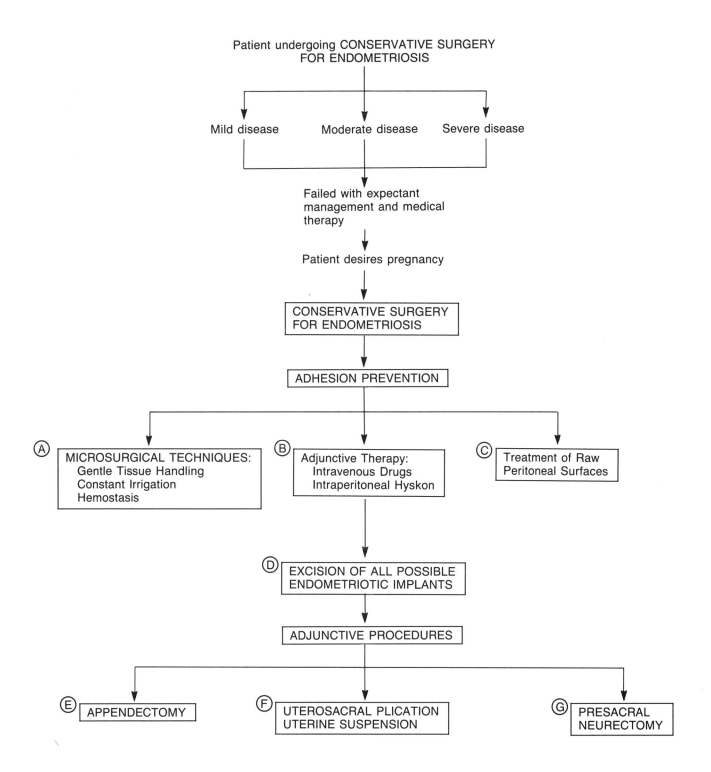

Patient undergoing CONSERVATIVE SURGERY
FOR ENDOMETRIOSIS

Mild disease   Moderate disease   Severe disease

Failed with expectant
management and medical
therapy

Patient desires pregnancy

CONSERVATIVE SURGERY
FOR ENDOMETRIOSIS

ADHESION PREVENTION

Ⓐ MICROSURGICAL TECHNIQUES:
Gentle Tissue Handling
Constant Irrigation
Hemostasis

Ⓑ Adjunctive Therapy:
Intravenous Drugs
Intraperitoneal Hyskon

Ⓒ Treatment of Raw
Peritoneal Surfaces

Ⓓ EXCISION OF ALL POSSIBLE
ENDOMETRIOTIC IMPLANTS

ADJUNCTIVE PROCEDURES

Ⓔ APPENDECTOMY

Ⓕ UTEROSACRAL PLICATION
UTERINE SUSPENSION

Ⓖ PRESACRAL
NEURECTOMY

FAILED SURGICAL THERAPY

Gad Lavy, M.D.
Mary Lake Polan, M.D., Ph.D.

A. When surgical and medical therapy have failed and pain persists, a more extensive surgical procedure is needed. Removal of the uterus, which is the likely source of new endometriotic implants and in addition can be a source of pain, and removal of the ovaries, which supply the hormonal support for the disease process, are highly effective in achieving pain relief. At the time of surgery all accessible endometrial implants and adhesions are removed.

B. When pregnancy fails to occur after a conservative surgical procedure, reassessment of the pelvis is needed. Even when it is clear that endometriosis has recurred, a repeat laparotomy may not be the procedure of choice, since the incidence of pregnancy following repeat surgery is low. A laparoscopy performed at this time reveals the degree of recurrence and allows assessment of the prognosis for pregnancy without subjecting the patient to a major surgical procedure.

C. Small endometrial implants and filmy adhesions that have not been totally removed at laparotomy or that have reformed following surgery can be treated via the laparoscope. The use of the laser makes the procedure safer and more effective. The pregnancy incidence following laparoscopic surgery is still low.

D. The finding of dense pelvic adhesions at laparoscopy makes the possibility of pregnancy unlikely. In preparation for in vitro fertilization–embryo transfer (IVF-ET), the accessibility of the ovaries for laparoscopic aspiration of follicles can be determined.

E. When dense adhesions are present in the pelvis, the ovaries are often obscured and access for follicle aspiration for IVF-ET could be risky or impossible. Release of these dense adhesions often requires a laparotomy. The ovaries are freed, and to ensure adequate access, ovarian suspension is performed by reefing the uterine-ovarian ligament up to the posterior uterine wall with a nonabsorbable suture.

References

DeCherney AH, Tarlatzis BC, Laufer N, Naftolin F. A simple technique of ovarian suspension in preparation for in vitro fertilization. Fertil Steril 1985; 43:659–661.

Laufer N, Tarlatzis BC, Naftolin F. In vitro fertilization: state of the art. Semin Reprod Endocrinol 1984; 2:197.

Polan ML. Endometriosis. Semin Reprod Endocrinol 1984; 2:186.

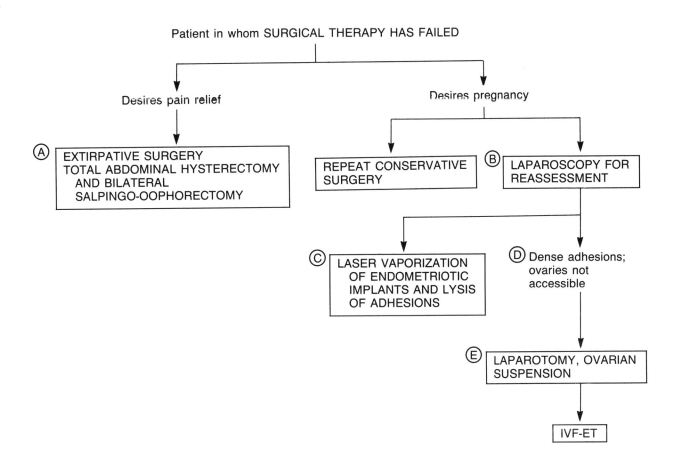

Patient in whom SURGICAL THERAPY HAS FAILED

Desires pain relief

Desires pregnancy

Ⓐ EXTIRPATIVE SURGERY
TOTAL ABDOMINAL HYSTERECTOMY
AND BILATERAL
SALPINGO-OOPHORECTOMY

REPEAT CONSERVATIVE
SURGERY

Ⓑ LAPAROSCOPY FOR
REASSESSMENT

Ⓒ LASER VAPORIZATION
OF ENDOMETRIOTIC
IMPLANTS AND LYSIS
OF ADHESIONS

Ⓓ Dense adhesions;
ovaries not
accessible

Ⓔ LAPAROTOMY, OVARIAN
SUSPENSION

IVF-ET

LAPAROSCOPY: DIAGNOSIS

Michael P. Diamond, M.D.
Mary Lake Polan, M.D., Ph.D.

A. Laparoscopy is usually performed under general anesthesia, although it can be performed using local or regional anesthesia. Difficulties associated with local or regional anesthesia include patient anxiety, diaphragmatic pressure when respiration is not being controlled mechanically, and the discomfort created by intra-abdominal gas. Diagnostic laparoscopy is usually performed in the dorsal lithotomy position to allow placement of instruments into the uterus for manipulation (Fig. 1). This allows greater visualization of pelvic structures.

B. In preparation for standard diagnostic laparoscopy, the abdomen, perineum, and vagina are prepared. After placement of a speculum in the vagina, an instrument is placed on the cervix for uterine manipulation. If a Conn cannula is to be used, a tenaculum is placed first, followed by insertion of the cannula into the cervical os. Humi, Hui, or Foley catheters may also be used. Any of these instruments allows chromotubation for assessment of tubal patency. If assessment of tubal patency is not desired during the diagnostic laparoscopy, greater uterine manipulation can be obtained by placing a tenaculum on the cervix, followed by a blunt curette nearly to the top of the uterine fundus, and taping these instruments together.

C. Insufflation of the abdominal cavity is performed after placement of the Verres needle periumbilically. The most common placement of the incision, approximately 1 cm in length, is just below the umbilicus. A more cosmetic alternative is placement of the incision in the umbilicus itself; this also allows placement of the needle and trocar through the thinnest portion of the abdominal wall. The initial incision can be made large enough to place the laparoscopic trocar, thus avoiding extending a very small incision for the Verres needle. The Verres needle must be grasped properly on its upper portion above the spring to benefit from the spring activated, blunt tip safety mechanism. If it is grasped improperly at its tip, the blunt tip cannot extend beyond the sharp point after entering the abdominal cavity, thus increasing the risk of damage to intra-abdominal structures.

D. The gas most commonly used for abdominal cavity insufflation is carbon dioxide. Usually the total volume of 2 to 3 liters is placed prior to insertion of the laparoscopic trocar. The correct amount for each patient varies with the size of the abdominal cavity and can be estimated by noting the loss of liver dullness and the extent of abdominal distention; this is difficult to determine in obese women.

E. After the abdominal cavity is appropriately insufflated, the Verres needle is removed and the laparoscopic trocar placed. This is most commonly done blindly, pointing the trocar toward the hollow of the pelvis. Care must be taken to avoid the sacral promontory. An alternative is open laparoscopy in which the laparoscopic trocar is placed after dissecting down through the layers of the abdominal wall into the abdominal cavity. This potentially reduces the risk of damage to underlying structures inherent in blind placement of the laparoscopic trocar. Such a risk is increased in individuals who have had previous abdominal surgery and those at risk for adhesion of abdominal structures to the anterior abdominal wall.

F. Following placement of the laparoscopic trocar and the laparoscope, the abdominal cavity is examined for injuries due to placement of the Verres needle and trocar. It is important to examine the area immediately beneath the incision. Subsequently the anterior abdominal wall is examined for the presence of adhesions that would impair placement of the second puncture probe.

G. Diagnostic laparoscopy requires placement of a second puncture probe in order to allow visualization of all surfaces of the pelvic structures by elevating the ovaries and manipulating the tubes. Visualization is also facilitated by manipulation of the instruments in the uterine cavity.

H. The pelvis should be examined in a systematic fashion. This can be done in any sequence, which should become a routine for the surgeon and should include the ovarian surfaces, uterus, tubes, cul de sac, and peritoneal surfaces.

I. Chromotubation is performed with diluted indigo carmine dye in order to evaluate tubal patency. It is important to visualize the distal end of each tube and not merely the presence of dye in the posterior cul de sac. Additionally the tubes can be examined for evidence of sacculation or partial fimbrial occlusion.

References

Gomel V. Laparoscopy and hysteroscopy in gynecologic practice. Chicago: Year Book, 1986.

Hulka JF, ed. Textbook of laparoscopy. Orlando: Grune & Stratton, 1985.

Wheeless CR. Laparoscopy. In: Mattingly RF, ed. Te Linde's operative laparoscopy. 5th ed. Philadelphia: JB Lippincott, 1977.

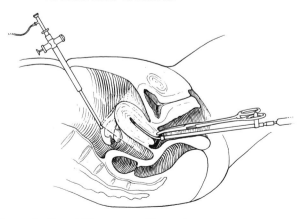

Figure 1 Dorsal lithotomy position at laparoscopy.

Patient undergoing LAPAROSCOPY FOR DIAGNOSIS

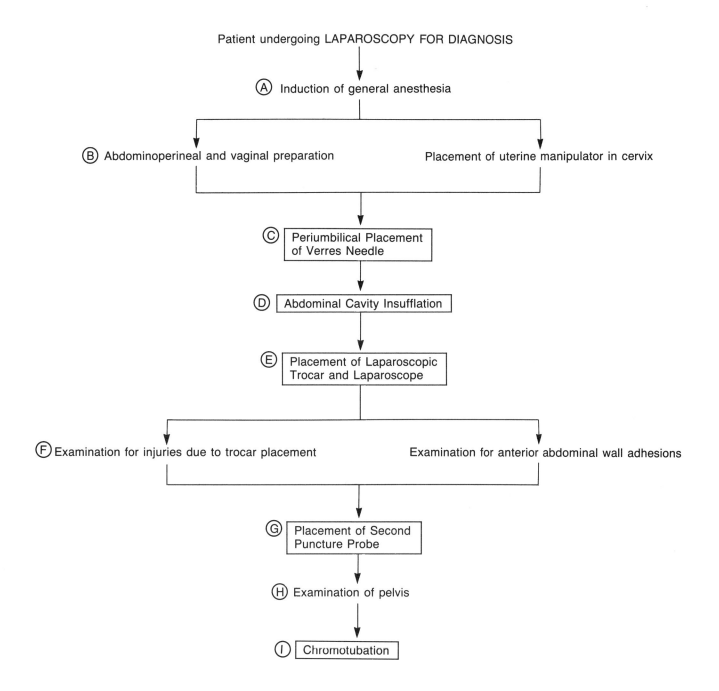

Ⓐ Induction of general anesthesia

Ⓑ Abdominoperineal and vaginal preparation

Placement of uterine manipulator in cervix

Ⓒ Periumbilical Placement of Verres Needle

Ⓓ Abdominal Cavity Insufflation

Ⓔ Placement of Laparoscopic Trocar and Laparoscope

Ⓕ Examination for injuries due to trocar placement

Examination for anterior abdominal wall adhesions

Ⓖ Placement of Second Puncture Probe

Ⓗ Examination of pelvis

Ⓘ Chromotubation

LAPAROSCOPY: TREATMENT

Michael P. Diamond, M.D.
Mary Lake Polan, M.D., Ph.D.

A. After a single puncture laparoscopy has been performed, a second puncture instrument should be placed in order to allow visualization of all surfaces of pelvic structures.

B. Pelvic disease is identified throughout the pelvis. This evaluation should be done in a systematic fashion so as not to overlook any area of disease. An estimate of the severity of lesions is critical to the subsequent decision to treat laparoscopically. Options include laparoscopic treatment at that time, laparoscopic treatment at a later time after discussion of the findings with the patient, or treatment at laparotomy. Discussion should be held with the patient prior to the procedure to aid the physician in making this therapeutic decision. Operative laparoscopy for the treatment of tuboperitoneal disease is becoming increasingly widespread. However, some of the techniques are beyond the capabilities of many surgeons or require instruments that are not available in all hospitals. Patients with extensive pelvic disease can be referred to surgeons who undertake more advanced laparoscopic surgery. Alternatively the pelvic disease can be treated at laparotomy.

C. If the decision is to perform laparoscopic correction of the tuboperitoneal disease, additional punctures may be necessary. If so, third, fourth, or even fifth puncture sites are placed. Their placement depends on the pelvic disease identified. They are used to facilitate manipulation of the pelvic structures to allow access to individual areas or to provide traction for surgical treatment. Procedures can be performed by viewing directly through the laparoscope, with an attachment made via a beam splitter to allow video monitoring if desired. Alternatively the entire procedure can be viewed through the video system. Use of the video system has the advantage of allowing the other personnel in the operating room to observe the procedure. It also allows operating room personnel who are manipulating the instruments in the additional puncture sites to participate directly, rather than relying solely on instructions from the surgeon. Diseases amenable to laparoscopic treatment include adhesions, endometriosis, fimbrial occlusion (either complete or partial), ovarian cysts, and ectopic pregnancies. Doyle procedures (transection of uterosacral ligaments) also can be undertaken. Unknown lesions should be subjected to biopsy for pathologic diagnosis.

D. Adhesions can be lysed using blunt dissection, cautery, lasers, scissors, or thermal instruments. Lasers available for the performance of these procedures include carbon dioxide, argon, KTP-532, and the Nd:Yag lasers.

E. After identification or biopsy, endometriosis can be ablated or vaporized using cautery or laser (Fig. 1). Copious irrigation of the pelvis is required to remove any of the chocolate cyst-like material from endometriomas.

F. Treatment of fimbrial occlusion, whether partial or complete, can be performed using laser, cautery, or scissors. If a complete obstruction is present, it helps to distend the fallopian tube with dye from the cervical cannula in order to facilitate performance of the procedure.

G. Ovarian cysts can be drained through the laparoscope using cautery, laser, or a needle. Such a technique is also utilized in in vitro fertilization and gamete intrafallopian transfer procedures.

H. The uterosacral ligaments can be transected using electrocautery or laser as a potential way of treating pelvic pain.

I. Ectopic pregnancies can be identified by diagnostic laparoscopy and subsequently can be treated by operative laparoscopy. This procedure can be performed either with or without placement of Pitressin at the proximal and distal margins of the ectopic gestation followed by antimesenteric incisions. These incisions can be made using cautery or one of the lasers.

J. If an unknown lesion is identified at the time of laparoscopy, biopsy should be done for pathologic identification to rule out malignant disease.

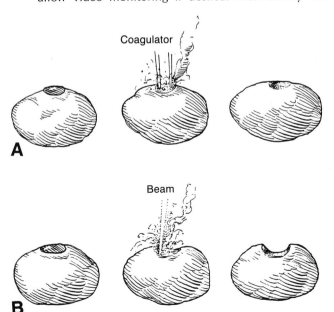

Figure 1 Techniques for laparoscopic treatment of a surface endometrioma: *A*, coagulation; *B*, vaporization. (After Martin DC, ed. Intra-abdominal laser surgery. Memphis: Resurge Press, 1986.)

References

Diamond MP, DeCherney AH. Ovulation induction and oocyte recovery for in vitro fertilization. In: Sciarra JJ, ed. Gynecology and obstetrics. Philadelphia: Harper & Row, 1987.

Martin DC, Diamond MP. Operative laparoscopy: comparison of lasers with other techniques. Curr Probl Obstet Gynecol Fertil 1986; 9(12).

Polan ML. Endoscopy in infertility. In: Sciarra JJ, ed. Gynecology and obstetrics. Philadelphia: Harper & Row, 1987.

Patient undergoing LAPAROSCOPY FOR TREATMENT

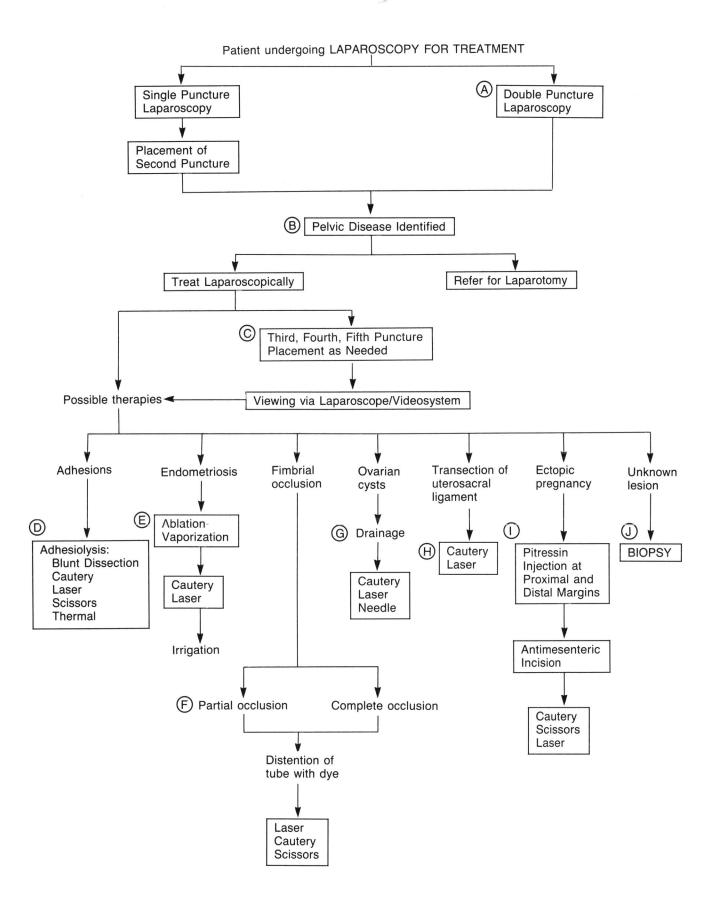

HYSTEROSCOPY: DIAGNOSIS

Michael P. Diamond, M.D.
Mary Lake Polan, M.D., Ph.D.

A. Hysteroscopy is performed to evaluate the uterine cavity. It is most often performed with the patient in the dorsal lithotomy position. Depending on the type of hysteroscope and the distending medium to be utilized, the procedure can be performed in either an office or an operating room.

B. Office hysteroscopy preparation involves vaginal preparation and placement of a vaginal speculum. Anesthesia can be either local or paracervical, although in many cases none is used. Hysteroscopes amenable to use in the office are the Hamou colpohysteroscope and the ambient light hysteroscope. These instruments allow visualization of the uterine cavity but do not permit operative hysteroscopy to be performed.

C. Performance of hysteroscopy in the operating room gives greater latitude with respect to instruments and the distending media that can be utilized. Depending on the instruments chosen, the procedure can be performed with local or paracervical anesthesia or no anesthesia. Operative hysteroscopy is usually done under general anesthesia. After induction of anesthesia and placement of the patient in the dorsal lithotomy position, the vagina is prepared and the speculum is placed.

D. The three most commonly used distending media are carbon dioxide gas, water or dextrose 5 percent in water (D5W), and Hyskon (32 percent dextran 70). Hyskon is often used because it mixes poorly with blood, and thus the field is less likely to be obscured during operative procedures than with the use of water or D5W. Additionally, Hyskon, being more viscous, is less likely to flow out of the cervix around the hysteroscope. Hyskon can be used with electrocautery, as with the urologic resectoscope. A potential complication of the use of carbon dioxide as a distending medium is embolization of the gas.

E. The hysteroscopes that are available include viewing or diagnostic hysteroscopes as well as operative hysteroscopes. The advantage of the diagnostic hysteroscope is that it is of small diameter and thus requires less dilation of the cervix. However, if the decision is then made to use an operative hysteroscope, it requires removal of the diagnostic scope followed by placement of the operating scope. As new instrumentation becomes available, this problem may be overcome.

F. After decisions about the distending medium and hysteroscope have been made, a tenaculum is placed on the cervix, the cervix is dilated if needed, and the hysteroscope is placed in the cervical canal cavity (Fig. 1). It is advanced under direct visualization to allow viewing of the uterine cavity, including both tubal ostia.

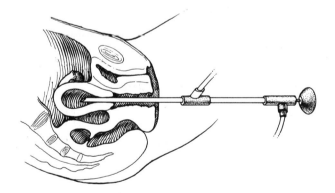

Figure 1 Hysteroscopy performed in the dorsal lithotomy position.

References

Hamou J, Taylor PJ. Panoramic, contact, and microcolpohysteroscopy in gynecologic practice. Curr Probl Obstet Gynecol 1982; 6:2.

Sugimoto O. Diagnostic and therapeutic hysteroscopy for traumatic intrauterine adhesions. Am J Obstet Gynecol 1978; 131:539–547.

Valle RF. Hysteroscopy in the evaluation of female infertility. Am J Obstet Gynecol 1980; 137:425–431.

Patient undergoing HYSTEROSCOPY: DIAGNOSIS

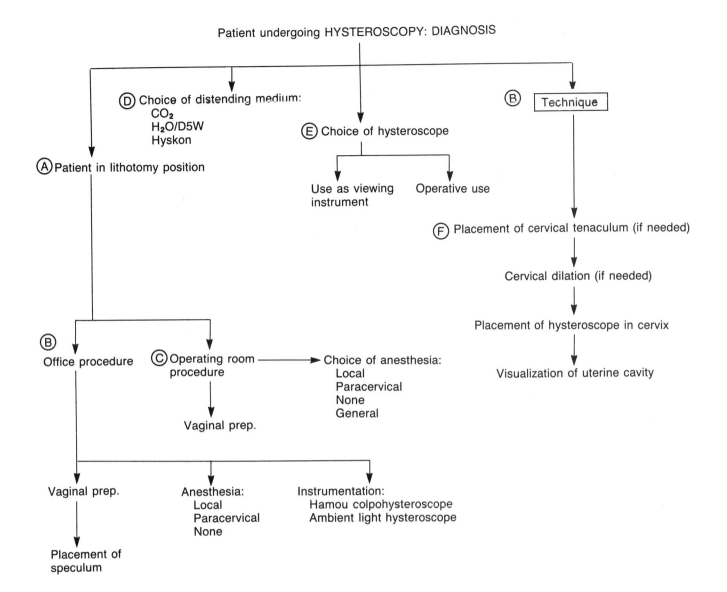

Ⓓ Choice of distending medium:
  CO_2
  H_2O/D5W
  Hyskon

Ⓐ Patient in lithotomy position

Ⓔ Choice of hysteroscope

Use as viewing instrument

Operative use

Ⓑ Technique

Ⓕ Placement of cervical tenaculum (if needed)

Cervical dilation (if needed)

Placement of hysteroscope in cervix

Visualization of uterine cavity

Ⓑ Office procedure

Ⓒ Operating room procedure ⟶ Choice of anesthesia:
  Local
  Paracervical
  None
  General

Vaginal prep.

Vaginal prep.

Anesthesia:
  Local
  Paracervical
  None

Instrumentation:
  Hamou colpohysteroscope
  Ambient light hysteroscope

Placement of speculum

HYSTEROSCOPY: TREATMENT

Michael P. Diamond, M.D.
Mary Lake Polan, M.D., Ph.D.

A. A variety of uterine diseases can be identified hysteroscopically, including uterine synechiae (adhesions), intrauterine devices (IUD), myomas, polyps, uterine septa, products of conception, and malignant disease.

B. Uterine synechiae can be lysed by using the hysteroscope itself as a blunt instrument or by employing hysteroscopic instruments such as scissors, a resectoscope, or a laser. The most commonly used laser is the Nd:Yag laser with or without a sapphire tip. Much of this work is now experimental.

C. Intrauterine devices can be identified by using the hysteroscope. If they are free in the uterine cavity, they can be grasped and removed. If they appear to have perforated the myometrium, diagnostic laparoscopy is advisable in order to assess the location intra-abdominally.

D. Intracavitary myomas or uterine polyps can be identified hysteroscopically. The polyp base can be difficult to identify. These lesions can be removed either by dilation and curettage (D&C) of the uterus or by using hysteroscopic resectoscope or laser techniques. If resectoscopic techniques are utilized, it is advantageous to perform concomitant laparoscopy. This has the advantage of revealing whether uterine perforation occurs, thereby minimizing the risk of damage to other pelvic structures.

E. Uterine septa can be treated hysteroscopically as well. This has been accomplished using either the resectoscope, scissors, or laser techniques. It is safest to perform concomitant laparoscopy to detect perforation if it occurs. If this procedure is performed, the septum should be divided down to the level of the adjacent uterine walls.

F. On occasion nonviable pregnancies are identified by the clinical setting, ultrasound scans, and human chorionic gonadotropin levels. However, localization of these pregnancies to the uterine cavity, fallopian tube, or elsewhere is often difficult. These potentially can be identified by hysterosalpingography or hysteroscopy. If the products of conception are identified in the uterine cavity, they can be evacuated by dilation and curettage of the uterus.

G. Abnormal appearing tissue identified at the time of hysteroscopy should be subjected to biopsy examination to rule out the possibility of malignant disease.

References

DeCherney AH, Diamond MP. Therapeutic hysteroscopy. Postgrad Obstet Gynecol 1986; 6:1.

Siegler AM, Kemmann E. Hysteroscopy. Obstet Gynecol Surv 1975; 30:567–588.

Valle RF, Sciarra JJ. Current status of hysteroscopy in gynecologic practice. Fertil Steril 1979; 32:619–632.

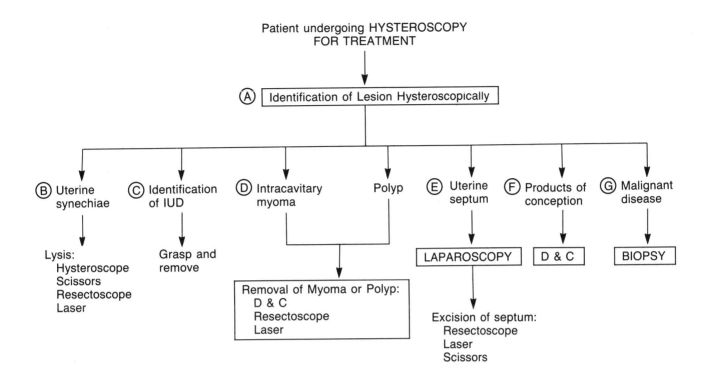

LASER LAPAROSCOPY

Michael P. Diamond, M.D.
Mary Lake Polan, M.D., Ph.D.

A. Laser laparoscopy, or for that matter any form of operative laparoscopy, requires acceptance by the operating room staff and other physicians that the procedure will take longer than routine diagnostic laparoscopy. This requires changes in booking the operating room as well as changes in attitude of all the individuals utilizing the operating room.

B. A wide variety of reproductive pelvic surgical procedures can be performed laparoscopically. The lasers currently available are the carbon dioxide, argon, Nd:Yag, and KTP-532 lasers. In the latter three types of lasers the beam travels through a fiber, in contrast with the carbon dioxide laser, which does not use a fiber (Figs. 1,2). Sapphire tips have recently been introduced for attachment to the three fiber lasers, but they are used primarily with the Nd:Yag laser. They have the advantage of converting the tissue effects of the Nd:Yag laser so that the degree of tissue penetration is reduced.

C. Whether utilizing the carbon dioxide, argon, KTP, or Nd:Yag laser, the laser can be introduced either from the operating channel of an operating laparoscope or through a second puncture site. The choice depends primarily on individual preference.

D. Operative laparoscopy, including operative laser laparoscopy, often requires the use of third, fourth, or even fifth puncture sites. This is necessary in order to manipulate pelvic structures to reduce the risk of injury to them. As with procedures performed at laparotomy, traction on tissues to be incised is helpful. This can be established in laparoscopic procedures by manipulation of the uterus with an instrument that has been placed through the cervical canal into the uterine cavity and by the additional puncture sites.

E. Although not essential, it is useful to have a video system available when performing operative laparoscopy. This allows operating room personnel to visualize the procedure as it is performed, reducing boredom and increasing attentiveness of the operative assistants. Finally, the surgeon can perform the procedure while viewing it through the video system. This obviates the need to continually view through the laparoscope and reduces back strain. On the other hand, depth perception is lost. A potential difficulty that arises with the use of these lasers is the development of smoke in the abdominal cavity. This must be removed in order to allow appropriate visualization of pelvic structures if extensive work is to be performed. Filter systems specifically designed for smoke evacuation are available commercially.

F. Procedures performed using lasers laparoscopically include adhesiolysis, vaporization of endometriosis, fimbrioplasty, neosalpingostomy, linear salpingostomy, drainage of ovarian cysts, and Doyle procedures (transection of the uterosacral ligaments).

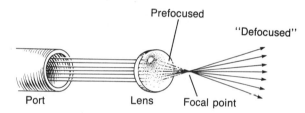

Figure 1 Focusing of the laser beam. (After Martin DC. Laser physics and practice. In: Hunt RB, ed. Atlas of female infertility surgery. Chicago: Year Book, 1985).

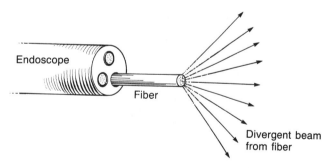

Figure 2 The laser beam diverges as it exits from the endoscopic fiber. (After Martin DC. Diamond MP. Operative laparoscopy: the role of the CO_2 laser. In: Martin DC, ed. Intra-abdominal laser surgery. Memphis: Resurge Press, 1986).

References

Daniell JF. Laparoscopic salpingostomy: early clinical results. Lasers Surg Med 1983; 3:161 (abstract).

Diamond MP, DeCherney AH, Polan ML. Laparoscopic use of the argon laser in nonendometriotic reproductive pelvic surgery. J Reprod Med 1986; 31:1011–1013.

Keye WR, Dixon J. Photocoagulation of endometriosis with the argon laser through the laparoscope. Obstet Gynecol 1984; 62:383–388.

Martin DC, Diamond MP. Operative laparoscopy: comparison of lasers with other techniques. Curr Probl Obstet Gynecol Fertil 1986; 9 (12).

USE OF LASERS IN LAPAROSCOPY

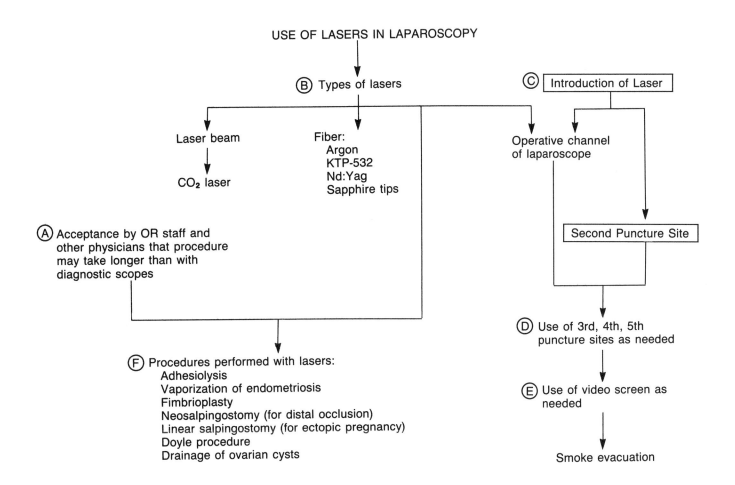

Ⓐ Acceptance by OR staff and
   other physicians that procedure
   may take longer than with
   diagnostic scopes

Ⓕ Procedures performed with lasers:
   Adhesiolysis
   Vaporization of endometriosis
   Fimbrioplasty
   Neosalpingostomy (for distal occlusion)
   Linear salpingostomy (for ectopic pregnancy)
   Doyle procedure
   Drainage of ovarian cysts

Ⓓ Use of 3rd, 4th, 5th
   puncture sites as needed

Ⓔ Use of video screen as
   needed

Smoke evacuation

LASER LAPAROTOMY

Michael P. Diamond, M.D.
Mary Lake Polan, M.D., Ph.D.

A. Regardless of whether the laser is used for reproductive pelvic surgical procedures, the tenets of microsurgery should be observed. These include the use of magnification when necessary, minimization of tissue handling, meticulous attention to hemostasis, careful approximation of tissue planes, prevention of tissue drying, and avoidance of the introduction of foreign bodies.

B. A wide variety of reproductive pelvic surgical procedures can be performed at laparotomy. These include adhesiolysis, vaporization of endometriosis, fimbrioplasty, neosalpingostomy, linear salpingostomy, the Doyle procedure (transection of the uterosacral ligaments), and drainage of ovarian cysts. These procedures also can be performed using nonlaser techniques (e.g., electrocautery and sharp dissection). To date the use of lasers at laparotomy in reproductive pelvic surgical procedures has not improved pregnancy outcome. Thus, it appears to be up to the operator whether to use laser or nonlaser techniques. Easy access to deep areas of the pelvis and the posterior cul de sac, which are often difficult to reach using other techniques, is a potential advantage of lasers.

C. The primary laser utilized at the time of laparotomy is the carbon dioxide laser. The desired tissue effect can be altered by varying the wattage, spot size, use of the laser at the focal point, the length of time the laser is discharged, and the use of "superpulse" modalities. The laser can be utilized either free-hand or by attachment to a microscope via a micromanipulator. The advantage of the free-hand technique is that it allows rapid movement from one portion of the pelvis to another and also allows quick adjustments of the beam from a focused to a defocused mode. Attachment of the laser to a microscope provides the magnification often utilized in microsurgical procedures. In addition it allows more precise delivery of the laser beam. New couplers are now being developed that allow simple defocusing of the laser attached to the microscope.

D. Potentially all lasers used in laser laparoscopy could also be used at laparotomy. In practice, however, the argon, KTP, and Nd:Yag lasers (with or without the sapphire tips) have been used infrequently at the time of laparotomy.

E. Depending on the disease identified, the procedures described can be performed using the carbon dioxide laser. Smoke that develops from the use of the laser should be evacuated. Failure to do so has been associated with the development of a bronchitis-like syndrome.

F. Utilization of surgical adjuvants preoperatively, intraoperatively, and postoperatively is a controversial topic. The hypothesis is that such agents reduce the likelihood of postoperative adhesion formation.

G. An early second-look laparoscopy to evaluate the state of the pelvis postoperatively is performed by many surgeons. Its capacity to improve the chances for pregnancy has not been demonstrated. However, it does allow assessment of the outcome of the procedure. This information can be of importance to the patient, because if extensive adhesions have re-formed, she can be advised to consider in vitro fertilization or adoption. Additionally it allows the surgeon to evaluate the outcome of the surgical procedure performed.

References

Daniell JF. The role of lasers in infertility surgery. Fertil Steril 1984; 42:815–823.

Daniell JF, Diamond MP, McLaughlin DS, et al. Clinical results of terminal salpingostomy using the CO₂ laser: report of the Intra-abdominal Laser Study Group. Fertil Steril 1986; 45:175–178.

Kelly RW, Roberts DK. Experience with the carbon dioxide laser in gynecologic microsurgery. Am J Obstet Gynecol 1983; 146:585–588.

Tulandi T, Farag R, McInnes RA, et al. Reconstructive surgery of hydrosalpinx with and without the carbon dioxide laser. Fertil Steril 1984; 42:839–842.

USE OF LASERS FOR LAPAROTOMY

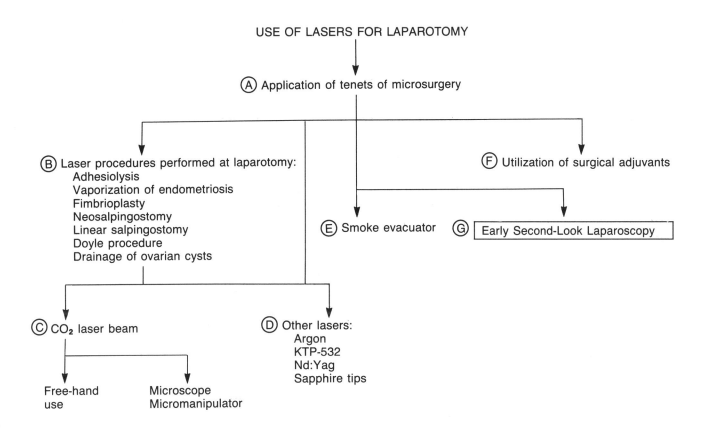

Ⓐ Application of tenets of microsurgery

Ⓑ Laser procedures performed at laparotomy:
  Adhesiolysis
  Vaporization of endometriosis
  Fimbrioplasty
  Neosalpingostomy
  Linear salpingostomy
  Doyle procedure
  Drainage of ovarian cysts

Ⓕ Utilization of surgical adjuvants

Ⓔ Smoke evacuator

Ⓖ Early Second-Look Laparoscopy

Ⓒ CO_2 laser beam

Ⓓ Other lasers:
  Argon
  KTP-532
  Nd:Yag
  Sapphire tips

Free-hand
use

Microscope
Micromanipulator

EVALUATION OF THE MALE

Stephen P. Boyers, M.D.
Gad Lavy, M.D.

A. Male factors account for up to 50 percent of all cases of infertility. The mainstay of the evaluation is semen analysis. Modern semen analysis should include an objective assessment of the proportion and velocity of motile spermatozoa and a careful assessment of sperm morphology, such as that provided by multiple exposure photography and videomicrography. Normal semen should have a sperm concentration of 20 million per milliliter or higher, 40 percent motile or greater, mean velocity of 20 μm per second or higher, and 60 percent or more oval forms.

B. Although there is substantial variation in semen quality between samples in the same male, it is unlikely that the fertility assessment (fertile versus subfertile) will change with repeated sampling. Nonetheless an abnormal semen analysis result should be confirmed by at least one repeat test before deciding that male factor infertility exists. The male with abnormal results in two or more semen tests should undergo a complete urologic evaluation, including endocrinologic assessment. When no specific etiology is found, or when therapy fails to restore normal semen parameters, a trial of artificial insemination may be considered, using either husband or donor sperm, depending on the severity of the semen abnormality and the couple's wishes.

C. The postcoital test (PCT) is an indispensable companion to the semen analysis, regardless of whether the latter yields normal or abnormal results. The presence of any sperm in the vaginal vault or cervical mucus at least implies potency and ejaculatory competence. A normal PCT correlates with the sperm concentration at semen analysis. Male factor infertility is unlikely when the results of both the semen analysis and the PCT are normal, and a thorough evaluation of the female partner becomes essential. When results of the female evaluation are also normal and infertility remains unexplained after a complete work-up, a search for antisperm antibodies may be worthwhile. Head-directed immunoglobulins can interfere with fertilization even though standard semen parameters and motility in cervical mucus are normal. The zona-free hamster oocyte sperm penetration test is another method of assessing the fertilizing capability of sperm when conventional assessments of the male yield normal results. A normal PCT with abnormal semen analysis results does not exclude male factors, but assessment of the female should proceed in parallel with the male evaluation.

D. When the PCT is abnormal, an in vitro test of sperm-mucus penetration may be helpful in distinguishing sperm from mucus abnormalities, particularly when done as a cross reaction test with donor mucus and donor sperm. When the husband's sperm penetrate both the wife's and the donor's mucus poorly and donor sperm penetrate both well, immunologic male factors should be suspected and tested by the immunobead technique.

E. When artificial insemination by husband (AIH) is being considered, a technique for concentrating sperm in a small volume of seminal plasma should be considered. The migration test involves washing sperm free of seminal plasma and allowing motile sperm to swim or migrate into an overlayer of tissue culture medium, such as Ham's F-10 medium. Washed migrated sperm may be used for intrauterine insemination in a way that seminal plasma sperm cannot, because seminal prostaglandins may provoke uterine contractions and pain and even an anaphylactic reaction. If sperm migration is not available, the first portion of a split ejaculate may provide a concentrated specimen for intracervical AIH.

F. Failure to conceive after four to six cycles of well timed, periovulatory inseminations with the husband's sperm leaves two therapeutic options. Donor artificial insemination is highly successful in isolated cases of male factor infertility and is the only option other than adoption for men with complete azoospermia. In vitro fertilization may be successful even in severe oligoasthenospermia.

References

Alexander NJ. Male evaluation and semen analysis. Clin Obstet Gynecol 1982; 25:463-482.

Bronson R, Cooper G, Rosenfeld D. Sperm antibodies: their role in infertility. Fertil Steril 1984; 42:171-183.

Bronson RA, Cooper GW, Rosenfeld DL. Sperm-specific isoantibodies and autoantibodies inhibit the binding of human sperm to the human zona pellucida. Fertil Steril 1982; 38:724-729.

Dubin L, Amelar RD. Etiologic factors in 1294 consecutive cases of male infertility. Fertil Steril 1971; 22:469-474.

Hargreave TB, Nilson S. Semenology. In: Hargreave TB, ed. Male infertility. New York: Springer-Verlag, 1983:56.

Katz DF, Overstreet JW. Sperm motility assessment by videomicrography. Fertil Steril 1981; 35:188-193.

Katz DF, Overstreet JW, Hanson FW. A new quantitative test for sperm penetration into cervical mucus. Fertil Steril 1980; 33:179-186.

Makler A. A new multiple exposure photography method for objective human spermatozoal motility determination. Fertil Steril 1978; 30:192-199.

Makler A. Use of the elaborated multiple exposure photography method in routine sperm motility analysis and for research purposes. Fertil Steril 1980; 33:160-166.

Rogers BJ. The sperm penetration assay: its usefulness reevaluated. Fertil Steril 1985; 43:821-840.

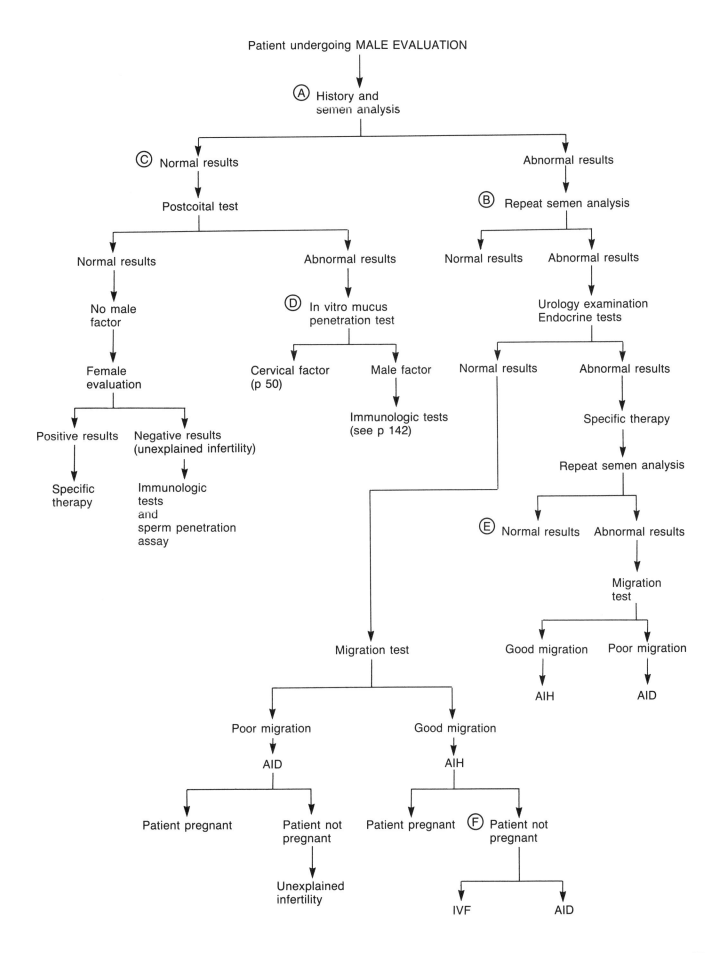

Patient undergoing MALE EVALUATION

Ⓐ History and semen analysis

Ⓒ Normal results

Abnormal results

Postcoital test

Ⓑ Repeat semen analysis

Normal results

Abnormal results

Normal results

Abnormal results

No male factor

Ⓓ In vitro mucus penetration test

Urology examination
Endocrine tests

Female evaluation

Cervical factor (p 50)

Male factor

Normal results

Abnormal results

Positive results

Negative results (unexplained infertility)

Immunologic tests (see p 142)

Specific therapy

Specific therapy

Immunologic tests and sperm penetration assay

Repeat semen analysis

Ⓔ Normal results

Abnormal results

Migration test

Migration test

Good migration

Poor migration

AIH

AID

Poor migration

Good migration

AID

AIH

Patient pregnant

Patient not pregnant

Patient pregnant

Ⓕ Patient not pregnant

Unexplained infertility

IVF

AID

135

ROUTINE SEMEN ANALYSIS

Gad Lavy, M.D.
Stephen P. Boyers, M.D.

A. Both partners of an infertile couple should be evaluated in parallel. The mainstay of the male evaluation is the semen analysis. It should be performed early in the course of the infertility evaluation. Abnormal results on semen analysis indicate the need for repetition of the analysis at least once for confirmation before initiating a more extensive male work-up.

B. To insure standardization, patients should be carefully instructed regarding preparation for the test, method of semen collection, and transport of the sample to the laboratory. We advise 2 to 3 days of abstinence to replete extragonadal reserves. Prolonged abstinence is not recommended. Coitus interruptus is not a reliable technique for semen collection. We instruct the patient to masturbate into a wide mouthed, clean, urine collection cup, taking care to avoid contaminating the sample with lubricants that might impair sperm survival. The sample should be transported to the laboratory within 1 hour, keeping the sample at body temperature during transport. When the patient cannot or will not collect a sample by masturbation, a special condom (seminal collection device) may be used.

C. Normal semen forms a coagulum immediately after ejaculation and then liquefies over the next 20 to 30 minutes. When liquefaction fails to occur, the semen sample should be aspirated into a syringe and ejected through a 19 gauge needle back into the semen container. Adequate liquefaction is a prerequisite to dividing the sample for microscopic and macroscopic evaluations.

D. Macroscopic evaluation includes an assessment of semen color, volume, and viscosity. Normal semen has a pearly, opalescent color. Blood tinged or purulent semen is abnormal. The mean normal semen volume is 3.0 ml, but a range of 0.1 to 9.0 ml has been reported in fertile males. A low semen volume suggests incomplete sample collection. Repeatedly low volumes might indicate male factor infertility when postcoital testing indicates inadequate sperm penetration of cervical mucus.

E. Modern semen analysis uses objective reproducible methods, either multiple exposure photography (MEP) or videomicrography, to assess sperm density, motility, and morphology (Fig. 1). We routinely use the MEP method. The Makler chamber provides a constant volume chamber for the semen sample, along with an integral calibrated grid for rapid calculation of the sperm concentration in an undiluted sample and an optical quality coverglass, which facilitates MEP. The essential parameters of semen quality are the sperm density, the percentage motile, the mean velocity, and the percentage with normal oval morphology.

F. Sperm density should be 20 million or more sperm per milliliter. Oligospermia is defined as less than 20 million sperm per milliliter. Ninety-five percent of fertile males have sperm concentrations higher than 20 million sperm per milliliter. Azoospermia is designed as the absence of spermatozoa in the ejaculate. Both oligospermia and azoospermia can be caused by a variety of disorders, and thorough urologic and endocrine evaluations are mandatory.

G. Before the advent of MEP or videomicrography for semen analysis, motility was subjectively measured and sperm progression was graded 0 to 4+. Modern semen analysis allows precise quantitation of the mean sperm velocity in microns per second. Normally 40 percent or more of the sperm are motile, and the mean sperm velocity is 20 μm per second or greater. Asthenospermia is defined as less than 40 percent motility, frequently with subnormal velocity. Sperm morphology also can be assessed by videomicrography or simple photography. At least 60 percent of the sperm should be of normal oval shape and size. Abnormalities include small sperm (microcephalic), large sperm (macrocephalic), tapered sperm, amorphous sperm, and those with midpiece and tail defects. Teratospermia is defined as more than 40 percent abnormal forms. The detection of asthenospermia or teratospermia should also be followed by a thorough urologic evaluation.

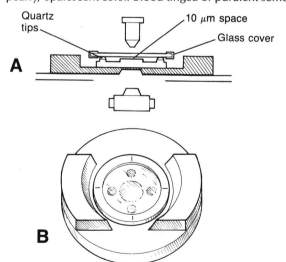

Figure 1 *A,* Cross section of the improved 10-μm chamber; four quartz tips insure the 10-μm space below the glass cover. *B,* Correct coverglass placement is seen by the appearance of rainbow colors at the four points of contact between the quartz tips and the coverglass.

References

Katz DF, Overstreet JW. Sperm motility assessment by videomicrography. Fertil Steril 1981; 35:188–193.

MacLeod J. Semen quality in one thousand men of known fertility and in eight hundred cases of infertile marriage. Fertil Steril 1951; 2:115–139.

Makler A. Use of the elaborated multiple exposure photography (MEP) method in routine sperm motility analysis and for

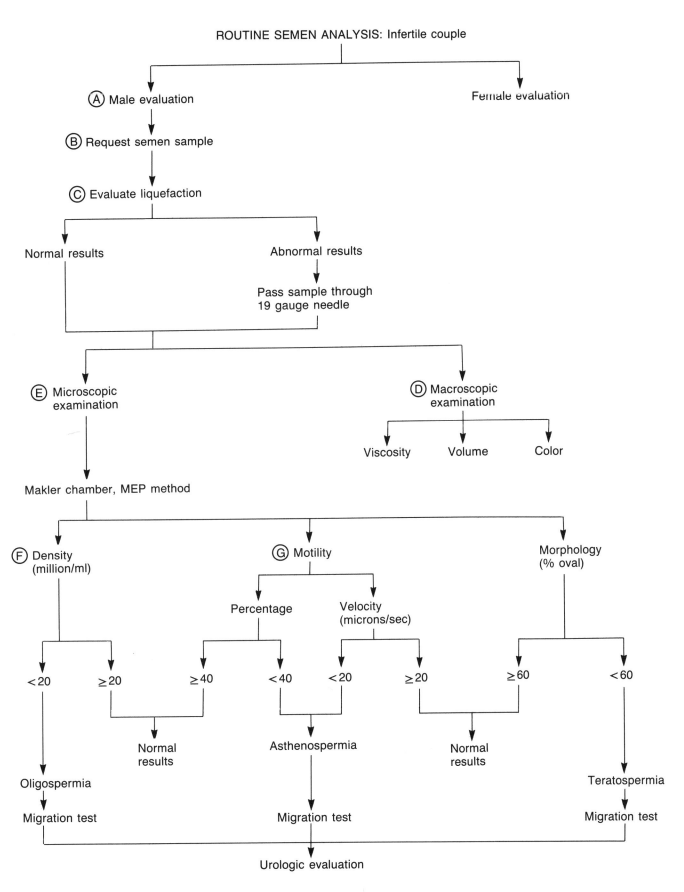

ROUTINE SEMEN ANALYSIS: Infertile couple

(A) Male evaluation

Female evaluation

(B) Request semen sample

(C) Evaluate liquefaction

Normal results

Abnormal results

Pass sample through
19 gauge needle

(E) Microscopic
examination

(D) Macroscopic
examination

Viscosity   Volume   Color

Makler chamber, MEP method

(F) Density
(million/ml)

(G) Motility

Morphology
(% oval)

Percentage   Velocity
(microns/sec)

<20   ≥20   ≥40   <40   <20   ≥20   ≥60   <60

Normal
results

Asthenospermia

Normal
results

Oligospermia

Teratospermia

Migration test

Migration test

Migration test

Urologic evaluation

research purposes. Fertil Steril 1980; 33:160–166.
Rehan NE, Sobrero AJ, Fertig JW. The semen of fertile men: statistical analysis of 1300 men. Fertil Steril 1975; 26:492–502.

Sobrero AJ, Rehan NE. The semen of fertile men. II. Semen characteristics of 100 fertile men. Fertil Steril 1975; 26:1048–1056.

MIGRATION TEST

Gad Lavy, M.D.
Stephen P. Boyers, M.D.

A. The most common type of male factor infertility is idiopathic infertility in which oligoasthenoteratospermia exists in repeated semen samples with no apparent anatomic or endocrinologic cause and, therefore, with no specific therapy. Artificial insemination with the husband's sperm remains one of the most common empiric therapies, its goal being to place the maximal number of motile sperm high in the female reproductive tract at the precise time of ovulation, a "boost up" to avoid the attrition that naturally befalls vaginal sperm. Intrauterine insemination (IUI) places the sperm beyond the cervical barrier, making it useful in cases of both cervical and male factor infertility.

B. Whole semen cannot be placed into the uterine cavity without producing uterine contractions and pain, the consequence of high levels of prostaglandins in the seminal fluid. Sperm washing and migration constitute a method of concentrating motile sperm in a prostaglandin-free medium that can be used for IUI. The first step involves incubation of the fresh whole ejaculate at room temperature for 20 minutes to allow liquefaction. Hyperviscous samples that fail to liquefy

spontaneously can be forced several times by syringe through a 19 gauge needle.

C. Liquefied sperm is diluted 1:4 with Ham's F-10 tissue culture medium containing 20 percent cord serum. The diluted sample is mixed thoroughly before centrifugation.

D. Washing is completed by a process called soft centrifugation. The diluted sample is layered over a cushion of Lipiodol, which increases the surface area at the base of the sample, providing a soft cushion to absorb some of the gravitational forces associated with centrifugation and facilitating migration of motile sperm from a layer of sperm cells spun down to the semen-oil interface. Soft centrifugation decreases the sperm damage normally caused by centrifugation. The sample is spun at 300× gravity for 10 minutes (Fig. 1). Excess supernatant is aspirated, leaving 0.5 ml behind without disturbing the sperm layer below.

E. The centrifuge tube is tilted gently to 45 degrees to further increase the surface area above the oil cushion and is incubated at 37° C in an atmosphere of 5 percent carbon dioxide for 15 minutes. During this time motile sperm "swim-up" from the layer of spun cells into the Ham's medium above. Motile sperm that have successfully migrated are harvested by gently aspirating 0.3 ml of the Ham's F-10 layer, care being taken not to disturb the immotile cells at the base. Thus, the motile sperm are concentrated in a small volume of prostaglandin-free fluid that is ideal for IUI.

F. The result of the washing and migration procedure is evaluated by standard multiple exposure photography (MEP) semen analysis, the migrated sample being analyzed for sperm count, motility, mean velocity, and morphology. The migrated sample usually shows a significant increase in motility and mean velocity and a decrease in abnormal forms. Two million motile sperm are considered the minimum for intrauterine insemination. If the level is below this minimum, donor sperm should be considered as an alternative to artificial insemination by husband (AIH).

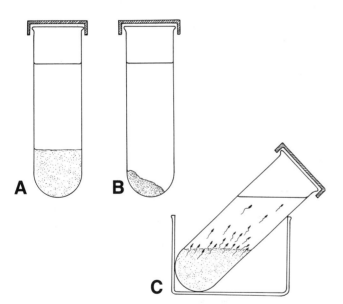

Figure 1 *A*, Sperm is mixed with culture medium and, after being gently mixed by inversion, is centrifuged to 200 G for 5 to 10 minutes. *B*, Discard the supernatant, retaining the sperm pellet. *C*, After two sperm washings, gently layer the pellet with 1 to 3 milliliters of culture medium. The highly motile spermatozoa swim to the top and can be harvested.

References

Makler A, Murillo O, Huszar G, et al. Improved techniques for collecting motile spermatozoa from human semen. I. A self-migratory method. Int J Androl 1984; 7:61–70.

Makler A, Murillo O, Huszar G, et al. Improved techniques for separating motile spermatozoa from human semen. II. An atraumatic centrifugation method. Int J Androl 1984; 7:71–78.

MIGRATION TEST

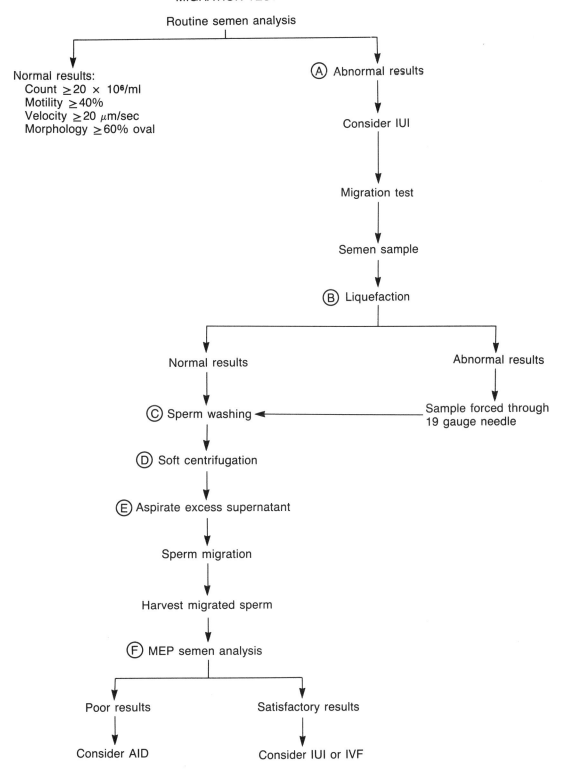

Routine semen analysis

Normal results:
Count $\geq 20 \times 10^6$/ml
Motility $\geq 40\%$
Velocity $\geq 20\ \mu$m/sec
Morphology $\geq 60\%$ oval

(A) Abnormal results

Consider IUI

Migration test

Semen sample

(B) Liquefaction

Normal results

Abnormal results

Sample forced through 19 gauge needle

(C) Sperm washing

(D) Soft centrifugation

(E) Aspirate excess supernatant

Sperm migration

Harvest migrated sperm

(F) MEP semen analysis

Poor results

Satisfactory results

Consider AID

Consider IUI or IVF

SPLIT EJACULATE

Gad Lavy, M.D.
Stephen P. Boyers, M.D.

A. The split ejaculate method allows preparation of a semen sample for either intrauterine or intracervical AIH when facilities for sperm washing and migration are not available. The goal, as for sperm migration, is the concentration of motile sperm in a small fluid volume. The technique involves fractionating the ejaculate by collecting first and subsequent spurts of semen in two separate containers. The sample is collected by masturbation following 2 to 3 days of abstinence. The patient is instructed to collect the first spurt of semen in one container and all subsequent spurts in a second container. Both are submitted for multiple exposure photography (MEP) semen analysis.

B. The first portion of the ejaculate is made up of products of the testis, epididymis, vas deferens, and prostate, whereas the second portion contains fluid from the seminal vesicles. In 90 percent of men the first portion of a split ejaculate is the sperm-rich fraction. This, and the fact that the first portion contains relatively low levels of prostaglandin, make it suitable for intrauterine insemination. It should be emphasized that both fractions of the split ejaculate need to be analyzed, since in 5 percent of men, the second fraction contains more sperm than the first and in another 5 percent sperm density is equal in the two fractions.

C. The high volume, low density fraction is discarded and the low volume, high density fraction is used for insemination. In the absence of cervical factors, the entire first fraction may be used for intracervical insemination. When intrauterine insemination is desired, 0.1 to 0.3 ml of the first fraction may be placed into the uterine cavity.

References

Amelar RD, Hotchkiss RS. The split ejaculate: its use in the management of male infertility. Fertil Steril 1965; 16:46–60.

Eliasson R, Lindholmer C. Distribution and properties of sperm in different fractions of split ejaculates. Fertil Steril 1972; 23:252–256.

Farris EJ, Murphy DP. The characteristics of the two parts of the partitioned ejaculate and the advantages of its use for intrauterine insemination: a study of 100 ejaculates. Fertil Steril 1960; 11:465–469.

Harvey C, Jackson MH. A method of concentrating spermatozoa in human semen. J Clin Pathal 1955; 8:341–342.

Kotoulas I-GB, Burgos-Briceno LA, Arana J, Balmaceda JP, Asch RH. Human sperm penetration in bovine cervical mucus clinical studies. II. Use of split ejaculates. Fertil Steril 1984; 42:268–273.

Perez-Pelaez M, Cohen MR. The split ejaculate in homologous insemination. Int J Fertil 1965; 10:25–30.

SPLIT EJACULATE

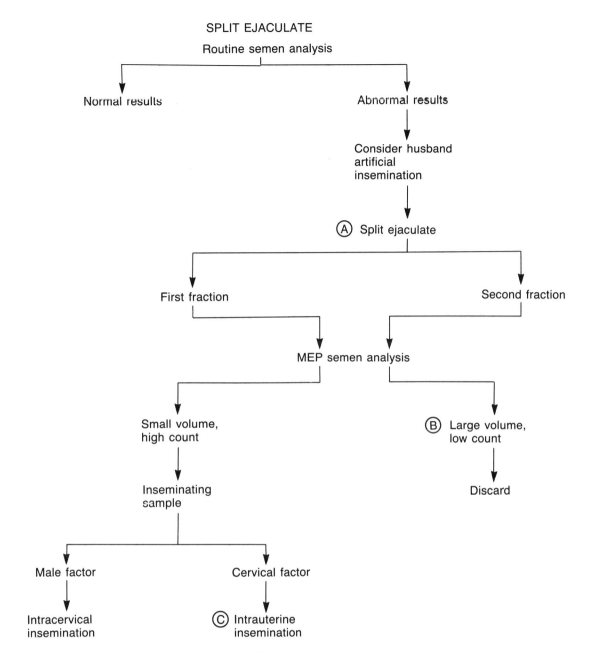

Routine semen analysis

Normal results

Abnormal results

Consider husband
artificial
insemination

Ⓐ Split ejaculate

First fraction

Second fraction

MEP semen analysis

Small volume,
high count

Ⓑ Large volume,
low count

Inseminating
sample

Discard

Male factor

Cervical factor

Intracervical
insemination

Ⓒ Intrauterine
insemination

ANTISPERM ANTIBODIES

Bruce S. Shapiro, M.D.
Gad Lavy, M.D.
Stephen P. Boyers, M.D.

A. The presence of antisperm antibodies should be suspected in men who have a history of vasectomy and vasovasostomy or other testicular surgery or injury and when spontaneous sperm agglutination or severe asthenospermia is observed at routine semen analysis. A postcoital test showing poor sperm penetration despite apparently normal cervical mucus quality and normal semen parameters also suggests immunologic factors. An in vitro mucus cross penetration test can more specifically point to antibodies in the semen or cervical mucus. Finally, the incidence of antisperm antibodies is increased in couples with otherwise unexplained infertility.

B. The human spermatozoon is a complex cell with a variety of surface antigens. Antibodies against the sperm head, midpiece, tail, and tail-tip have been identified. Some antibodies, such as those against the tail-tip only, appear to have little if any functional significance, whereas head directed antibodies clearly can interfere with sperm-oocyte interaction. Until recently tests for antisperm antibodies have been relatively nonspecific, and much of the confusion regarding immunologic factors and infertility has stemmed from lack of a standardized method for quantitating specific antibodies. The immunobead test overcomes many of these difficulties (Fig. 1). Micronized polyacrylamide spheres are coated with rabbit antihuman antiglobulin, which is specific for either immunoglobulin G (IgG), immunoglobulin A (IgA), or immunoglobulin M (IgM). Sperm bound antibodies are identified by incubating sperm and beads. Serum antibodies are identified by incubating serum with antibody-free sperm cells and then incubating those sperm with immunobeads. Binding of sperm to immunobeads is identified and quantitated microscopically by counting bound and unbound sperm, classified by site of binding and class of immunoglobulin.

C. When antisperm antibodies are suspected in the male, both serum and semen can be tested by the immunobead method. In practical terms, only the semen need be evaluated, since the presence of antibodies in serum only, without sperm bound antibodies, is thought not to have functional significance. Sperm bound and circulating antibodies are not always correlated.

D. When antisperm antibodies are suspected in the female, both serum and cervical mucus can be tested by the immunobead method. In practical terms only the serum is routinely evaluated because the assay is technically more difficult in cervical mucus. If antisperm antibodies are positively identified in female serum, and the postcoital and in vitro cervical mucus cross penetration tests point to a cervical factor, the presence of antisperm antibodies in cervical mucus is generally assumed.

E. Just as our understanding of the genesis of antisperm antibodies remains limited, so are the options for therapy. In the male, treatment has been primarily directed at immunosuppression with glucocorticoids. Several protocols have been described, including dexamethasone 2 to 3 mg per day for 9 to 13 weeks, prednisone 60 mg per day for 7 to 21 days, and methylprednisolone 96 mg per day for 7 days, repeated cyclically. There are no well controlled trials that demonstrate an unequivocal benefit of steroid therapy on immunologic infertility, and the side effects are significant, including scattered reports of aseptic necrosis of the femoral head. Artificial insemination by husband (AIH) after rapid semen dilution and sperm washing, after immunoabsorption, and in vitro fertilization (IVF) are options currently being explored. Donor artificial insemination (AID) is an effective option for many couples.

F. In the female with antisperm antibodies, treatment has been equally disappointing. Donor sperm is of no use because antisperm antibodies appear to be generic rather than human leukocyte antigen specific. Condom therapy has been advocated to prevent further exposure to sperm antigens, in the hope that antibody titers would decline, but this approach is extremely frustrating to couples wanting to conceive and offers no guarantee of success. Glucocorticoids have been used as for the male, with no better results. Intrauterine insemination (IUI) may be helpful when antibodies are limited to the cervical mucus, but there is no way to confirm the absence of similar antibodies in uterine, tubal, or follicular fluids. As a last resort, in vitro fertilization has been used to circumvent antisperm antibodies in the female, washing oocytes in Ham's F-10 medium to remove follicular fluid, avoiding maternal serum in the insemination medium, and dispersing the cumulus with hyaluronidase, all in an effort to make the oocyte more accessible to sperm. Pregnancies have been reported with these techniques.

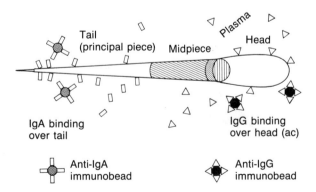

Figure 1 Washed motile sperm are mixed with a suspension of immunobeads that detect antibodies by binding to the sperm surface (to which immunoglobulins have bound). Thus, both the regional specificity of the binding of antisperm antibodies and the proportion of sperm in the ejaculate bound by immunoglobulins may be determined. Immunobead bending detects IgAs bound to the tail and IgGs bound to the head of the sperm.

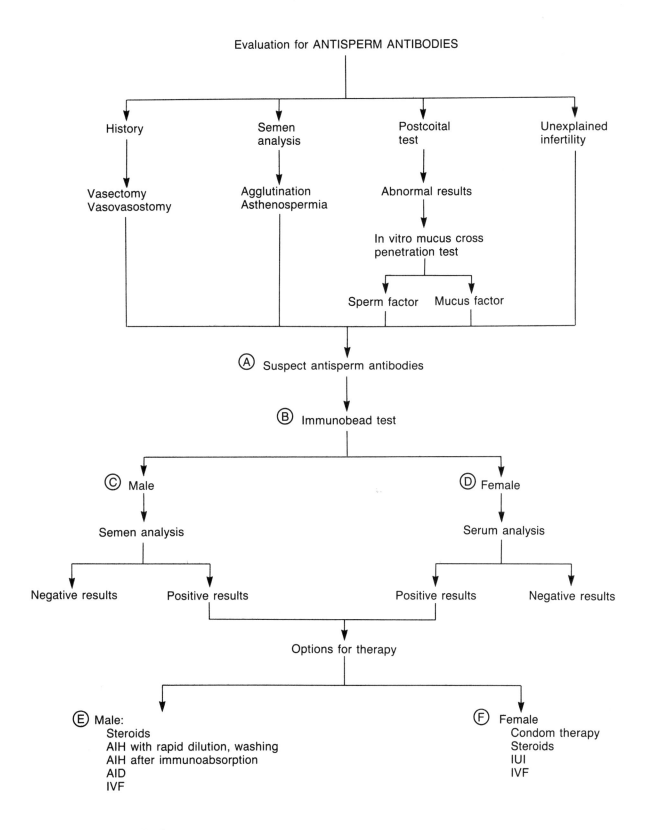

Evaluation for ANTISPERM ANTIBODIES

History → Vasectomy / Vasovasostomy

Semen analysis → Agglutination / Asthenospermia

Postcoital test → Abnormal results → In vitro mucus cross penetration test → Sperm factor / Mucus factor

Unexplained infertility

(A) Suspect antisperm antibodies

(B) Immunobead test

(C) Male → Semen analysis → Negative results / Positive results

(D) Female → Serum analysis → Positive results / Negative results

Options for therapy

(E) Male:
Steroids
AIH with rapid dilution, washing
AIH after immunoabsorption
AID
IVF

(F) Female
Condom therapy
Steroids
IUI
IVF

References

Alexander NJ, Sampson JH, Fulgham DL. Pregnancy rates in patients treated for antisperm antibodies with prednisone. Int J Fertil 1983; 28:63–67.

Bronson RA, Cooper GW, Rosenfeld DL. Autoimmunity to spermatozoa: effect on sperm penetration of cervical mucus as reflected by postcoital testing. Fertil Steril 1984; 41:609-614.

Bronson RA, Cooper GW, Rosenfeld DL. Sperm antibodies: their role in infertility. Fertil Steril 1984; 42:171-183.

Bronson RA, Cooper GW, Rosenfeld DL. Use of freeze-thawed sonicated human sperm as an in vitro immunoabsorbant. Am J Reprod Immunol 1982; 2:162.

DeAlmeida M, Feneuyl D, Rignaud C, Jouannet P. Steroid therapy for male infertility associated with antisperm antibodies. Results of a small randomized clinical trial. Int J Androl 1985; 8:111–117.

POSTCOITAL TEST: MALE EVALUATION

Gad Lavy, M.D.
Stephen P. Boyers, M.D.

A. The postcoital test (PCT) is an important part of the evaluation of male factors in an infertility investigation. It is simple to perform, is inexpensive, and provides valuable information concerning coital performance of the male as well as about sperm, cervical mucus, and sperm-mucus interaction. It should be performed early in the course of evaluating the infertile couple. Semen analysis should be done separately, as the two tests provide complementary data. Periovulatory timing is essential. The test has little or no value and is difficult to schedule in anovulatory or oligoovulatory women; regular ovulation should be documented before planning a PCT.

B. To be interpreted properly, the PCT must be done in the periovulatory portion of the menstrual cycle. In the normal female, cervical mucus is most favorable for sperm survival and sperm penetration at midcycle, when the endocervical glands are stimulated by high preovulatory levels of estradiol. Earlier or later in the cycle, cervical mucus is scant, cellular, viscous, and impenetrable, acting as a barrier to the uterine cavity. A poorly timed test provides little information about either cervical mucus or sperm. For purposes of this algorithm, we assume optimal timing and good quality midcycle cervical mucus. In another section we review the PCT in more detail, particularly as it applies to evaluating cervical factors (p 46).

C. When microscopic examination of cervical mucus 1 to 6 hours after intercourse reveals no spermatozoa whatsoever, a specimen of fluid from the posterior vaginal fornix should be examined. The absence of sperm in the vagina indicates a coital problem. Coital technique (vaginal versus anal penetration) should be assessed. Husbands frequently fail to perform under the pressure of scheduled and graded intercourse, and couples should be reassured that this is a common transient problem. Other problems include impotence, retrograde ejaculation, and azoospermia.

D. The absence of motile sperm in cervical mucus despite normal ejaculation and a normal semen analysis suggests a problem with sperm-mucus interaction. An in vitro mucus cross penetration test can help distinguish between cervical mucus and sperm factors.

E. A normal postcoital test result is defined as more than 10 progressively motile sperm per high power microscopic field in a midcycle cervical mucus sample examined after coitus. The time interval after coitus has not been standardized. We prefer to do the PCT 1 to 6 hours after intercourse.

References

Davajan V, Kunitake G. Fractional in vivo and in vitro examination of postcoital cervical mucus in the human. Fertil Steril 1969; 20:197–210.

Fredricsson B, Bjork G. Morphology of postcoital spermatozoa in the cervical secretion and its clinical significance. Fertil Steril 1977; 28:841–845.

Templeton AA. The female partner. In: Hargreave TB, ed. Male infertility. New York: Springer-Verlag, 1983:188.

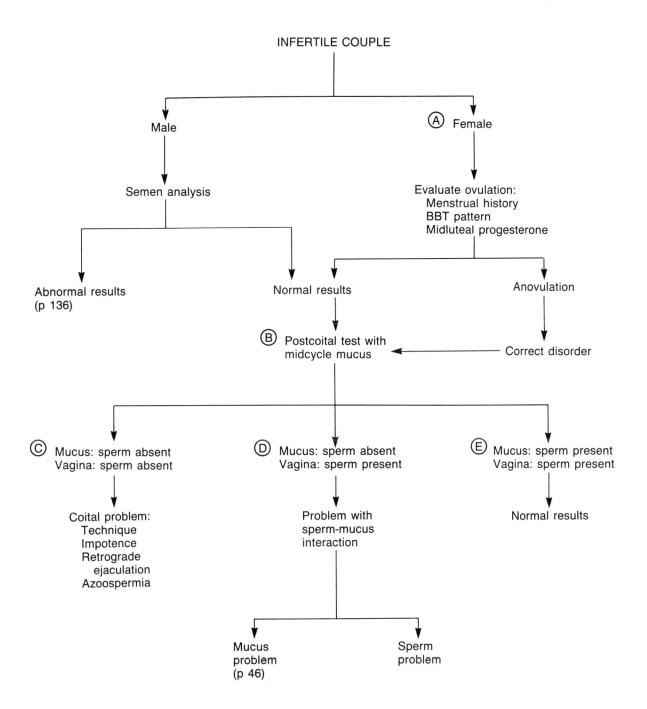

INFERTILE COUPLE

Male

Semen analysis

Abnormal results
(p 136)

Normal results

Ⓐ Female

Evaluate ovulation:
    Menstrual history
    BBT pattern
    Midluteal progesterone

Anovulation

Correct disorder

Ⓑ Postcoital test with
    midcycle mucus

Ⓒ Mucus: sperm absent
    Vagina: sperm absent

Coital problem:
    Technique
    Impotence
    Retrograde
        ejaculation
    Azoospermia

Ⓓ Mucus: sperm absent
    Vagina: sperm present

Problem with
sperm-mucus
interaction

Mucus
problem
(p 46)

Sperm
problem

Ⓔ Mucus: sperm present
    Vagina: sperm present

Normal results

ENDOCRINE EVALUATION OF THE MALE

Gad Lavy, M.D.
Stephen P. Boyers, M.D.

A. Semen abnormalities may reflect underlying endocrine disease in the male. Patients with oligospermia (sperm count less than 20 million per milliliter) or asthenospermia (motility less than 40 percent) should have a thorough history and physical examination with particular attention to substance abuse, exposure to toxins, sexual performance, and evidence of genital abnormality or hypoandrogenization. Testicular size and consistency should be noted and the scrotum examined for varicoceles. Hormonal testing should include measurement of the serum follicle stimulating hormone (FSH), luteinizing hormone (LH), and testosterone (T) levels.

B. The combination of high FSH and LH and low testosterone levels confirms the presence of testicular failure. These patients are azoospermic with both Leydig cell and germinal cell failure. Donor artificial insemination (AID) and adoption are alternatives for infertile couples. There is no therapy to restore testicular function.

C. A high FSH level with normal LH and testosterone levels implies isolated germinal cell failure. These patients have normal Leydig cell function and are normally androgenized but have azoospermia or oligospermia. Depending on the degree of semen abnormality and the outcome of the migration test, these couples may be candidates for either husband artificial insemination (AIH) or AID, in vitro fertilization (IVF), or adoption. Again there is no known therapy to restore germinal cell function.

D. Low FSH, LH, and testosterone levels (hypogonadotropic hypogonadism) often reflect hypothalamic-pituitary disease, including pituitary tumors and hyperprolactinemia. A thorough neurologic examination and drug history followed by measurement of the serum prolactin level and evaluation of a computed tomography (CT) scan of the pituitary lead to a diagnosis.

E. Hyperprolactinemia may be caused by a variety of antidopaminergic drugs. A pituitary CT scan can distinguish patients with pituitary tumors from those with idiopathic hyperprolactinemia. Those with normal results on CT scanning should be treated with bromocriptine. Follow-up x-ray views should be obtained in 6 months, since small microadenomas may cause hyperprolactinemia without initially being visible on the CT scan. When the CT scan demonstrates a tumor, options include bromocriptine or surgery.

F. Normoprolactinemic men with hypogonadotropic hypogonadism may also have central nervous system tumors, and a CT scan is again indicated. The identification of a tumor warrants further testing of the pituitary-thyroid and pituitary-adrenal axes if these have not already been tested. Measurement of the serum thyroxine (T₄) level, thyroxine binding capacity (RT₃ uptake), and thyroid stimulating hormone (TSH) level identifies patients with pituitary hypothyroidism. An ACTH (adrenocorticotropic hormone, Cortrosyn) stimulation test serves to evaluate adrenal integrity. When both prolactin levels and the CT scan results are normal, the diagnosis is idiopathic hypogonadotropic hypogonadism. Severe weight loss, as in anorexia nervosa, or stress, as in strenuous exercise, may be causally related to this syndrome. Testicular stimulation with human menopausal gonadotropins (Pergonal) may restore normal spermatogenesis and androgen biosynthesis.

G. Most men with semen abnormalities have no identifiable endocrinopathy, and FSH, LH, and testosterone levels are normal. Azoospermic patients should be evaluated for ejaculatory duct agenesis or obstruction and for complete retrograde ejaculation. Absence of seminal fluid fructose suggests the former, while examination of a postejaculation urine specimen identifies those with retrograde ejaculation. Oligospermic patients should be carefully evaluated for varicocele. Therapeutic options for infertility include AIH, AID, IVF, and adoption.

H. Men with androgen insensitivity have normal FSH levels and increased LH and testosterone levels. Many of these patients have genital abnormalities, such as hypospadias, which reflect inadequate fetal androgenization, and gynecomastia, the consequence of elevated estradiol levels and an increased estradiol: testosterone ratio. No specific therapy is effective. AIH, AID, IVF, and adoption are options.

References

DeKretser DM. The endocrinology of male infertility. Br Med Bull 1979; 35:187-192.

Means AR, Fakunding JL, Huckins L, Tindall DJ, Vitale R. Follicle stimulating hormone, the Sertoli cell and spermatogenesis. Recent Prog Horm Res 1976; 32:447-527.

Nieschlag E, Wickings EJ, Mauss J. Endocrine testicular function in infertility. In: Fabbrini A, Steinberger E, eds. Recent progress in andrology. Proceedings of Serono symposium. Vol 14. London: Academic Press, 1979:101.

Swerdloff RS, Boyers SP. Evaluation of the male partner of an infertile couple: an algorithmic approach. JAMA 1982; 247:2418-2422.

Wu F. Endocrinology of male infertility and fertility. In: Hargreave TB, ed. Male infertility. New York: Springer-Verlag, 1983:87.

Patient with
ABNORMAL SEMEN ANALYSIS

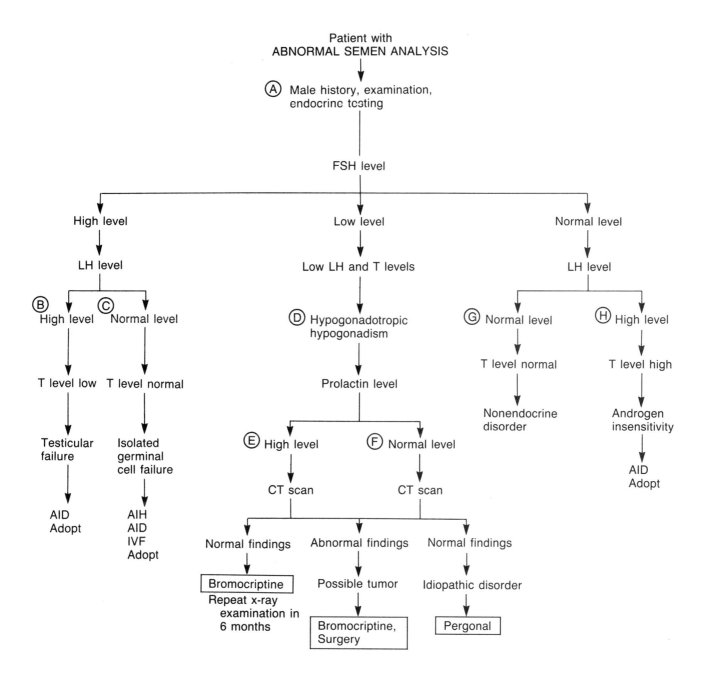

Ⓐ Male history, examination, endocrine testing

FSH level

High level — LH level
- Ⓑ High level → T level low → Testicular failure → AID / Adopt
- Ⓒ Normal level → T level normal → Isolated germinal cell failure → AIH / AID / IVF / Adopt

Low level — Low LH and T levels
- Ⓓ Hypogonadotropic hypogonadism → Prolactin level
  - Ⓔ High level → CT scan
    - Normal findings → Bromocriptine / Repeat x-ray examination in 6 months
    - Abnormal findings → Possible tumor → Bromocriptine, Surgery
  - Ⓕ Normal level → CT scan
    - Normal findings → Idiopathic disorder → Pergonal

Normal level — LH level
- Ⓖ Normal level → T level normal → Nonendocrine disorder
- Ⓗ High level → T level high → Androgen insensitivity → AID / Adopt

ARTIFICIAL INSEMINATION: HUSBAND

Gad Lavy, M.D.
Stephen P. Boyers, M.D.

A. The only absolute indications for artificial insemination by husband (AIH) are coital failure (vaginismus, impotence, or complete retrograde ejaculation) and the availability of only cryopreserved sperm. The benefit of AIH for immunologic or cervical infertility or for oligoasthenospermia has not been proven by controlled studies, and each of those disorders has a significant treatment-independent pregnancy incidence. Pending the results of controlled studies, a limited trial of AIH is warranted as long as other factors are not neglected.

B. Couples considering AIH should be informed of its relatively infrequent success, the need to place limits on an AIH trial, and the advisability of thoroughly exploring other fertility factors if a limited trial is unsuccessful. The risks of AIH are minimal. Intrauterine insemination may cause some crampy uterine pain and spotting; infection has not been a problem with washed migrated specimens. Husbands may have difficulty producing adequate semen samples "on demand," and many couples find the regimentation and mechanical nature of AIH psychologically disturbing and disruptive of spontaneous sexual activity.

C. As with most infertility therapy, the success of AIH is directly related to patient selection. Regular ovulatory cycles with an adequate luteal phase in women with tubal patency have the best chance of leading to pregnancy. The basal body temperature (BBT) chart is a useful tool for documenting regular ovulatory cycles and allows at least a retrospective assessment of the adequacy of insemination timing.

D. Semen may be supplied as either whole or split ejaculates. When sperm washing and migration are available, the whole ejaculate is used. When a migrated sample cannot be prepared, intrauterine insemination is probably contraindicated, since seminal prostaglandins can cause severe uterine discomfort and even an anaphylactic reaction. When intracervical insemination is planned, the first portion of a split ejaculate may provide a sperm-rich fraction in a small volume. Regardless of the technique used, the inseminating sample should be subjected to routine analysis of sperm density, motility, and velocity in an effort to keep track of semen quality over time. Three techniques of insemination, cervical cap, intracervical, and intrauterine, are shown in Figure 1.

E. The most critical part of AIH is its timing. For scheduling purposes the midcycle may be predicted on the basis of cycle length and BBT pattern. AIH is planned for the day of ovulation, generally a day or two before the BBT rise. Urinary luteinizing hormone (LH) kits are helpful in fine-tuning this schedule, as is the cervical score in couples with other than cervical infertility. If there is no distinct BBT rise by 48 hours after the first insemination, we re-examine the patient's cervix and reinseminate if the cervical score is still good. Using this protocol, we seldom inseminate more than twice in any normal cycle.

F. Most couples who conceive through AIH do so within the first four to six cycles of insemination. Failure to conceive with a limited trial is an indication to consider other infertility factors. Laparoscopy is indicated to detect occult peritubal-periovarian disease, including endometriosis, provided the work-up has already documented normal ovulatory function, luteal phase adequacy, and tubal patency by hysterosalpingography. In the absence of coexisting fertility factors, options to AIH should be considered, including artificial insemination by donor (AID), in vitro fertilization (IVF), and adoption.

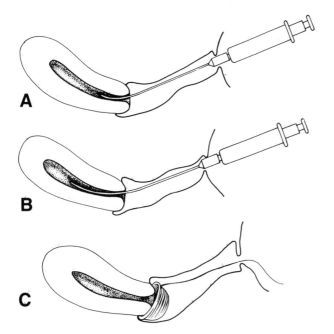

Figure 1 Insemination techniques: *A*, intracervical technique; *B*, intrauterine technique; *C*, cap technique.

References

Insler V, Melmed H, Eichenbrenner I, Serr DM, Lunenfeld B. The cervical score. Int J Gynaecol Obstet 1972; 10:223–228.

Nunley WC, Kitchin JD III, Thiagarajah S. Homologous insemination. Fertil Steril 1978; 30:510-515.

Steiman RP, Taymor ML. Artificial insemination homologous and its role in the management of infertility. Fertil Steril 1977; 28:146–150.

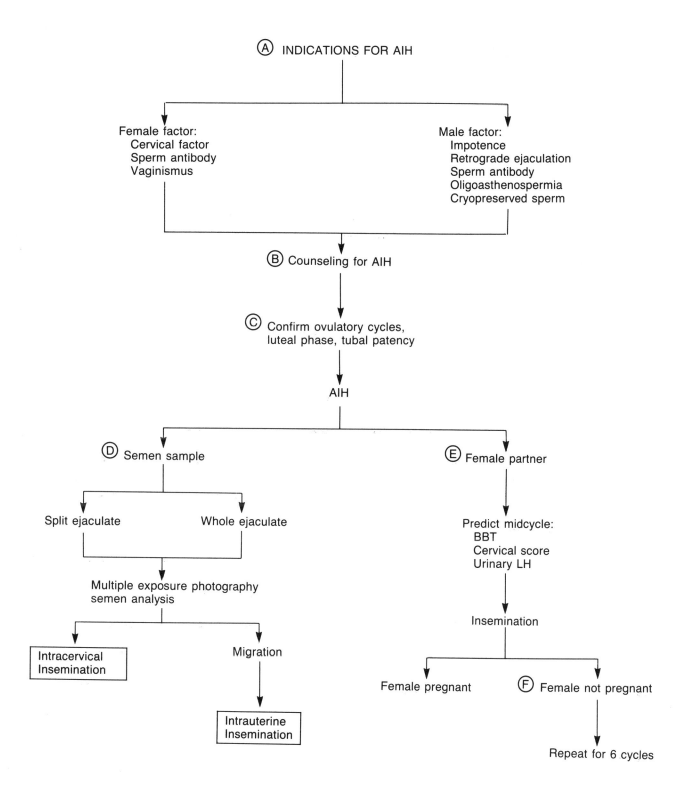

INTRAUTERINE INSEMINATION

Gad Lavy, M.D.
Stephen P. Boyers, M.D.

A. Both male factor infertility (oligoasthenoteratospermia) and cervical factor infertility can be treated by intrauterine insemination (IUI). In male infertility the goal of IUI is to place a sample containing motile sperm high in the reproductive tract about the time of ovulation. After intercourse many sperm are lost as they strive to ascend from the vagina to the tubal ampullae. Sperm survive in the vagina only a few hours, and the cervix acts as a selective filter, which relatively few sperm cross. With oligoasthenospermia, deposition of migrated sperm high in the reproductive tract may increase the likelihood that at least some sperm will reach the oocyte. In cases of cervical infertility the cervix or cervical mucus represents a barrier that can be breached by IUI.

B. Patient selection is the most important determinant of success with intrauterine insemination. Regular ovulatory cycles and patency of at least one fallopian tube are minimal requirements for IUI. Hysterosalpingography is our choice for initial assessment of tubal patency, and ovulation and luteal phase adequacy are assessed by the basal body temperature (BBT) pattern, the midluteal serum progesterone level, and late luteal endometrial biopsy for histologic dating.

C. The timing of intrauterine insemination is critical, perhaps more so than with intracervical insemination. Normal cervical mucus acts as a reservoir for sperm release into the upper reproductive tract over at least 48 hours. When cervical mucus is abnormal or is bypassed by IUI, the timed release function of the cervix may be lost, making insemination timing more critical. For scheduling purposes the patient calls at the onset of menses, and the first IUI is planned for days 12 to 14 of a 28-day cycle, adjusted earlier or later on the basis of the range of actual cycle lengths for each patient.

D. The date predicted for midcycle may be changed on the basis of the BBT pattern, the urinary luteinizing hormone (LH) level, and the cervical score (although the latter is not helpful in patients who have abnormal cervical mucus as the indication for IUI).

E. Sperm washing and migration remove motile sperm from the seminal fluid, concentrating them in a small volume of prostaglandin-free fluid for IUI. This procedure requires about 2 hours; thus the semen sample should be delivered fresh, within 1 hour after ejaculation, 2 hours prior to insemination. Semen quality is evaluated by multiple exposure photography (MEP) semen analysis, both before and after migration.

F. Insemination is done with the patient in the lithotomy position. The cervix is visualized with a bivalve speculum and is cleansed with a cotton swab moistened with warm Ham's F-10 medium. No local anesthesia or tenaculum is necessary. The 0.3 ml migrated sample is injected via a small Teflon catheter and tuberculin syringe through the internal cervical os into the fundal uterine cavity and the catheter is withdrawn slowly. The patient remains supine for 20 minutes. No antibiotics or prostaglandin inhibitors are used.

G. After insemination the patient continues to follow the BBT levels and returns in 24 to 48 hours for a possible repeat insemination, depending on the BBT and the cervical score. If the BBT remains low, with no distinct rise, and the cervical score remains high, a repeat IUI is recommended. If the BBT shifts upward and the cervical score declines after the initial insemination, a repeat procedure is not necessary. Patients who fail to conceive after six well timed cycles of IUI should be evaluated further for coexisting female infertility factors. Laparoscopy should be considered to rule out peritubal adhesions or pelvic endometriosis in these patients.

References

Glass RH, Ericsson RJ. Intrauterine insemination of isolated motile sperm. Fertil Steril 1978; 29:535–538.

Hull ME, Magyar DM, Vasquez JM, Hayes MF, Moghissi KS. Experience with intrauterine insemination for cervical factor and oligospermia. Am J Obstet Gynecol 1986; 154:1333-1338.

Kerin JFP, Peek J, Warnes GM, et al. Improved conception rate after intrauterine insemination of washed spermatozoa from men with poor quality semen. Lancet 1984; 1:533-534.

Makler A, DeCherney A, Naftolin F. A device for injecting and retaining a small volume of concentrated spermatozoa in the uterine cavity and cervical canal. Fertil Steril 1984; 42:306-308.

Makler A, Murillo O, Huszar G, et al. Improved techniques for separating motile spermatozoa from human semen. II. An atraumatic centrifugation method. Int J Androl 1978; 7:71-78.

INTRAUTERINE INSEMINATION

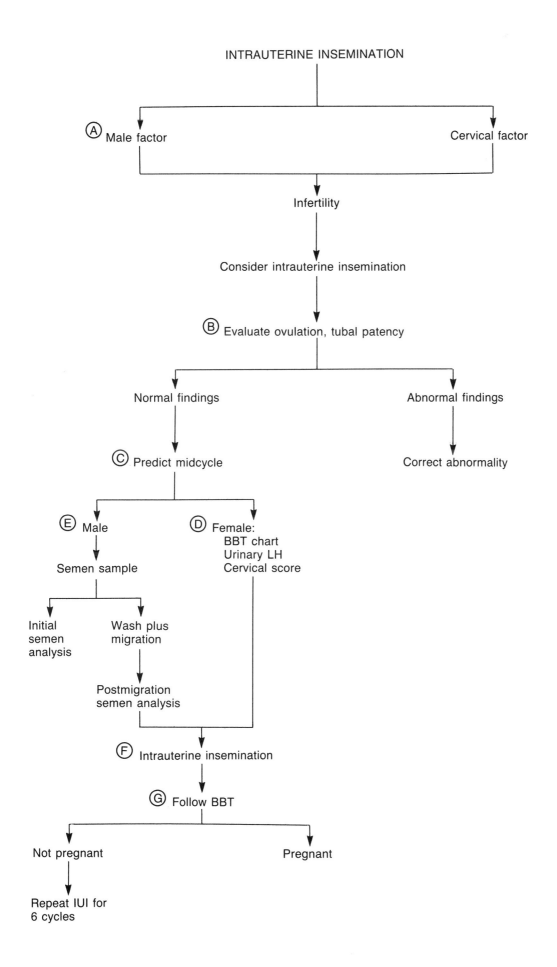

ARTIFICIAL INSEMINATION: DONOR

Gad Lavy, M.D.
Stephen P. Boyers, M.D.

A. Donor artificial insemination (AID) should be offered to couples with azoospermia and those with oligoasthenoteratospermia who fail to conceive despite an adequate trial of artificial insemination by husband (AIH). It should also be considered in order to circumvent heritable male transmitted genetic disorders and blood group incompatibility in previously sensitized patients. Other options include adoption and, for semen abnormalities other than azoospermia, in vitro fertilization.

B. Ovulation and luteal function should be evaluated by the basal body temperature (BBT), the midluteal serum progesterone level, and late luteal endometrial biopsy. In women at high risk for tubal disease (a history of pelvic infection, ectopic pregnancy, intrauterine device use, previous endometriosis) at least unilateral tubal patency should be documented by a hysterosalpingogram. In patients without risk factors for tubal disease, a trial of AID is warranted after documenting ovulation alone, as long as the trial is limited and a complete female fertility assessment is done for patients who fail to conceive after three to six well timed AID cycles. Anovulation should be evaluated and corrected before beginning AID.

C. Couples considering AID should be counseled concerning the medical, ethical, and legal aspects of the procedure. They should have a clear understanding of the donor screening process and should understand that their risk of conceiving a child with a birth defect is the same as that of couples conceiving spontaneously. The risk of acquiring a sexually transmitted disease should be explained along with the usual precautions for preventing such transmission. Donor-recipient anonymity should also be discussed. The couple should have a clear overview of the technical aspects of the procedure. The BBT pattern, urinary luteinizing hormone (LH) level, and cervical score are all used to pinpoint the midcycle for scheduling insemination.

D. Donors are thoroughly screened before being accepted. Screening includes a complete medical-genetic history and testing for semen quality and sexually transmissible diseases. Donors are matched to the infertile male for race, stature, eye color, and blood type and Rh (see donor screening algorithm, p 154).

E. Insemination is timed as for intrauterine insemination. Frozen semen allows the donor to be tested for sexually transmissible diseases at the time the sample is collected, with results available before the sample is used. The disadvantage of cryopreservation is that a significant fraction of the sperm are killed by the freeze-thaw process, decreasing semen quality. A normal sample with a sperm density greater than 60 million sperm per milliliter and more than 50 percent motility should withstand the freeze-thaw process well. Normal children have been born following AID with sperm frozen for as long as 10 years. Whether fresh or frozen, each donor sample should be evaluated before use. More than a few white cells in a fresh sample should signal possible infection, and the sample should be cultured and the insemination canceled or a different donor used.

F. AID may be done intracervically unless there is a specific indication for intrauterine insemination. Most couples who conceive with AID do so within the first three insemination cycles and 95 percent conceive within six cycles. There is no need to abandon AID if the patient fails to conceive after six cycles, but a thorough evaluation for coexisting female factors should be completed, including laparoscopy.

References

Aiman J. Factors affecting the success of donor insemination. Fertil Steril 1982; 37:94-99.

Behrman SJ. Artificial insemination. Fertil Steril 1959; 10:248-258.

Kleegman SJ. Therapeutic donor insemination. Fertil Steril 1954; 5:7-31.

Richter MA, Haning RV Jr, Shapiro SS. Artificial donor insemination: fresh versus frozen semen; the patient as her own control. Fertil Steril 1984; 41:277-280.

Virro MR, Shewchuk AB. Pregnancy outcome in 242 conceptions after artificial insemination with donor sperm and effects of maternal age on the prognosis for successful pregnancy. Am J Obstet Gynecol 1984; 148:518-524.

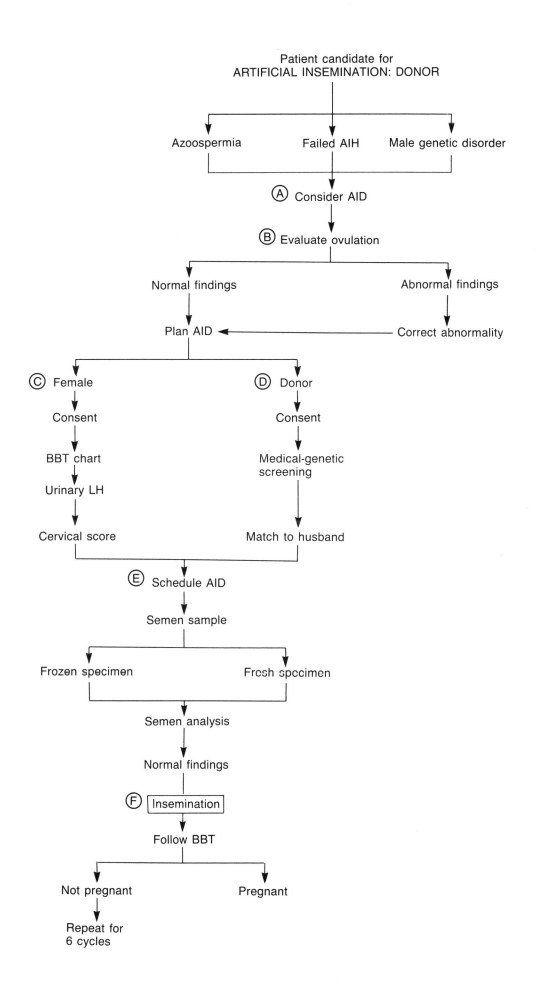

Patient candidate for
ARTIFICIAL INSEMINATION: DONOR

Azoospermia   Failed AIH   Male genetic disorder

Ⓐ Consider AID

Ⓑ Evaluate ovulation

Normal findings   Abnormal findings

Plan AID ◄──────────────────── Correct abnormality

Ⓒ Female   Ⓓ Donor

Consent   Consent

BBT chart   Medical-genetic
                               screening

Urinary LH

Cervical score   Match to husband

Ⓔ Schedule AID

Semen sample

Frozen specimen   Fresh specimen

Semen analysis

Normal findings

Ⓕ │Insemination│

Follow BBT

Not pregnant   Pregnant

Repeat for
6 cycles

DONOR SCREENING FOR ARTIFICIAL INSEMINATION

Gad Lavy, M.D.
Stephen P. Boyers, M.D.

A. Prospective donors are interviewed to evaluate their reliability, availability, and psychologic stability. The screening requirements are thoroughly explained, as is the therapeutic value of artificial insemination by donor (AID), the need to avoid sexual disease transmission, and the policy of strict confidentiality and anonymity. It is our policy not to disclose the success or failure of AID to donors, but simply to give them copies of the results of their screening laboratory and semen analyses for future reference.

B. The first step in donor screening is to obtain a complete medical and genetic history that records information concerning the health of the donor and his first degree relatives (mother, father, siblings, and children). Donors with special risks (Tay-Sachs disease, thalassemia, sickle cell disease) are screened specifically for those traits in addition to routine screening. It is not possible to completely eliminate the risk of transmitting genetic disease, because, first, almost all disease has a genetic component and, second, a truly complete medical-genetic history relies on the donor's knowledge and memory, which are not always accurate. Although donors with special risks can be excluded, couples should understand that in the general population without special risk 2 to 3 percent of babies still have major birth defects and several percent more have learning disabilities or behavioral problems. Donor screening cannot eliminate these risks. The yield of abnormal findings with routine karyotyping of donors is so low that it is not worthwhile. The medical history and physical examination are also designed to detect donors who have acute or chronic undiagnosed disease, such as hepatitis, which would make them ineligible until resolution of the problem.

C. Laboratory screening is primarily designed to detect carriers of transmissible diseases, especially those transmissible by semen. Laboratory tests include a Venereal Disease Research Laboratory (VDRL) test, a hepatitis screen, and the Western blot test for human immune deficiency virus (HIV). Homosexual men and drug abusers are not eligible under any circumstance because of their high risk for AIDS. Prospective donors with abnormal laboratory findings are referred for therapy.

D. A routine multiple exposure photographic semen analysis is required of all prospective donors, regardless of whether they have been proven fertile or not. Donors should have high quality semen with counts of 60 million per milliliter or higher, motility of 50 percent or greater, mean velocity of 20 μm per second or higher, and 60 percent normal forms or more. Abnormal results warrant repeating the semen analysis. Men with persistently abnormal semen analysis results may desire urologic follow-up. A semen analysis with normal findings should be followed by semen cultures for gonococcus and *Chlamydia*, and culture positive individuals should be treated and cured prior to acceptance.

E. To facilitate matching to the infertile husband, donors are asked to record information concerning race, height, and hair and eye color for themselves and first degree relatives. The ABO type and Rh are determined. A confidential file is maintained for each donor.

References

Jennings RT, Dixon RE, Nettles JB. The risks and prevention of Neisseria gonorrhoeae transfer in fresh ejaculate donor insemination. Fertil Steril 1977; 28:554-556.

Johnson WG, Schwartz RC, Chutorian AM. Artificial insemination by donors: the need for genetic screening. N Engl J Med 1981; 304:755-757.

Joyce EN. Recruitment, selection and management of donors. In: Brudenal M, Mclaren A, Short R, Symonds M, eds. Artificial insemination: proceedings of the fourth study group of the Royal College of Obstetricians and Gynecologists. London: Royal College of Obstetricians and Gynecologists, 1976: 60.

Report of the ad hoc committee on artificial insemination. Birmingham, AL: The American Fertility Society, 1980:1-28.

Schoysman R. Problems of selecting donors for artificial insemination. J Med Ethics 1975; 1:34-35.

Stewart GJ, Cunningham AL, Driscoll GL, et al. Transmission of human T-cell lymphotropic virus type III (HTLV-III) by artificial insemination by donor. Lancet 1985; 2:581-584.

Templeton AA, Triseliotis J. AID and adoption. In: Hargreave TB, ed. Male infertility. New York: Springer-Verlag, 1983:310.

Verp MS, Cohen MR, Simpson JL. Necessity of formal genetic screening in artificial insemination by donor. Obstet Gynecol 1983; 62:474-479.

DONOR RECRUITMENT

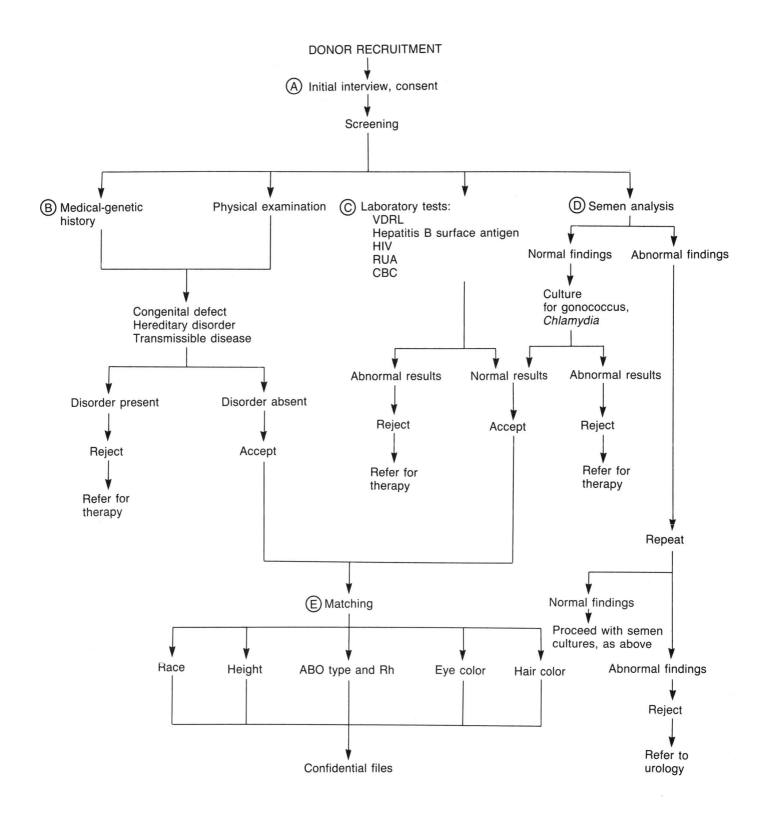

RETROGRADE EJACULATION

Gad Lavy, M.D.
Stephen P. Boyers, M.D.

A. Retrograde ejaculation means that semen passes into the urinary bladder instead of the penile urethra at the time of ejaculation. Patients usually complain of an absence, or a very small volume, of ejaculate or present with small semen volumes and azoospermia or severe oligospermia. Patients may also note turbid urine after intercourse. The diagnosis should be suspected when the endocrinologic work-up reveals normal gonadotropin and testosterone levels and a very low semen volume (less than 0.5 ml). A history of genitourinary surgery, diabetes, or a neurologic disorder should strengthen the suspicion in regard to retrograde ejaculation.

B. The diagnosis is made by finding sperm in a postejaculation urine sample. If the sperm are recovered from urine immediately after ejaculation, centrifuged, washed, and resuspended in Ham's F-10 medium, sperm density, motility, velocity, and morphology can be evaluated. When no sperm are seen in the postejaculation urine sample, an obstructive etiology for azoospermia should be considered and the seminal fluid fructose level should be measured.

C. The major etiologies of this condition are bladder neck incompetence, either congenital (bladder extrophy) or acquired (prostatectomy, bladder neck resection); neurogenic-neuropathic disorders (diabetes, multiple sclerosis, spinal cord injuries, surgical sympathectomy, or adrenergic blocking drugs); obstruction (urethral valves and strictures); and idiopathic disorders. Determination of the etiology requires a thorough neurologic examination and occasionally cystometric measurements, cystography, and vasography. Such a patient ultimately should be referred to a urologist for evaluation and treatment.

D. Some causes of retrograde ejaculation are correctable by surgery or drug therapy. Antihistamines and anticholinergic drugs may be helpful. All too often, however, permanent correction is not possible and artificial insemination is indicated. Alkalinization of the urine is accomplished with oral bicarbonate administration (1 teaspoon of baking soda in water or Kool-Aid) four times daily, starting 48 hours before a semen sample is needed. Sometimes ejaculation with a full bladder is enough to reverse the direction of the ejaculate, and the couple may have intercourse with that technique as a trial before beginning artificial insemination by husband. Otherwise the patient is instructed to void before intercourse to minimize the volume of urine that must be centrifuged to recover sperm. The bladder is emptied again immediately after ejaculation. The urine sample is centrifuged and the sperm pellet is resuspended in Ham's F-10 medium. After mixing and repeated centrifugation, the sperm pellet is resuspended and analyzed by multiple exposure photographic semen analysis prior to insemination, which may be either intrauterine or intracervical, depending on the quality of the cervical mucus and the quality of the inseminating sample.

References

Abrahams J, Solish G, Boorajian P, Waterhouse K. The surgical correction of retrograde ejaculation. J Urol 1975;114:888-890.

Collins JP. Retrograde ejaculation. In: Bain J, Schill WB, Scharzstein L, eds. Treatment of male infertility. New York: Springer-Verlag, 1982.

Crich JP, Jequier AM. Infertility in men with retrograde ejaculation: the action of urine on sperm motility, and a simple method for achieving antegrade ejaculation. Fertil Steril 1978; 30:572-576.

Hotchkiss R, Pinto A, Kleegman S. Artificial insemination with semen recovered from the bladder. Fertil Steril 1955; 6:37-40.

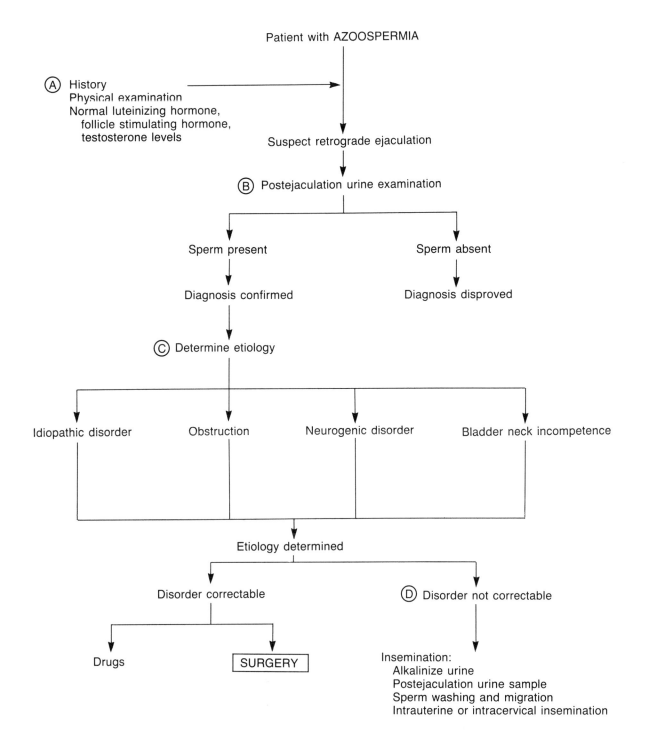

Patient with AZOOSPERMIA

A History
   Physical examination
   Normal luteinizing hormone,
     follicle stimulating hormone,
     testosterone levels

Suspect retrograde ejaculation

B Postejaculation urine examination

Sperm present

Sperm absent

Diagnosis confirmed

Diagnosis disproved

C Determine etiology

Idiopathic disorder

Obstruction

Neurogenic disorder

Bladder neck incompetence

Etiology determined

Disorder correctable

D Disorder not correctable

Drugs

SURGERY

Insemination:
   Alkalinize urine
   Postejaculation urine sample
   Sperm washing and migration
   Intrauterine or intracervical insemination

MALE INFERTILITY EVALUATION

Ronald D. Lee, M.D.

In 30 percent of infertile couples a significant male factor is the cause of the infertility. In an additional 20 percent there is a contributing male factor. Obviously an attempt to improve the "fertility potential" of a couple will be inadequate only if the female is treated and a concomitant male factor exists. Typically the woman begins the infertility evaluation with a visit to her family physician or gynecologist. An appropriate referral to an andrologist may be made at this time or after results of a "screening" semen analysis have been noted to be abnormal. Several advantages occur when the man and woman are seen and treated simultaneously. Early evaluation of the man may avoid unnecessary diagnostic studies for the woman if there is an insurmountable male factor. Second, concurrent evaluation of the couple most often leads to improved chances for fertility. Third, optimal timing of various diagnostic procedures or treatment modalities for either partner can best be managed when the couple are treated together. Lastly, synchronous evaluation may have positive psychologic benefits in that the couple share the burden of infertility rather than blaming the partner who is being evaluated.

A. A thorough history is taken with an emphasis on eliciting childhood illnesses, infectious diseases, exposure to gonadotoxins, hereditary problems, sexual dysfunction, the medical and surgical history, and a thorough review of systems. Physical examination focuses on body habitus and limb length, hair distribution, presence or absence of gynecomastia, penile abnormalities, palpable thyroid, the scrotal contents, and a thorough rectal examination.

B. Next appropriate laboratory testing is performed. Although the semen analysis remains the "gold standard" for the evaluation of the male factor, it is not a test for fertility but rather a set of parameters that are useful in assessing the potential obstacles the male may present in initiating a pregnancy. Semen analysis may be performed by several different methods, each yielding slightly different results. It is important to standardize the method of collection, number of days of abstinence, and technique of analysis in order to be able to interpret results for a given laboratory. At least two semen samples should be obtained for baseline data, since it has been estimated that an error of 10 to 15 percent is inherent in performing semen analysis.

C. Additional laboratory studies may be needed during evaluation of the male factor. These might include urinalysis, endocrine tests, cultures of appropriate fluids, tests of sperm function, tests for the presence of antisperm antibodies, genetic studies, and tests of Sertoli cell function.

D. Therapy of the infertile man may be divided into three main types: surgical, medical, and sperm enhancement or processing procedures. Each category of treatment has its own advantages and disadvantages, and no single type of treatment may be applicable to a particular problem. By using a thorough history and physical examination along with at least two semen analyses as the starting point, the evaluation and treatment of the infertile man may proceed.

References

Greenberg SH, Lipshultz LI, Wein AJ. Experience with 425 subfertile male patients. J Urol 1978; 119:507–510.

Lee RD, Lipshultz LI. Male infertility. In: Resnick MI, ed. Current trends in urology. Vol 3. Baltimore: Williams & Wilkins, 1985:30.

Sherins RJ, Howards SS. Male infertility. In: Walsh PC, ed. Campbell's urology. 5th ed. Philadelphia: WB Saunders, 1986:639.

Evaluation of the INFERTILE MAN

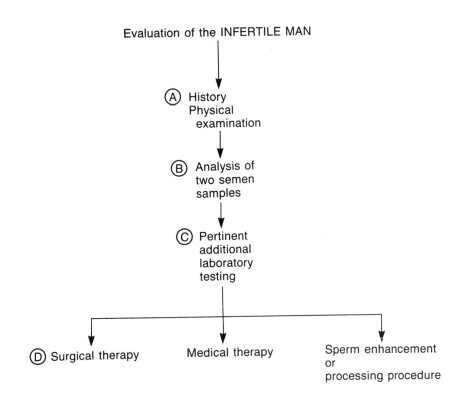

Ⓐ History
Physical
examination

Ⓑ Analysis of
two semen
samples

Ⓒ Pertinent
additional
laboratory
testing

Ⓓ Surgical therapy   Medical therapy   Sperm enhancement
or
processing procedure

SEMEN ANALYSIS

Ronald D. Lee, M.D.

A. After a complete history and physical examination, at least two semen analyses are conducted using a standard abstinence period of 2 to 3 days. On the basis of the results of these semen analyses, patients may be divided into four groups.

B. When all seminal parameters appear to be normal, the infertility evaluation should focus on further defining any female factor. If there seems to be no apparent female factor, consideration for further investigation of the male factor through specialized testing such as the sperm penetration assay or tests of Sertoli cell function should be made.

C. When azoospermia is present on two occasions, "decision making" is continued using the appropriate algorithm. In some series the incidence of azoospermia in men seen for evaluation of infertility is approximately 10 percent.

D. Multiple abnormal seminal parameters are approached both as group abnormalities and also by looking at the most "abnormal" parameter to determine therapy. Evaluation and treatment should proceed as outlined.

E. Abnormalities in the semen analysis involving a single parameter (e.g., density, motility, morphology, volume, viscosity) are commonly encountered. They may be approached in a systematic fashion as outlined.

References

Greenberg SH, Lipshultz LI, Wein AJ. Experience with 425 subfertile male patients. J Urol 1978; 119:507–510.

Lipshultz LI, Kaufman JJ, eds. Current urologic therapy. Philadelphia: WB Saunders, 1980.

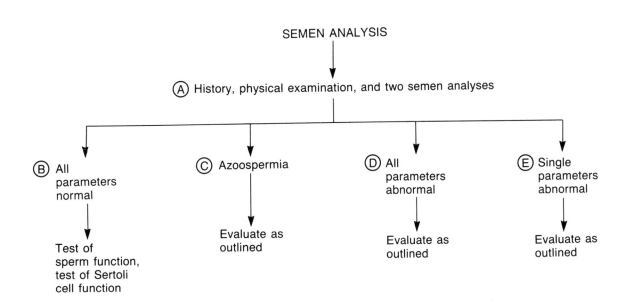

SEMEN ANALYSIS

A History, physical examination, and two semen analyses

B All parameters normal

Test of sperm function, test of Sertoli cell function

C Azoospermia

Evaluate as outlined

D All parameters abnormal

Evaluate as outlined

E Single parameters abnormal

Evaluate as outlined

AZOOSPERMIA

Ronald D. Lee, M.D.

Azoospermia is present in approximately 10 percent of the men being evaluated for infertility. It should be confirmed on at least two occasions. Many etiologies for azoospermia exist, some being amenable to therapy and others representing irreparable disease.

A. A simple office test, the postejaculation urine examination, is done to rule out the possibility of retrograde ejaculation. Usually in these patients semen collections are of very small volume and high pH. Often there may be clues from the history, such as bladder neck surgery, diabetes mellitus, or treatment with medications known to affect bladder neck competence, such as alpha-adrenergic antagonists. If numerous sperm are present in the postejaculation urine, attempts to convert to antegrade ejaculation are made or, failing this, harvesting of the bladder sperm is performed. When no sperm are seen in the postejaculation urine, a serum level of follicle stimulating hormone (FSH) is obtained.

B. When the serum level of follicle stimulating hormone is markedly elevated, i.e., greater than twice normal, the couple is encouraged to pursue alternate methods to increase their family size. If FSH levels are below normal limits, further endocrinologic evaluation is indicated. The spectrum of hypogonadotropic hypogonadism, with its numerous etiologies, may be encountered, including both hypothalamic and pituitary abnormalities.

C. Serum FSH levels less than or equal to twice the normal level are followed by seminal fructose testing. This may be done qualitatively in the office, using a resorcinol-hydrochloric acid solution and testing for colorimetric changes. If the results of physical examination are consistent with aplasia of the vasa deferentia, seminal fructose testing helps to confirm the absence of a complete efferent duct system. In conjunction with normal results on physical examination, seminal fructose testing helps direct the type of therapy for these patients.

D. Testicular biopsy with vasography is considered next. Several outcomes are possible. With normal testicular histologic findings and aplasia or absence of the vas deferens, an epididymal reservoir (artificial spermatocele) may be placed. This experimental procedure on occasion has yielded collections of sperm that have been used to successfully initiate pregnancy through insemination. "Open" epididymal aspiration may also be considered. Excurrent duct obstruction with normal testicular histologic findings may be present from the testis to the ejaculatory duct. We prefer to diagnose epididymal obstruction by visually inspecting the epididymis for dilated "tubules." This is done in conjunction with vasography. Retrograde vasography (i.e., contrast injection toward the epididymis from the vasotomy injection site) rarely defines the location of the obstruction and has the potential for causing inflammatory reactions or "blow-out" lesions of the epididymis. For these reasons, we do not advocate it. Vasal obstruction may be noted on vasography and, if present and In an easily accessible location, may be approached for vasovasostomy. Visual inspection of the epididymis may reveal a level of epididymal obstruction, and epididymovasostomy may be considered. Young's syndrome, a combination of obstructive azoospermia and chronic sinopulmonary infections, may also respond to epididymovasostomy or alternatively to ductal lavage. Vasography, when ejaculatory duct obstruction is present, shows dilated seminal vesicles and ampullas without contrast medium entering the prostatic urethra or bladder. This condition may respond to transurethral incision of the ejaculatory ducts, although recurrent scarring is a problem. With mildly abnormal testicular histologic findings and no evidence of obstruction on vasography, patients with varicoceles may respond to varicocele ligation. Also in these patients attempts to define any gonadotoxin exposure should be carried out, with removal of the gonadotoxin if feasible. With markedly abnormal testicular biopsy findings the couple is encouraged to seek other methods of increasing the family size.

References

Handelsman DJ, Conway AJ, Boylan LM, Turtle JR. Young's syndrome: obstructive azoospermia and chronic sinopulmonary infections. N Engl J Med 1984; 310:3–9.

Hendry WF. The long-term results of surgery for obstructive azoospermia. Br J Urol 1981; 53:664–668.

Mehan DJ. Results of ligation of internal spermatic vein in the treatment of infertility in azoospermic patients. Fertil Steril 1976; 27:110–114.

Wagenknecht LV. Modern trends of surgical treatment in male infertility: alloplastic spermatocele in cases of excretory azoospermia. Eur Urol 1976; 2:37.

Weintraub CM. Transurethral drainage of the seminal tract for obstruction, infection and infertility. Br J Urol 1980; 52:220–225.

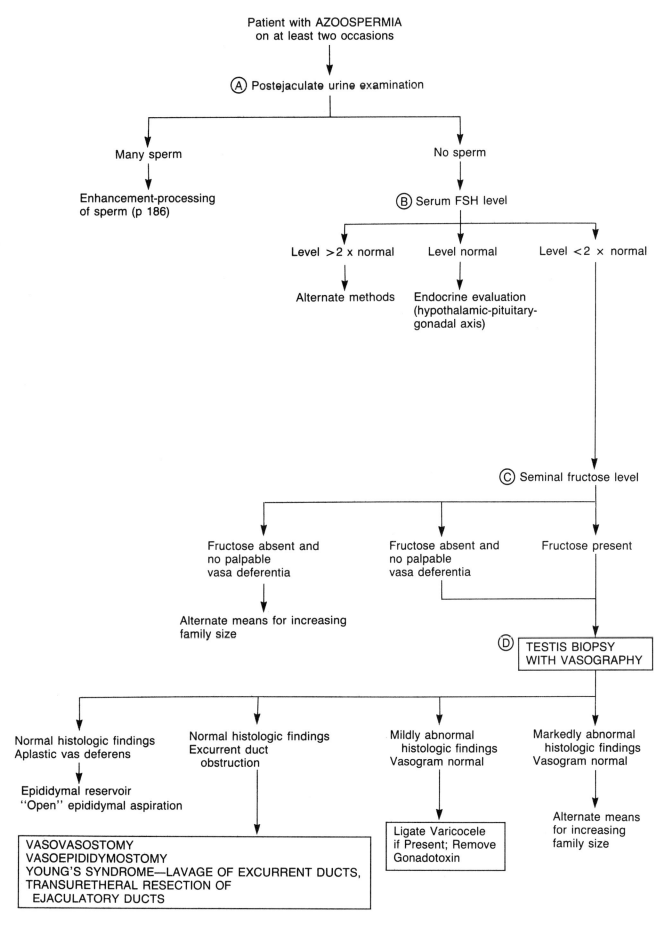

Patient with AZOOSPERMIA
on at least two occasions

(A) Postejaculate urine examination

Many sperm

Enhancement-processing
of sperm (p 186)

No sperm

(B) Serum FSH level

Level >2 x normal

Alternate methods

Level normal

Endocrine evaluation
(hypothalamic-pituitary-
gonadal axis)

Level <2 x normal

(C) Seminal fructose level

Fructose absent and
no palpable
vasa deferentia

Alternate means for increasing
family size

Fructose absent and
no palpable
vasa deferentia

Fructose present

(D) TESTIS BIOPSY
WITH VASOGRAPHY

Normal histologic findings
Aplastic vas deferens

Epididymal reservoir
"Open" epididymal aspiration

Normal histologic findings
Excurrent duct
obstruction

Mildly abnormal
histologic findings
Vasogram normal

Markedly abnormal
histologic findings
Vasogram normal

Alternate means
for increasing
family size

Ligate Varicocele
if Present; Remove
Gonadotoxin

VASOVASOSTOMY
VASOEPIDIDYMOSTOMY
YOUNG'S SYNDROME—LAVAGE OF EXCURRENT DUCTS,
TRANSURETHERAL RESECTION OF
EJACULATORY DUCTS

ALL SEMINAL PARAMETERS ABNORMAL

Ronald D. Lee, M.D.

A. Simultaneous abnormalities of several or all of the bulk seminal parameters are the most commonly encountered semen abnormalities in infertile men. They may be approached as group abnormalities or by evaluating the "most abnormal" parameter if a particular parameter is markedly abnormal. When multiple seminal abnormalities are seen, serum follicle stimulating hormone levels (FSH) are obtained, and if they are more than twice the normal level, other methods for increasing family size are considered. If the FSH level is less than normal, an endocrine work-up to evaluate the hypothalamic-pituitary-gonadal axis is performed. Serum testosterone (T), luteinizing hormone (LH), and prolactin (PRL) levels are obtained. Additional tests to assess other pituitary hormones and imaging studies of the sella turcica are performed. Therapy may include human chorionic gonadotropin–human menopausal gonadotropin (hCG-hMG) stimulation, bromocriptine administration, or pituitary surgery.

B. When the FSH level is normal or slightly elevated (less than twice the normal level), a careful review of the history is undertaken with an emphasis on eliciting possible transient problems from gonadotoxin exposure.

These might include exposure to certain drugs known to impair spermatogenesis, such as sulfasalazine, cimetidine, nitrofurantoin, and possibly alcohol, nicotine, and tetrahydrocannabinol; heat exposure either externally through occupational or recreational contacts or internally from febrile illness; a history of "stress;" or a history of exposure to environmental toxins. A repeat semen analysis 3 months after removal from gonadotoxin exposure may show marked "spontaneous" improvement.

C. Varicocele is the most common cause of male subfertility (Fig. 1). Typically it presents with alterations in sperm motility accompanied by decreases in sperm density and in the percentage of sperm of normal morphology. Improvement in seminal quality after varicocele ligation ranges from 40 to 70 percent, with pregnancy incidences of approximately 25 to 50 percent. In selected cases the addition of postoperative hormonal therapy may improve conception incidences even further.

D. An immunologic cause for infertility may be considered. Antisperm antibody levels are measured and treatment instituted if appropriate (see p 184).

E. Multiple abnormal seminal parameters should also raise the possibility of endocrine dysfunction. Serum LH, PRL, and testosterone levels should be obtained to further evaluate this. Treatment may consist of either hormonal replacement or suppression.

F. There may be no obvious cause for the abnormal seminal parameters. In such cases empirical therapy has been employed with some success. Such therapy might consist of hormonal stimulation or scrotal hypothermia. In addition, the use of intrauterine insemination with a washed or "swim-up" specimen has been encouraging.

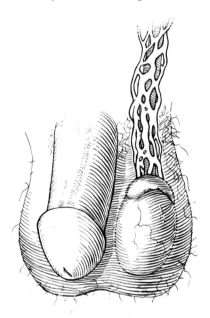

Figure 1 An enlarged scrotal vein, or varicocele, may cause a rise in temperature and subsequent reduction in sperm production.

References

Allen NC, Herbert CM, Maxson WS, et al. Intrauterine insemination: a critical review. Fertil Steril 1985; 44:569–580.

Greenberg SH. Varicocele and male fertility. Fertil Steril 1977; 28:699–706.

Sorbie PJ, Perez-Marrero R. The use of clomiphene citrate in male infertility. J Urol 1984; 131:425–429.

Swerdloff RS, Boyers SP. Evaluation of the male partner of an infertile couple: an algorithmic approach. JAMA 1982; 247:2418–2422.

Zorgniotti AW, Sealfon AI. Scrotal hypothermia: new therapy for poor semen. Urology 1984; 23:439–441.

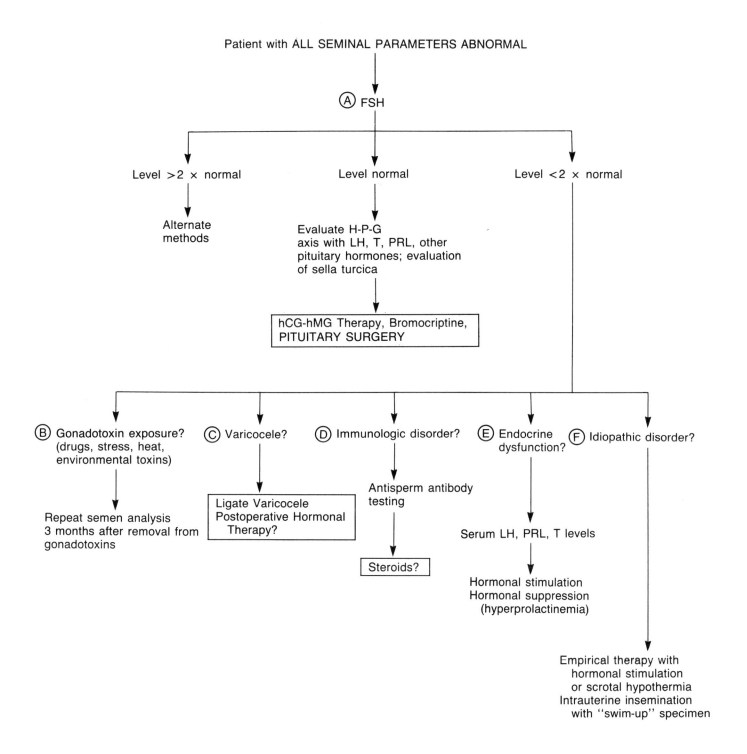

Patient with ALL SEMINAL PARAMETERS ABNORMAL

Ⓐ FSH

Level >2 × normal

Alternate methods

Level normal

Evaluate H-P-G axis with LH, T, PRL, other pituitary hormones; evaluation of sella turcica

hCG-hMG Therapy, Bromocriptine, PITUITARY SURGERY

Level <2 × normal

Ⓑ Gonadotoxin exposure? (drugs, stress, heat, environmental toxins)

Repeat semen analysis 3 months after removal from gonadotoxins

Ⓒ Varicocele?

Ligate Varicocele Postoperative Hormonal Therapy?

Ⓓ Immunologic disorder?

Antisperm antibody testing

Steroids?

Ⓔ Endocrine dysfunction?

Serum LH, PRL, T levels

Hormonal stimulation Hormonal suppression (hyperprolactinemia)

Ⓕ Idiopathic disorder?

Empirical therapy with hormonal stimulation or scrotal hypothermia Intrauterine insemination with "swim-up" specimen

SINGLE ABNORMAL SEMINAL PARAMETER

Ronald D. Lee, M.D.

A. Although multiple abnormal seminal parameters are most often encountered in evaluation of the infertile man, patients may have isolated disturbances in any of these parameters. Aberrations in motility are the most common (26 percent), while morphologic abnormalities are the least common (1 percent). We evaluate volume, viscosity, morphology, motility–forward progression, and sperm density when examining the semen, and although there is no absolute order for reviewing the parameters, we have found it helpful to review density and motility–forward progression last so as not to overlook a problem in the other seminal parameters.

B. A simple test is to measure semen volume. When it is low, that is, less than 1.5 ml, it is necessary to rule out a possible collection error, retrograde ejaculation, a hypoandrogenic state, or inflammation of the accessory sex glands. Appropriate therapy might include a repeat semen analysis if a collection error is suspected; sympathomimetic drugs or urine alkalinization and concentration with homologous insemination if retrograde ejaculation is documented and does not respond to sympathomimetic therapy; hormonal replacement if a true hypoandrogenic state exists; treatment with antimicrobial drugs if a diagnosis of accessory sex gland infection can be made; and finally use of homologous insemination for consistently low semen volumes. Conversely, when semen volumes are high, that is, greater than 5 ml, split ejaculation semen analysis (SA) is performed. The "better" fraction may then be used for homologous insemination. If the first fraction is the "better" one, as is the case 90 percent of the time, withdrawal coitus may also be employed. The use of mechanical concentration, with resuspension of the sperm pellet in a small amount of fluid medium, in conjunction with homologous insemination may also be considered.

C. Hyperviscous semen is not uncommonly seen during semen analysis and may be an impediment to sperm migration. We do not consider it to be of clinical significance, however, unless the postcoital test (PCT) findings are also abnormal, with a low number of sperm present or decreased sperm motility. It is important to differentiate between hyperviscosity and delayed liquefaction (see pp 174, 176). Appropriate therapy might include amylase liquefaction for delayed seminal liquefaction or mucolytic drugs, split ejaculate insemination, or mechanical thinning for hyperviscous semen.

D. An increased number of abnormal sperm forms may be seen in a variety of conditions. These might include stress or following gonadotoxin exposure or in association with varicocele or idiopathic disorders. Usually there are abnormalities in other seminal parameters, but on rare occasion isolated morphologic aberrations are seen. If this is the only abnormality seen in the semen, a repeat semen analysis in 2 to 3 months is indicated since this may be a transient phenomenon. Removal of the gonadotoxin or source of stress may also be helpful. Varicocele ligation with abnormal morphology as the only problem in the seminal parameters is controversial.

E. Decreases in sperm density below 20×10^6 per ml have been associated with an increased incidence of infertility. If due to endocrine abnormalities such as hypogonadotropic hypogonadism or hyperprolactinemia, treatment with hormonal supplementation or hormonal suppression often is helpful. When oligospermia is due to volume abnormalities, either high or low, consideration should be made for the use of split ejaculate insemination or mechanical concentration, respectively. Often no identifiable cause for oligospermia is found—so-called idiopathic oligospermia. A variety of treatment options may be used in an attempt to improve sperm density. Empirical hormonal therapy, scrotal hypothermia, and homologous insemination using a washed or "swim-up" semen specimen have all been claimed to be of some benefit. Newer techniques such as gamete intrafallopian transfer and in vitro fertilization are possible options once less complex ones have been exhausted. Polyzoospermia may be treated with multiple daily ejaculates, split ejaculate insemination, or withdrawal coitus.

F. Motility forward progression abnormalities may be secondary to a variety of causes, including antisperm antibodies, nonimmunologic agglutination, genital tract infection, varicocele, and idiopathic causes. Treatment may be directed at a specific cause if it is identifiable. Antisperm antibodies may respond to high dose intermittent steroid therapy. Vitamin C has been used to decrease nonimmunologic sperm agglutination. Appropriate antimicrobial drugs may be used to treat genital gland infection. Varicocele ligation is performed when both asthenospermia and a varicocele are present. Therapy for idiopathic asthenospermia may include the empirical use of scrotal hypothermia or insemination with a washed or "swim-up" specimen.

References

Amelar RD. Coagulation, liquefaction and viscosity of human semen. J Urol 1962; 87:187–190.

Lee RD, Lipshultz LI. Infertility. In: Resnick MI, ed. Current trends in urology. Vol. 3. Baltimore: Williams & Wilkins, 1985:30.

Lipshultz LI, Howards SS. Evaluation of the subfertile man. In: Lipshultz LI, Howard SS, eds. Infertility in the male. New York: Churchill Livingstone, 1983:187.

MacLeod J. Human seminal cytology as a sensitive indicator of the germinal epithelium. Int J Fertil 1964; 9:281–295.

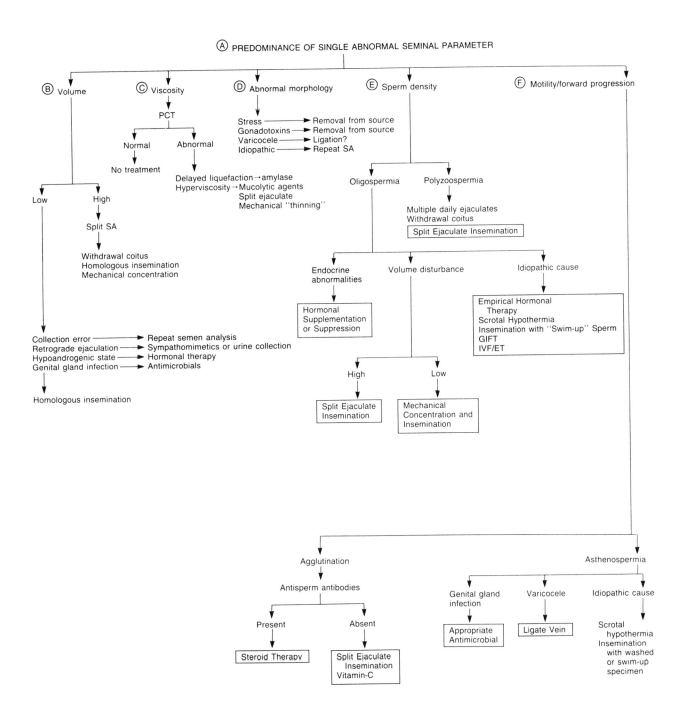

A PREDOMINANCE OF SINGLE ABNORMAL SEMINAL PARAMETER

B Volume

C Viscosity

PCT

Normal

Abnormal

No treatment

Low

High

Split SA

Withdrawal coitus
Homologous insemination
Mechanical concentration

Collection error ⟶ Repeat semen analysis
Retrograde ejaculation ⟶ Sympathomimetics or urine collection
Hypoandrogenic state ⟶ Hormonal therapy
Genital gland infection ⟶ Antimicrobials

Homologous insemination

D Abnormal morphology

Stress ⟶ Removal from source
Gonadotoxins ⟶ Removal from source
Varicocele ⟶ Ligation?
Idiopathic ⟶ Repeat SA

Delayed liquefaction→amylase
Hyperviscosity→Mucolytic agents
Split ejaculate
Mechanical ''thinning''

E Sperm density

Oligospermia

Polyzoospermia

Multiple daily ejaculates
Withdrawal coitus
Split Ejaculate Insemination

Endocrine
abnormalities

Volume disturbance

Idiopathic cause

Hormonal
Supplementation
or Suppression

Empirical Hormonal
   Therapy
Scrotal Hypothermia
Insemination with ''Swim-up'' Sperm
GIFT
IVF/ET

High

Low

Split Ejaculate
Insemination

Mechanical
Concentration and
Insemination

F Motility/forward progression

Agglutination

Antisperm antibodies

Present

Absent

Steroid Therapy

Split Ejaculate
Insemination
Vitamin-C

Asthenospermia

Genital gland
infection

Varicocele

Idiopathic cause

Appropriate
Antimicrobial

Ligate Vein

Scrotal
hypothermia
Insemination
with washed
or swim-up
specimen

ENDOCRINE EVALUATION

Ronald D. Lee, M.D.

A. Endocrine evaluation is performed, in most cases, at the same time as semen analysis. Typically it includes serum levels of follicle stimulating hormone (FSH), luteinizing hormone (LH), and testosterone (T), although for cost containment purposes a useful screening test might be determination of the serum FSH level alone. Estrogen (E_2) or prolactin (PRL) levels may be obtained in certain cases. In a simplistic sense the FSH level reflects activity in the seminiferous tubules, while the LH level is an indirect measurement of Leydig cell function (Fig. 1). The testosterone level also reflects Leydig cell function. Estrogen determinations are made if end organ resistance to testosterone is suspected or if gynecomastia or other signs of hyperestrogenism exist. Prolactin levels are obtained if there is associated galactorrhea, impotence, or visual field changes or if signs of renal failure or acromegaly exist.

B. A normal FSH level with elevated LH and testosterone levels represents an androgen insensitivity state. Serum estrogen levels are usually also elevated. Unfortunately no adequate therapy exists for this type of disorder. A normal FSH level with normal LH and testosterone levels is a common pattern encountered in evaluation of the infertile man. It can be seen with numerous disorders resulting in subfertility, including varicocele, genital tract infection, and immune infertility. Evaluation proceeds according to the pattern of abnormality seen on semen analysis. In azoospermic patients with this pattern one should suspect either ductal obstruction or retrograde ejaculation. When FSH and LH levels are normal but the testosterone level is low, suspect either a decrease in sex hormone binding protein or obesity as a possible cause.

C. A low serum FSH level may be seen as an isolated finding with normal LH and testosterone levels. Therapy may consist of replacement stimulation with human menopausal gonadotropin (hMG), indirect stimulation with clomiphene, or direct pituitary stimulation with gonadotropin releasing hormone (GnRH). A low serum FSH level may also be seen as part of a picture of hypogonadotropic hypogonadism with decreased serum LH and testosterone levels. It may be associated with anosmia as well as with deficiencies in other pituitary hormones. This combination may be seen secondary to hypothalamic or pituitary tumors, and on occasion associated hyperprolactinemia is discovered. GnRH formation or secretion may be impaired.

D. An elevated FSH level in association with an elevated LH level and a low to normal testosterone level represents primary testicular failure and is not amenable to therapy. Alternative means of increasing family size should be discussed with the couple. Likewise isolated FSH elevation with normal LH and testosterone levels represents spermatogenic failure without associated Leydig cell injury. Mild elevation of the FSH level may be seen with varicoceles. There have been occasional reports of decreasing FSH levels with improved seminal parameters following varicocele ligation in this setting.

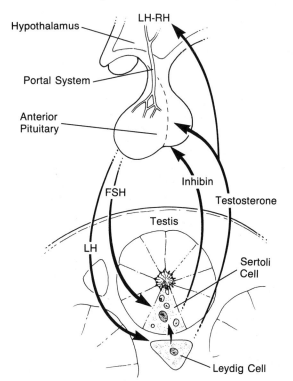

Figure 1 The normal feedback relationship of the hypothalamic pituitary testicular axis.

References

Aiman J, Griffin JE, Gazak JM, et al. Androgen insensitivity as a cause of infertility in otherwise normal men. N Engl J Med 1979; 300:223–227.

Glass AR, Swerdloff RS, Bray GA, Dahms WT, Atkinson RL. Low serum testosterone and sex-hormone-binding-globulin in massively obese men. J Clin Endocrinol Metab 1977; 45:1211–1219.

Maroulis GB, Parlow AF, Marshall JR. Isolated follicle-stimulating hormone deficiency in man. Fertil Steril 1977; 28:818–822.

Sherins RJ, Howards SS. Male infertility. In: Walsh PC, ed. Campbell's urology. 5th ed. Philadelphia: WB Saunders, 1986:639.

Vigersky RA. Endocrine evaluation and differential diagnosis of male infertility. In: Infertility seminar of the AUA. Lipshultz LI, Program Director. Dallas, 1984.

Patient undergoing ENDOCRINE EVALUATION

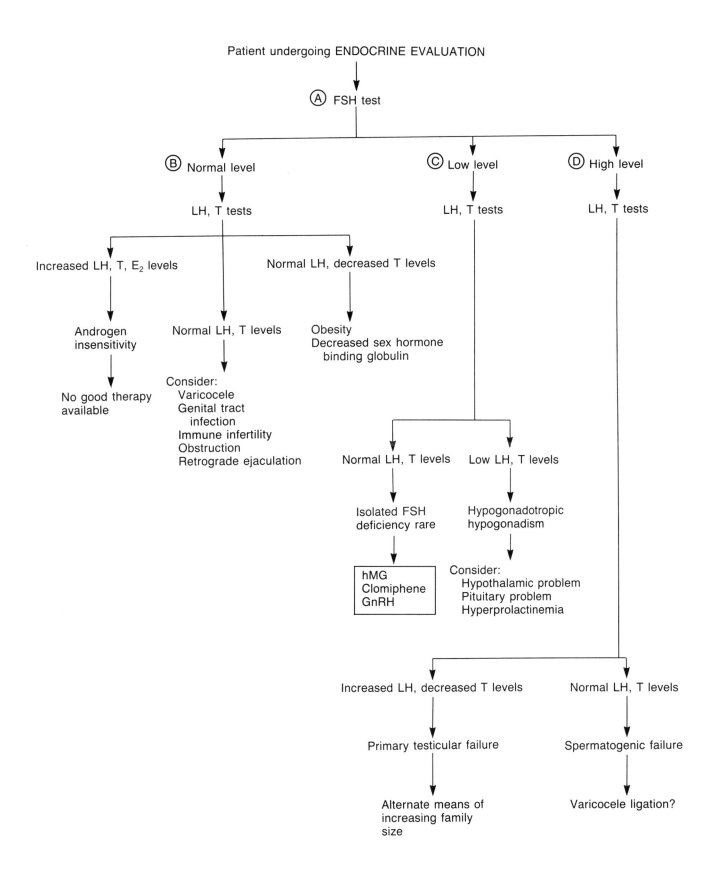

HYPERPROLACTINEMIA

Ronald D. Lee, M.D.

A. Although commonly seen in association with secondary amenorrhea and infertility in women, hyperprolactinemia has a less well defined role in male infertility. Hyperprolactinemia clearly may be seen in association with abnormal semen parameters. It has been suggested that return of the serum prolactin level to normal improves the results of semen analyses, although in fact this is not always true. Typically men who present with infertility and are found to have hyperprolactinemia also have associated symptoms and signs such as impotence, gynecomastia, hypogonadism, galactorrhea, visual field defects, or clinical findings consistent with hypothyroidism or renal insufficiency. When the physician is confronted with any of these clinical findings in association with male factor infertility, serum prolactin levels should be measured. Also, when the serum testosterone level is low and the serum follicle stimulating hormone (FSH) and luteinizing hormone (LH) levels are low or low normal, prolactin levels should be checked.

B. If the prolactin level is found to be elevated, the determination should be repeated to confirm the results, since they normally vary on a diurnal basis and are subject to fluctuation as a result of such elements as stress and nipple stimulation. A normal prolactin level on subsequent testing would lead one to search for other causes of male infertility. Repeated high levels of prolactin should prompt further investigation of the hypothalamic-pituitary-gonadal axis, after eliminating other possible causes of hyperprolactinemia, including medication (tranquilizers, alpha-methyldopa), renal insufficiency, hypothyroidism, and chest wall trauma.

C. Continued high levels of prolactin mandate inspection of the sella turcica with both plain films and computed tomographic scanning. In addition, visual field testing may be done to document compression of the optic chiasm (Fig. 1). When no abnormalities are noted on diagnostic imaging studies, treatment should commence with bromocriptine. Recent studies have suggested that pergolide may also be useful in this setting.

D. If a macroadenoma is documented on imaging studies, either surgical excision or bromocriptine therapy may be employed. Patients in whom medical failure is documented may be counseled to undergo surgical extirpation.

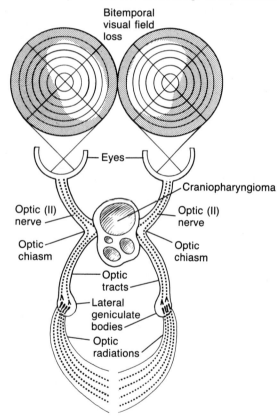

Figure 1 Bitemporal hemianopia caused by compression of the optic chiasm by a pituitary tumor or craniopharyngioma may signal the cause of infertility.

References

Carter JN, Tyson JE, Tolis G, et al. Prolactin-secreting tumors and hypogonadism in 22 men. N Engl J Med 1978; 299:847–852.

Murray FT, Cameron DF, Ketchum C. Return of gonadal function in men with prolactin-secreting pituitary tumors. J Clin Endocrinol Metab 1984; 59:79–85.

Saidi K, Wenn RV, Sharif F. Bromocriptine for male infertility. Lancet 1977; 1:250-251.

Segal S, Yaffe H, Laufer N, Ben-David M. Male hyperprolactinemia: effects on fertility. Fertil Steril 1979; 32:556–561.

Wong T-W, Jones TM. Hyperprolactinemia and male infertility. Arch Pathol Lab Med 1984; 108:35–39.

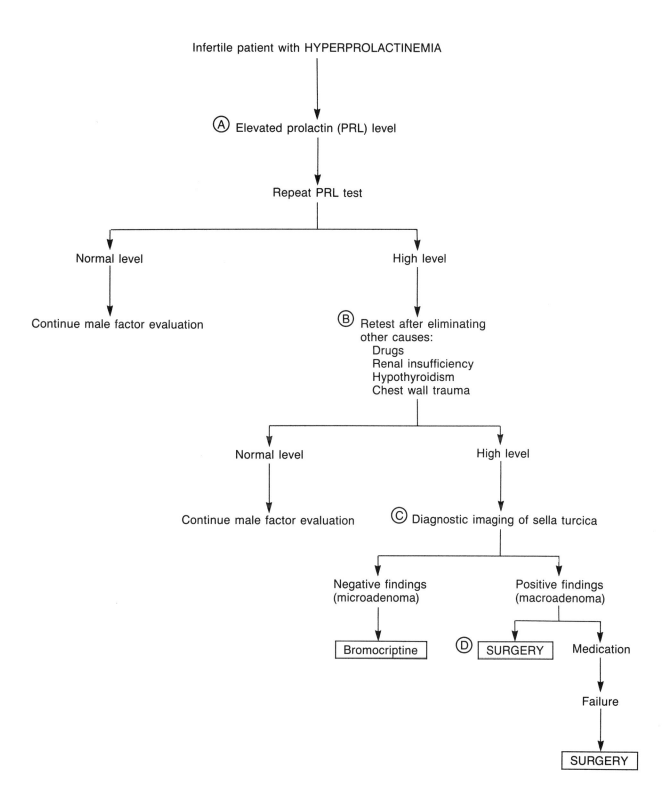

Infertile patient with HYPERPROLACTINEMIA

(A) Elevated prolactin (PRL) level

Repeat PRL test

Normal level

Continue male factor evaluation

High level

(B) Retest after eliminating
other causes:
Drugs
Renal insufficiency
Hypothyroidism
Chest wall trauma

Normal level

Continue male factor evaluation

High level

(C) Diagnostic imaging of sella turcica

Negative findings
(microadenoma)

Bromocriptine

Positive findings
(macroadenoma)

(D) SURGERY   Medication

Failure

SURGERY

SEMINAL VOLUME PROBLEM

Ronald D. Lee, M.D.

A. Seminal volume problems may be seen in up to 12 percent of men attending male infertility clinics. The normal range of semen volume, after 2 to 3 days of abstinence, is 1.5 to 5.0 ml. Problems may occur when the volume is either too low or too high.

Low Seminal Volume

B. The seminal volume is considered abnormally low when it is less than 1.5 ml. When one is confronted with specimens of low volume, it is important to exclude several sources of "collection error," including incomplete or spilled collection, a short abstinence period, or a specimen collected under "very stressful" conditions. These can all give spuriously low sample volumes and should be confirmed or denied using repeat semen analyses (SA). If the seminal volume on repeat studies is normal, continue evaluation of other seminal parameters as outlined.

C. If the seminal volume remains low, check the urine for the presence of retrograde ejaculation. A history of diabetes mellitus, bladder neck surgery, or ingestion of medications known to affect bladder neck competence, such as alpha-adrenergic antagonists, may raise the index of suspicion.

D. When retrograde ejaculation is present, appropriate therapy would include attempts to convert to antegrade ejaculation or, failing that, to harvest the sperm from collected urine that has been buffered and osmotically adjusted.

E. If there is no evidence for retrograde ejaculation, it is useful to obtain serum testosterone levels. Hypoandrogenic states may lead to decreased fluid production from the various genital glands. Hormonal replacement may have a salubrious effect on seminal volume. With a normal serum testosterone level the use of homologous insemination (AIH) with or without mechanical concentration may be considered.

High Seminal Volume

F. Seminal volumes greater than 5 ml are generally considered abnormal. If, however, sperm density, motility, and morphology are "normal" in the face of a large seminal volume, no further therapy may be needed. The semen volume should be evaluated with a standard 2 to 3 day abstinence period.

G. If seminal parameters other than volume are also abnormal, a split ejaculate specimen should be obtained. Roughly 90 percent of men show an increased number of motile sperm in the first portion as compared with the second fraction. This first fraction may be used either by insemination or by instructing the man to withdraw the penis from the vagina after the initial few spurts of ejaculate. Alternatively a "swim-up" migration technique may be employed to separate the motile sperm from the remainder, or more frequent ejaculations may be tried about the time of ovulation.

References

Amelar RD, Hotchkiss RS. The split ejaculate: its use in the management of male infertility. Fertil Steril 1965; 16:46–60.

Greenburg SH, Lipshultz LI, Wein AJ. Experience with 425 subfertile male patients. J Urol 1978; 119:507–510.

Murphy DP. The volume of the semen: a study of 3544 childless men. Fertil Steril 1967; 18:124–126.

Nachtigall RD, Faure N, Glass RH. Artificial insemination of husband's sperm. Fertil Steril 1979; 32:141–147.

Poland ML, Moghissi KS, Giblin PT, Ager JW, Olson JM. Variation of semen measures within normal men. Fertil Steril 1985; 44:396–400.

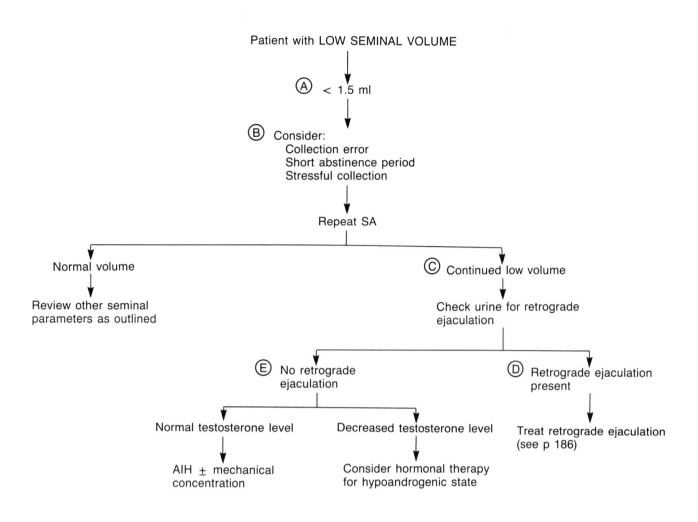

Patient with LOW SEMINAL VOLUME

Ⓐ < 1.5 ml

Ⓑ Consider:
   Collection error
   Short abstinence period
   Stressful collection

Repeat SA

Normal volume

Review other seminal
parameters as outlined

Ⓒ Continued low volume

Check urine for retrograde
ejaculation

Ⓔ No retrograde
   ejaculation

Ⓓ Retrograde ejaculation
   present

Normal testosterone level

Decreased testosterone level

Treat retrograde ejaculation
(see p 186)

AIH ± mechanical
concentration

Consider hormonal therapy
for hypoandrogenic state

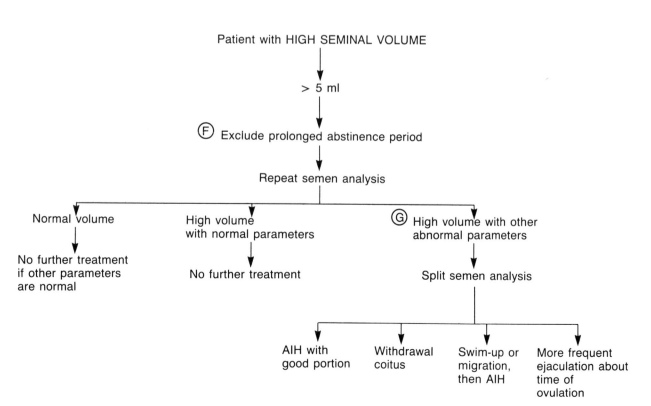

Patient with HIGH SEMINAL VOLUME

> 5 ml

Ⓕ Exclude prolonged abstinence period

Repeat semen analysis

Normal volume

High volume
with normal parameters

Ⓖ High volume with other
   abnormal parameters

No further treatment
if other parameters
are normal

No further treatment

Split semen analysis

AIH with
good portion

Withdrawal
coitus

Swim-up or
migration,
then AIH

More frequent
ejaculation about
time of
ovulation

HYPERVISCOUS SEMEN

Ronald D. Lee, M.D.

A. Normal semen, upon liquefaction, should be of such a consistency that it can be poured drop by drop. Conversely, hyperviscous semen is characterized by a thick, congealed appearance and a tendency to remain in clumps when poured. Viscous semen per se is not always associated with infertility; however, it is thought possibly to impede the movement of sperm through the female genital tract. When dealing with what appears to be hyperviscous semen, the clinician must be careful to differentiate the problem from that of delayed liquefaction. Re-evaluation of the sample after 60 minutes often shows a significant decrease in viscosity if delayed liquefaction is causative. If it appears that hyperviscosity is in fact present, postcoital testing (PCT) is done to evaluate the importance of this finding.

B. In the presence of normal PCT results, hyperviscous semen is not likely to be a problem. If, on the other hand, the postcoital test yields abnormal results, options for decreasing the seminal viscosity should be considered.

C. Methods for decreasing the seminal viscosity include mechanical disruption, chemical mucolysis, centrifugation with insemination, and split ejaculate insemination. Mechanical disruption consists of aspirating and injecting the seminal fluid through successively smaller needles, beginning with an 18 gauge and proceeding to a 23 gauge needle. Chemical mucolysis may be done using mucolytic agents such as acetylcysteine and adding a small amount of this agent to the semen sample. As an alternative, after centrifuging the hyperviscous semen, the "sperm pellet" may be removed and resuspended using an appropriate fluid medium such as a phosphate buffered solution in preparation for insemination. If the semen volume permits, a split ejaculate sample may be obtained and homologous insemination may be done using the initial (and usually less viscous) portion of the sample.

References

Amelar RD, Dubin L. A coital technique for promotion of fertility. Urology 1975; 5:228.

Bunge RG. Disorders other than endocrine and genetic. In: Cockett ATK, Urry RL, eds. Male infertility workup, treatment and research. New York: Grune & Stratton, 1976:97.

Tauber PF, Zaneveld LJD. Coagulation and liquefaction of human semen. In: Hafez ESE, ed. Human semen and fertility regulation in men. St. Louis: CV Mosby, 1976:153.

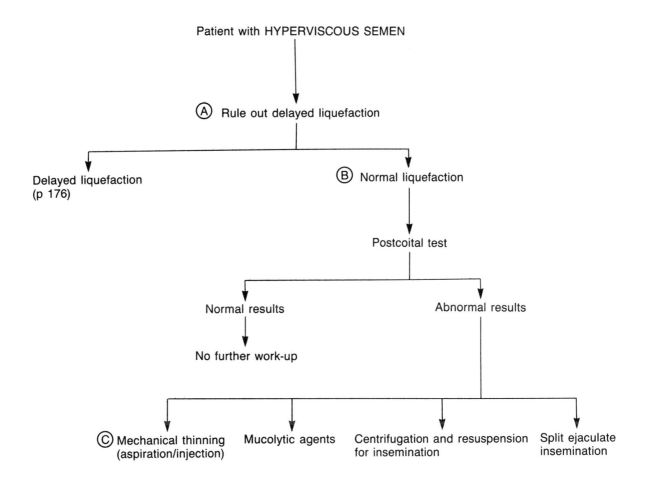

Patient with HYPERVISCOUS SEMEN

Ⓐ Rule out delayed liquefaction

Delayed liquefaction
(p 176)

Ⓑ Normal liquefaction

Postcoital test

Normal results

No further work-up

Abnormal results

Ⓒ Mechanical thinning
(aspiration/injection)

Mucolytic agents

Centrifugation and resuspension
for insemination

Split ejaculate
insemination

DELAYED SEMINAL LIQUEFACTION

Ronald D. Lee, M.D.

A. Semen typically coagulates following ejaculation and reliquefies up to 30 minutes later. If the semen remains coagulated, sperm motility may be affected. When semen fails to liquefy by 1 hour after ejaculation, post-coital testing (PCT) should be done to assess the clinical importance of delayed liquefaction. If the PCT result is normal, no further therapy for delayed liquefaction is needed.

B. When PCT results are abnormal, split ejaculate analysis should be performed. Here it is hoped that one of the two fractions will have both improved liquefaction and bulk seminal parameters. If the initial fraction contains the sperm-rich plasma with only small amounts of coagulating factors from the seminal vesicles, one might recommend either withdrawal coitus, i.e., the man withdrawing from the vagina after the initial ejaculatory spurts, or homologous insemination (AIH). If the second fraction has improved liquefaction with adequate seminal parameters, it may be used for insemination.

C. When neither portion is adequate in terms of improved liquefaction, the use of amylase vaginal suppositories is considered. They are constructed from the formula listed in the article by Amelar, and it should be remembered that some of the ingredients are not approved for use in humans.

References

Amelar RD. Questions and answers: infertility and non-liquifaction of semen. JAMA 1983; 250:1099.

Gerber WL. Management of delayed seminal liquefaction. In: Garcia C-R, Mastroianni L, Amelar RD, eds. Current therapy of infertility — 1984–85. St. Louis: CV Mosby, 1984.

Wilson VB, Bunge RG. Infertility and semen non-liquefaction. J Urol 1975; 113:509–510.

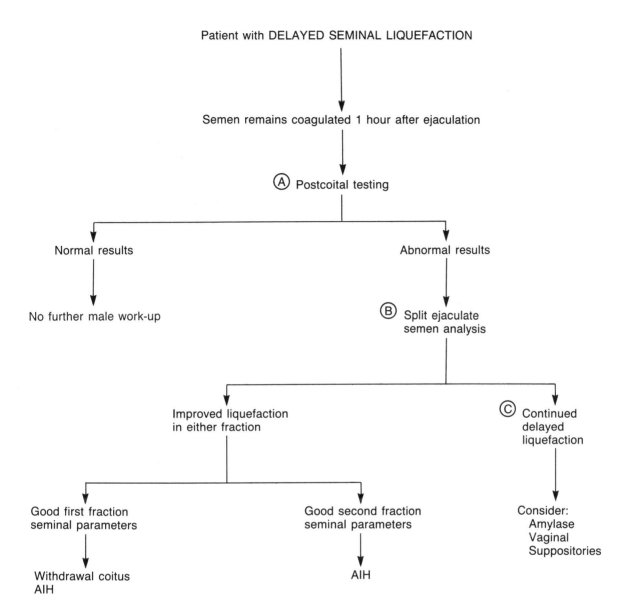

Patient with DELAYED SEMINAL LIQUEFACTION

Semen remains coagulated 1 hour after ejaculation

Ⓐ Postcoital testing

Normal results

No further male work-up

Abnormal results

Ⓑ Split ejaculate semen analysis

Improved liquefaction in either fraction

Good first fraction seminal parameters

Withdrawal coitus AIH

Good second fraction seminal parameters

AIH

Ⓒ Continued delayed liquefaction

Consider:
Amylase
Vaginal
Suppositories

POLYZOOSPERMIA

Ronald D. Lee, M.D.

A. Polyzoospermia is present when at least two semen analyses reveal more than 250 x 10⁶ sperm per milliliter. Its incidence ranges between 3 and 17 percent in the infertile male population. Its presence does not necessarily indicate a male infertility factor, but it has been associated with both an increased incidence of infertility and a higher incidence of spontaneous abortion. Evaluation for a possible female factor as a cause for the couple's infertility should always be carried out in cases of polyzoospermia.

B. Spontaneous pregnancy may occur with polyzoospermia but appears to do so at a reduced frequency. When evaluation rules out an obvious female factor, continued observation for several cycles is recommended. If pregnancy is not achieved, further therapy for polyzoospermia may be carried out.

C. When a female factor appears to be present, it warrants further investigation and treatment as indicated. Failure to initiate pregnancy after correction of the female factor should lead to re-evaluation of polyzoospermia as a potential negative element.

D. Semen volume is useful in dividing patients into groups for different treatment options. If the volume is less than normal, the ejaculate may be diluted with an appropriate diluent and homologous insemination (AIH) performed. With normal volumes multiple daily ejaculates about the time of ovulation may be useful. Volumes greater than normal may be further analyzed with split ejaculate semen analysis. If a good first fraction is present, a withdrawal coital technique may be employed. Alternatively insemination using the better fraction or a "swim-up" specimen can be done.

References

Amelar RD, Dubin L, Quigley MM, Schoenfeld C. Successful management of infertility due to polyzoospermia. Fertil Steril 1979; 31:521–524.

Barnea ER, Arronet GH, Weissenberg R, Lunenfeld B. Studies on polyspermia. Int J Fertil 1980; 25:303–306.

Glezerman M, Bernstein D, Zakut C, Misgav N, Insler V. Polyzoospermia: a definite pathologic entity. Fertil Steril 1982; 38:605–608.

Joël CA. New etiologic aspects of habitual abortion and infertility, with special reference to the male factor. Fertil Steril 1966; 17:374–380.

Rehan NE, Sobrero AJ, Fertig JW. The semen of fertile men: statistical analysis of 1300 men. Fertil Steril 1975; 26:492–502.

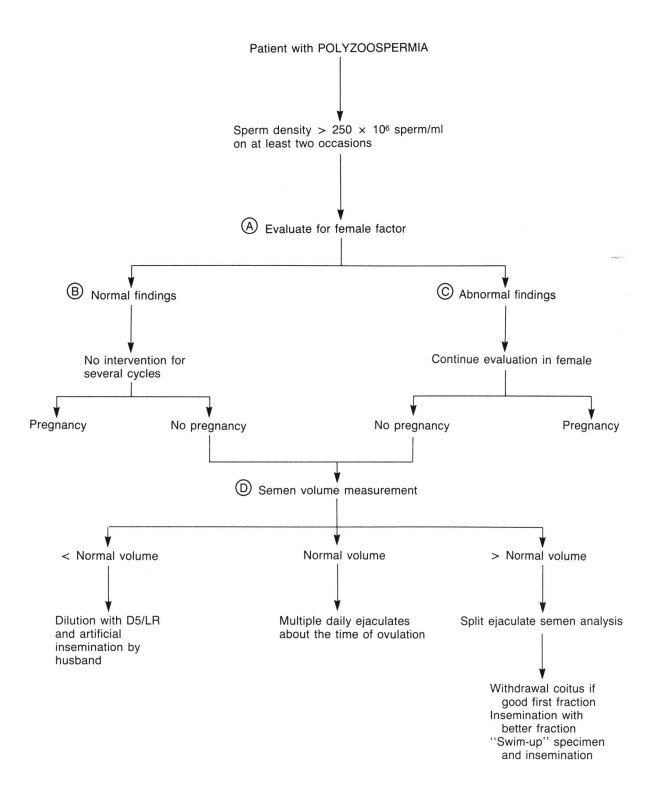

Patient with POLYZOOSPERMIA

Sperm density > 250 × 10⁶ sperm/ml
on at least two occasions

Ⓐ Evaluate for female factor

Ⓑ Normal findings

Ⓒ Abnormal findings

No intervention for
several cycles

Continue evaluation in female

Pregnancy

No pregnancy

No pregnancy

Pregnancy

Ⓓ Semen volume measurement

< Normal volume

Normal volume

> Normal volume

Dilution with D5/LR
and artificial
insemination by
husband

Multiple daily ejaculates
about the time of ovulation

Split ejaculate semen analysis

Withdrawal coitus if
good first fraction
Insemination with
better fraction
"Swim-up" specimen
and insemination

TESTICULAR BIOPSY—VASOGRAPHY

Ronald D. Lee, M.D.

A. Testicular biopsy is indicated in the evaluation of azoospermia, and rarely oligospermia, for aid in diagnosis and prognosis. Patients undergoing biopsy should have normal or only slightly elevated serum gonadotropin levels (FSH and LH) along with normal serum testosterone levels. The absence of retrograde ejaculation should be documented. The techniques of open versus closed biopsy (that is, percutaneous needle biopsy of the testis) both have their proponents (Fig. 1). We prefer open testicular biopsy, performed using local or general anesthesia, to which we add vasography and a thorough visual inspection of the epididymis. The open technique, we believe, is less traumatic than needle biopsy, and in view of the delicate tissue that the testes contain, this may be an important consideration. On the other hand, advocates of testicular percutaneous biopsy emphasize its simplicity and its capacity to provide the same information with less cost and discomfort to the patient.

B. Biopsy of one testis suffices if both are of approximately equal size. If there is a discrepancy in size, biopsy of both testes should be performed. In either case a mild fixative such as Bouin's solution should be used, since tissue architecture may be destroyed with formalin.

C. Several methods of evaluating testicular biopsy material exist. These include histopathologic examination, flow cytometry, and counting of spermatids. Each method yields different information that may be useful in planning treatment.

D. Vasography is performed to rule out the possibility of obstruction and, if present, to define the anatomic location of the lesion. Some clinicians prefer to perform vasography after histologic study results are known and, at the time of formal scrotal exploration, to decrease the formation of intrascrotal adhesions. Our preference is to do vasography at the time of testis biopsy. This information can be used in planning any surgery. Diluted contrast medium is injected through a small vasotomy, which is then repaired using magnification techniques. Attempt-

ing to place a small needle bluntly through the wall of the vas into the tiny lumen has not been consistently successful, and we have feared that the trauma of repeated punctures and attempts at injection of contrast medium, which may extravasate, would likely lead to scarring and compromise of luminal size. The choice of contrast agents does not appear to be crucial, although there is some suggestion that nonionic solutions may be less likely to cause inflammatory changes. Injection is made only toward the "abdominal side" of the vas and never toward the "testicular" side. Visualization of epididymal tubules with injected contrast medium is rarely complete and therefore is difficult to interpret. In addition, "blowout" of the epididymal tubules is a theoretical consideration with injections through the epididymis. When one is using fluoroscopy or pelvic radiography, contrast medium is injected into the vas until it enters either the prostatic urethra or the bladder. Visualization of the seminal vesicle is not sufficient, since obstruction distal to this may occur. Repair may be undertaken immediately if frozen sections reveal sperm, or repair may be delayed until permanent histologic sections are ready.

References

Bertram RA, Carson CC, Szpak C. Vasography: effect of various agents on vas deferens patency. J Urol 1985; 133:1087–1089.

Chan SL, Lipshultz LI, Schwartzendruber D. DNA flow cytometry: a new modality for quantitative analysis of testicular biopsies. Fertil Steril 1984; 41:485–487.

Posinovec J. The necessity for bilateral biopsy in oligo- and azoospermia. Int J Fertil 1976; 21:189–191.

Rodrigues-Netto N, Hayashi H, Hohne MP, Menezes de Goes G. Experimental comparative study of surgical and needle biopsies of the testis. Arch Androl 1979; 2:277.

Wong T-W, Straus FH, Warner NE. Testicular biopsy in the study of male infertility. I. Testicular causes of infertility. II. Post-testicular causes of infertility. Arch Pathol 1973; 95:151–159; 160–164.

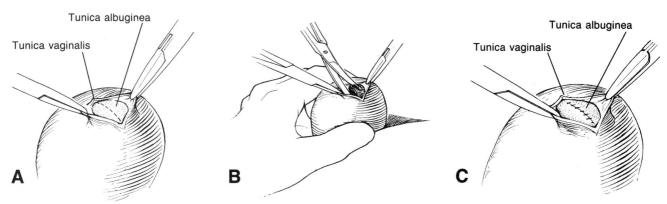

Figure 1 Method of testicular biopsy. *A*, The tunica vaginalis is incised, exposing the tunica albuginea. The edges of the tunica vaginalis are grasped with hemostats. *B*, A small bit of testicular stroma will extrude, and a 2 mm square portion is cut off with a small sharp pair of scissors. *C*, The tunica albuginea is closed with 4-0 chromic atraumatic sutures.

Patient undergoing TESTIS BIOPSY/VASOGRAPHY

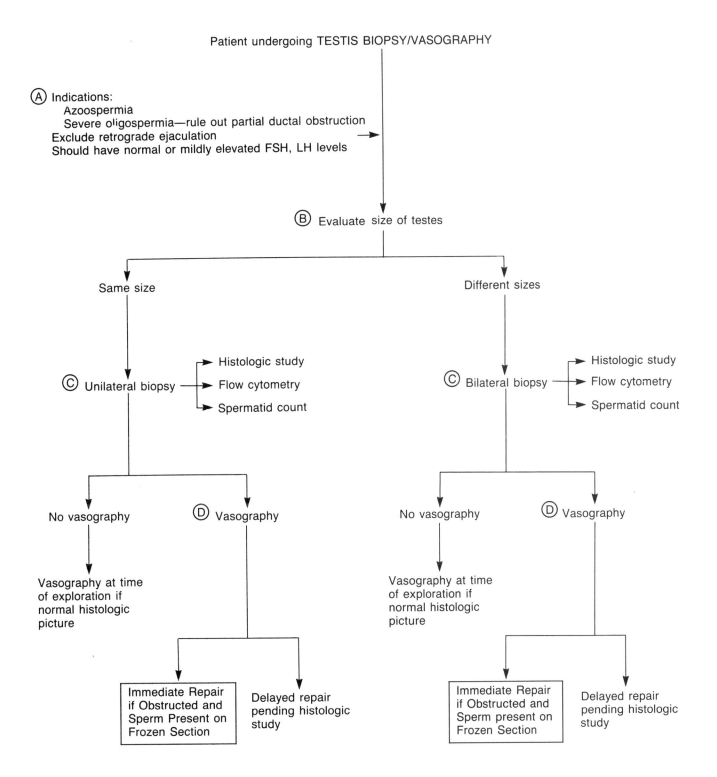

Ⓐ Indications:
    Azoospermia
    Severe oligospermia—rule out partial ductal obstruction
Exclude retrograde ejaculation
Should have normal or mildly elevated FSH, LH levels

Ⓑ Evaluate size of testes

Same size

Different sizes

Ⓒ Unilateral biopsy → Histologic study
→ Flow cytometry
→ Spermatid count

Ⓒ Bilateral biopsy → Histologic study
→ Flow cytometry
→ Spermatid count

No vasography

Ⓓ Vasography

No vasography

Ⓓ Vasography

Vasography at time
of exploration if
normal histologic
picture

Vasography at time
of exploration if
normal histologic
picture

Immediate Repair
if Obstructed and
Sperm Present on
Frozen Section

Delayed repair
pending histologic
study

Immediate Repair
if Obstructed and
Sperm present on
Frozen Section

Delayed repair
pending histologic
study

GENITAL TRACT INFECTION

Ronald D. Lee, M.D.

A. There is little argument that obvious cases of epididymitis can be precursors to the development of excurrent duct obstruction or testicular atrophy. What is not clear, however, is the effect that infection such as bacterial prostatitis has on fertility or, in a broader sense, the exact role that infectious organisms play when present in the male genital tract. There is no conclusive evidence linking the presence of microbes in semen cultures with infertility. There is little documentation supporting the roles of aerobic, anaerobic, and chlamydial organisms as primary causes of male factor infertility. Positive cultures for these organisms seem to bear varying relationships to seminal parameters.

B. Culturing semen specimens in men attending infertility clinics yields incidences of positive cultures as high as 100 percent. Clearly semen cultures performed in all men attending infertility clinics will be neither diagnostic nor cost effective. A clinical history or physical examination suggestive of genital tract infection, including a history of genital tract infection, scrotal or perineal pain, indurated epididymides, urethral discharge, or a tender prostate, defines a subgroup of men who might benefit from "three glass" urine cultures along with semen culture. In addition, men with "idiopathic" infertility or unexplained motility problems may be considered for microbe testing.

C. If the "three glass" urine culture or semen culture is positive and a urethral contaminant can be excluded, it seems worthwhile to treat with an appropriate antimicrobial. Additionally, if a clinical diagnosis of urethritis is confirmed by microbiologic testing, standard treatment regimens can be instituted. The organism that seems to be most strongly implicated as a primary cause of male factor infertility is *Ureaplasma urealyticum*. It appears to be capable of attaching to spermatozoa and impairing their motility. The data, however, are far from being unequivocal. Numerous studies show both greater numbers of this organism in infertile than in fertile men, and improvements in the pregnancy incidence in infertile couples treated with medications known to be active against Ureaplasma. However, abundant studies also fail to confirm these findings; in one of the few controlled studies carried out there was no significant difference in pregnancy incidence in couples treated with antimicrobial drugs to eradicate the disease and in control groups who were not treated.

D. If "three glass" testing and semen culture are negative, the evaluation should focus on other possible causes for male factor infertility. Although no good evidence exists to support the empirical use of antimicrobial drugs, they are often considered at this stage by the clinician in the hope of eradicating a "subclinical" infection by Ureaplasma or *Chlamydia*. Their use in this setting, however, must be carefully considered.

References

Desai S, Cohen MS, Khatamee M, Leiter E. Ureaplasma urealyticum (T-mycoplasma) infection: does it have a role in male infertility? J Urol 1980; 124:469–471.

Fowler JE. Genital tract infection and male infertility. In: Garcia C-R, Mastroianni L, Dubin RD, eds. Current therapy in infertility—1984–1985. Philadelphia: BC Decker, 1984.

Fowlkes DM, MacLeod J, O'Leary WM. T-mycoplasmas and human infertility: correlation of infection with alterations in seminal parameters. Fertil Steril 1975; 26:1212–1218.

Meare EM, Stamey TA. Bacteriologic localization patterns in bacterial prostatitis and urethritis. Invest Urol 1968; 5:492.

Naessens A, Foulon W, Debrucker P, Devroey P, Lauwers S. Recovery of microorganisms in semen and relationship to semen evaluation. Fertil Steril 1986; 45:101–105.

Patient with GENITAL TRACT INFECTION

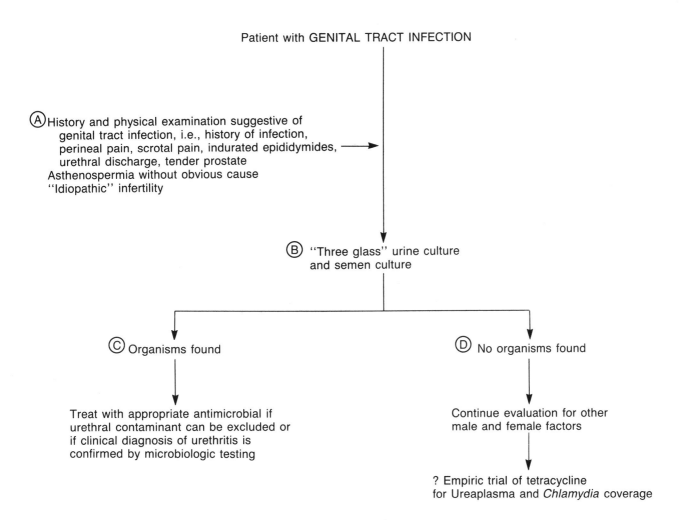

Ⓐ History and physical examination suggestive of
genital tract infection, i.e., history of infection,
perineal pain, scrotal pain, indurated epididymides,
urethral discharge, tender prostate
Asthenospermia without obvious cause
"Idiopathic" infertility

Ⓑ "Three glass" urine culture
and semen culture

Ⓒ Organisms found

Treat with appropriate antimicrobial if
urethral contaminant can be excluded or
if clinical diagnosis of urethritis is
confirmed by microbiologic testing

Ⓓ No organisms found

Continue evaluation for other
male and female factors

? Empiric trial of tetracycline
for Ureaplasma and *Chlamydia* coverage

IMMUNE INFERTILITY

Ronald D. Lee, M.D.

A. The role of antisperm antibodies and immune fertility in general has remained controversial. More vigorous definitions of the problem, the diagnostic testing involved, and the results of treatment have contributed to our increased understanding. Various estimates of the percentage of infertile couples affected by immune infertility range as high as 10 to 15 percent. It has become increasingly evident that serologic studies do not accurately reflect what takes place on a more "local" level. Several groups of infertile couples seem to be most at risk for an immune factor as a cause of infertility. These include cases in which the male has normal seminal parameters but the postcoital test (PCT) results are consistently poor; cases in which the seminal parameters indicate an isolated defect in sperm motility; and cases in which the semen appears to show a high level of sperm agglutination. Testing for antisperm antibodies (AB) may also be performed in couples with unexplained infertility (although the chances of finding antisperm antibodies in this group are not great) and in couples experiencing difficulty initiating pregnancy when the man has undergone vasectomy reversal.

B. In assessing the most appropriate method for antisperm antibody testing, it makes sense to choose a test that indicates whether actual antibodies are present on the sperm itself rather than circulating in the blood. When correlating the percentage of sperm affected by antibodies with the postcoital test results, it has been shown that if less than 50 percent of the sperm are antibody bound by immunobead testing, it is unlikely that there will be a significant change in the postcoital test results as compared with samples with no antibody binding. There may, however, still be effects of the antibodies on fertility at levels other than cervical mucus penetration, such as sperm-ovum binding or penetration and zygote development and transportation. It may be appropriate to treat men for this level of binding, although no good data are available. When no sperm are antibody bound, it is highly unlikely that empirical steroid therapy will be helpful. Conversely, when over 50 percent of the sperm are antibody bound, the institution of high dose steroid therapy is indicated.

C. Although long term low dose therapy has been suggested for a variety of reasons, it has not proved to be as useful as intermittent high dose steroid therapy. It is not clear why steroid therapy is in fact useful.

D. There are a significant number of men who develop side effects such as gastrointestinal bleeding, joint pain, and irritability while taking the medication. For these men a reduction of the original dose by half is undertaken and the therapy repeated for two additional cycles. If no improvement is seen as measured by improved semen analysis results, PCT results, or a decrease in the percentage of antibody bound sperm, steroid treatment is abandoned. When improvement is noted, however, therapy may continue for up to 6 months.

E. If no significant side effects are noted after the first cycle, two additional cycles of medication are given. Again, if no improvement is seen after the first three cycles, steroid therapy is abandoned; otherwise it may continue for up to six cycles if clinical improvement is noted. We use a daily total of 120 mg of prednisone given in two divided doses for 10 days, followed by a 3 day taper from the medication. Therapy may be instituted on either the first or the 21st day of the woman's cycle.

References

Bronson R, Cooper G, Rosenfeld D. Sperm antibodies: their role in infertility. Fertil Steril 1984; 42:171–183.

Haas GG, Cines DB, Schreiber AD. Immunologic infertility: identification of patients with antisperm antibody. N Engl J Med 1980; 303:722–727.

Hendry WF, Stedronska J, Parslow J, Hughes L. The results of intermittent high dose steroid therapy for male infertility due to antisperm antibodies. Fertil Steril 1981; 36:351–355.

Jones WR. Immunologic infertility—fact or fiction? Fertil Steril 1980; 33:577–586.

Mathur S, Baker ER, Williamson HO, et al. Clinical significance of sperm antibodies in infertility. Fertil Steril 1981; 36:486–495.

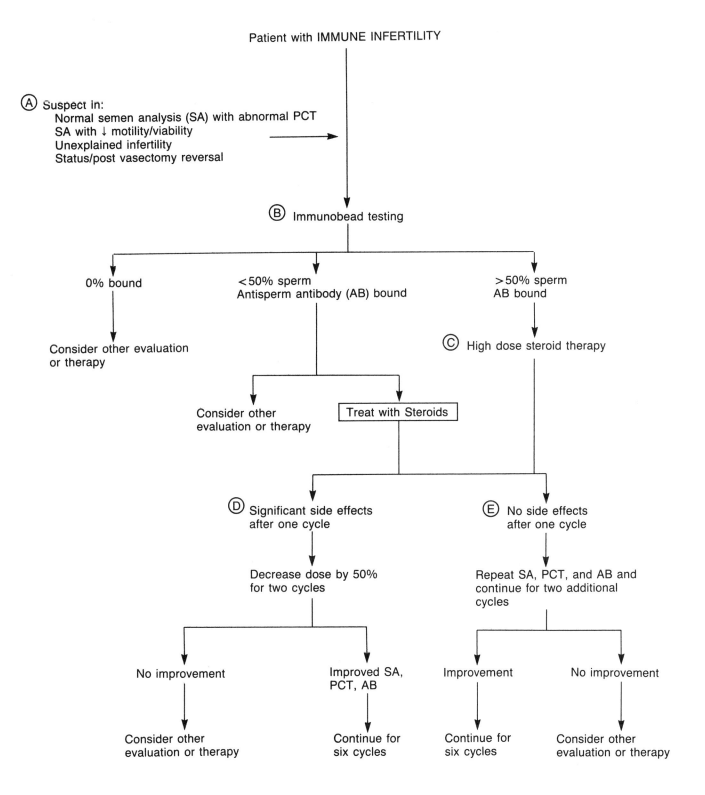

RETROGRADE EJACULATION

Ronald D. Lee, M.D.

A. Retrograde ejaculation may be caused by a number of diverse etiologies. They include inadequate chemical messenger, drug use (alpha-blockers), trauma or surgery, systemic disease (diabetes mellitus), disruption of nerve pathways, and idiopathic causes. It is not the same as lack of emission, which is also under control of the sympathetic nervous system. For antegrade ejaculation to occur there must be contraction of the bulbar urethral and pelvic floor muscles along with closure of the vesical neck and coordinated relaxation of the external urinary sphincter.

B. The diagnosis is suspected when semen analysis reveals a volume of less than 1 ml with a thin consistency and an acid pH. Azoospermia or severe oligospermia is present. A postejaculate urine specimen confirms the diagnosis by revealing numerous sperm in a centrifuged specimen. In this setting one must be sure to exclude an "incomplete" or spilled collection, a severe anxiety state with incomplete relaxation of the external urinary sphincter, a short time of abstinence after the previous ejaculation, and the absence of vasal aplasia, ejaculatory duct obstruction, or urethral stricture disease. If sperm are not identified in the postejaculate urine, one should continue with evaluation of the male factor as previously outlined.

C. When retrograde ejaculation is present, the goal is to convert it to antegrade ejaculation if possible. The male may be encouraged to participate in intercourse with a full bladder in the hope that the reflex stimulation of the bladder neck will keep it shut during ejaculation. If unsuccessful, the somewhat messy alternative of vaginal voiding may be tried, or a variety of medications, including alpha-adrenergics such as pseudoephedrine, phenylpropanolamine, imipramine, and brompheniramine, may be employed, always using a loading dose for several days. When vesical neck incompetence appears to be secondary to surgical procedures, surgical attempts to narrow the bladder neck have been reported to be successful.

D. If these methods fail to achieve an antegrade ejaculate, a voided or catheterized urine sample may be obtained and centrifuged, with the resultant sperm pellet resuspended in an appropriate medium for use in homologous insemination. Care must be taken to keep the urine pH as alkaline as possible and preferably higher than 7, using the oral administration of drugs such as sodium bicarbonate, and also to keep the urinary osmolality in a dilute range by increasing the patient's fluid intake beginning several hours prior to ejaculation.

References

Andaloro VA, Dube A. Treatment of retrograde ejaculation with brompheniramine. Urology 1975; 5:520.

Crich JP, Jequier AM. Infertility in men with retrograde ejaculation: the action of urine on sperm motility, and a simple method for achieving antegrade ejaculation. Fertil Steril 1978; 30:572–576.

Marmar JL, Prauss DE, DeBenedictis JJ. Post-coital voiding insemination: technique for patients with retrograde ejaculation and infertility. Urology 1977; 9:288.

Sandler B. Idiopathic retrograde ejaculation. Fertil Steril 1979; 32:474–475.

Thomas AJ. Ejaculatory dysfunction. Fertil Steril 1983; 39:445–454.

Patient with RETROGRADE EJACULATION

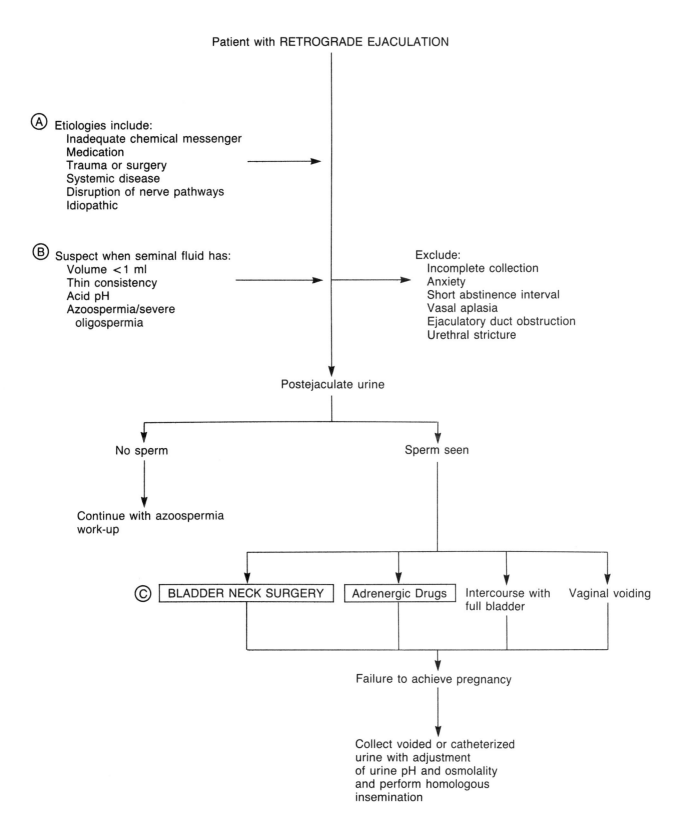

A Etiologies include:
    Inadequate chemical messenger
    Medication
    Trauma or surgery
    Systemic disease
    Disruption of nerve pathways
    Idiopathic

B Suspect when seminal fluid has:
    Volume <1 ml
    Thin consistency
    Acid pH
    Azoospermia/severe
      oligospermia

Exclude:
    Incomplete collection
    Anxiety
    Short abstinence interval
    Vasal aplasia
    Ejaculatory duct obstruction
    Urethral stricture

Postejaculate urine

No sperm

Sperm seen

Continue with azoospermia work-up

C BLADDER NECK SURGERY

Adrenergic Drugs

Intercourse with full bladder

Vaginal voiding

Failure to achieve pregnancy

Collect voided or catheterized urine with adjustment of urine pH and osmolality and perform homologous insemination

INFERTILITY IN THE PARAPLEGIC MALE

Ronald D. Lee, M.D.

The incidence of spinal cord injury in the United States is approximately 35 per 1,000,000. Of these, about 80 percent are males, many of whom are injured at a relatively young age. With advancements in medicine these men have been able to achieve reasonably long life expectancies, but often with the problems of sexual dysfunction and infertility. Probably less than 10 percent of the men with paraplegia are capable of initiating a pregnancy. Erectile dysfunction, ejaculatory dysfunction including aspermia, retrograde ejaculation, failure to ejaculate, and impaired spermatogenesis and sperm function secondary to testicular injury, hormonal abnormalities, infection, or medication may all contribute. It is useful to divide infertile paraplegic men into three groups based on their ability to have erections and to ejaculate.

A. Men with incomplete cord lesions may retain the ability to both erect and to ejaculate in an antegrade direction, or to ejaculate with a flaccid penis. If the seminal parameters are normal, continued evaluation of the female is indicated. When abnormal seminal parameters exist, as is most likely to be the case, continued evaluation is carried out as previously outlined.

B. In the paraplegic man who does not experience either erection or ejaculation, a thorough examination of the gonads is indicated, since if severe atrophy is present, alternate means of starting a family should be discussed. Assuming that the testes are of normal size (larger than 4 cm in longest dimension or more than 20 to 25 ml in volume) or very minimally decreased in size, a serum follicle stimulating hormone (FSH) level is obtained. If the FSH level is markedly elevated (that is, greater than twice normal), alternate means are discussed. A level of less than twice normal would lead next to testicular biopsy. Severe maturation arrest or hypospermatogenesis leads once more to a discussion of alternate methods. Normal histologic findings or mild hypospermatogenesis, seen in the testis biopsy specimen, makes the option of artificial ejaculation possible. Currently two methods of artificial ejaculation are being used. Electroejaculation is being done using an electrical stimulus conducted through a rectal probe to the area of the seminal vesicles. Approximately 60 to 70 percent of the men treated in this fashion are able to produce an ejaculate. Caution must be used to avoid rectal burns or epididymitis. Chemical ejaculation is carried out by injecting neostigmine into the intrathecal space. About 80 percent of the men so treated are able to ejaculate. These men must be monitored closely in an intensive care unit setting, since 60 percent experience autonomic dysreflexia that requires immediate treatment.

C. Some paraplegic men may experience erections but have no antegrade ejaculation. In these instances it is necessary to exclude retrograde ejaculation. This may be done using a voided or catheterized specimen after genital stimulation. If sperm are seen, an attempt is made to convert the ejaculate to an antegrade one using sympathomimetics. Failing this, the voided or catheterized urine may be appropriately "processed" and used for homologous insemination (AIH). If no sperm are seen, re-examination of the testes is performed with outcomes as delineated in B.

References

Amelar RD, Dubin L. Sexual function and fertility in paraplegic males. Urology 1982; 20:62.

Bennett CJ, McGuire EJ. Electroejaculation in neurologically impaired patients. Paper number 237, presented at AUA Meeting, New York, May 1986.

MacMahon RG, Lee RD, Lipshultz LI. Infertility in the paraplegic male. In: Garcia C-R, Mastroianni L Jr, Amelar RD, Dubin L, eds. Current therapy of infertility 1984–1985. Toronto: BC Decker, 1984:199.

Martin DE, Warner H, Crenshaw TL, et al. Initiation of erection and semen release by rectal probe electrostimulation (RPE). J Urol 1983; 129:637–642.

Perkash I, Martin DE, Warner H, Blank MS, Collins DC. Reproductive biopsy of paraplegics: results of semen collection, testicular biopsy and serum hormone evaluation. J Urol 1985; 134:284–288.

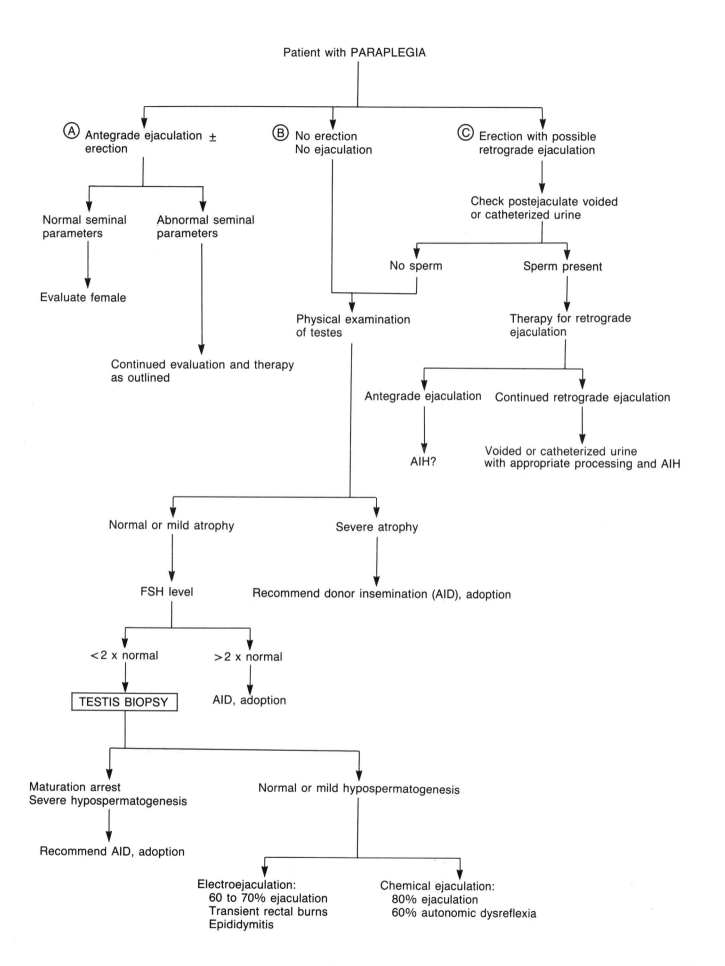

Patient with PARAPLEGIA

(A) Antegrade ejaculation ± erection

Normal seminal parameters

Evaluate female

Abnormal seminal parameters

Continued evaluation and therapy as outlined

(B) No erection No ejaculation

(C) Erection with possible retrograde ejaculation

Check postejaculate voided or catheterized urine

No sperm

Sperm present

Physical examination of testes

Therapy for retrograde ejaculation

Antegrade ejaculation

AIH?

Continued retrograde ejaculation

Voided or catheterized urine with appropriate processing and AIH

Normal or mild atrophy

Severe atrophy

FSH level

Recommend donor insemination (AID), adoption

<2 x normal

TESTIS BIOPSY

>2 x normal

AID, adoption

Maturation arrest Severe hypospermatogenesis

Recommend AID, adoption

Normal or mild hypospermatogenesis

Electroejaculation: 60 to 70% ejaculation Transient rectal burns Epididymitis

Chemical ejaculation: 80% ejaculation 60% autonomic dysreflexia

INFERTILITY AFTER VASECTOMY REVERSAL

Ronald D. Lee, M.D.

A. The incidence of pregnancy after vasovasostomy is usually in the 40 to 60 percent range. Inability to initiate a pregnancy after vasectomy reversal may be due to several factors, including an unresolved female factor, the presence of antisperm antibodies, loss of adequate sperm maturation as a result of epididymal or testicular changes, interruption of vasal innervation, or recurrent obstruction. By 6 months after vasovasostomy, semen analysis (SA) should reveal adequate sperm density and motility. If the results of semen analysis appear adequate in the presence of continued infertility, evaluation for a possible female factor should be considered.

B. If the results of semen analysis are abnormal, repeat analysis is performed in 3 months. At that time, if the results of analysis are normal, consideration should be given again to evaluation for a possible female factor. Repeat semen analysis, however, may still yield abnormal findings, revealing either azoospermia or oligoasthenospermia.

C. When azoospermia is seen 9 to 12 months after vasectomy reversal, the possibility of recurrent obstruction should be considered. If sperm were seen at the time of the initial vasectomy reversal, "re-do" vasectomy reversal, either vasovasostomy or epididymovasostomy, can be undertaken. If, on the other hand, no sperm were seen at the initial operation, testicular biopsy should be performed prior to any attempt at a "re-do" vasectomy reversal. With unfavorable testicular histologic findings the couple are advised to consider alternative means of increasing the family size. A more favorable histologic pic-

ture would make the option of "re-do" vasectomy reversal a reasonable one.

D. When the semen analysis reveals oligoasthenospermia, antisperm antibody studies are carried out. Steroid therapy may be instituted if antisperm antibody titers are elevated. If the titers are low or absent, continued evaluation and treatment of the abnormal parameters are carried out. Therapy should continue if the semen analysis shows improvement after several months. If, however, persistent oligospermia is seen, testicular biopsy may be recommended. Unfavorable histologic findings on biopsy should direct the couple toward alternate means of increasing the family size, but normal or slight hypospermatogenesis makes "re-do" vasectomy reversal an option.

References

Belker AM, Fuchs EF, Konnak JW, Sharlip ID, Thomas AJ. Transient fertility after vasovasostomy in 892 patients. J Urol 1985; 134:75–76.

Fuchs EF, Alexander NJ. Immunologic considerations before and after vasovasostomy. Fertil Steril 1983; 40:497–499.

Jarow JP, Budin RE, Dym M, et al. Quantitative pathologic changes in the human testis after vasectomy: a controlled study. N Engl J Med 1985; 313:1252–1256.

Knapp RM, Konnak JW, Lee RD. Evaluation and treatment of infertility following vasovasostomy. (Submitted for publication.)

Marshall S. Transient fertility after vasovasostomy. Urology 1978; 11:492.

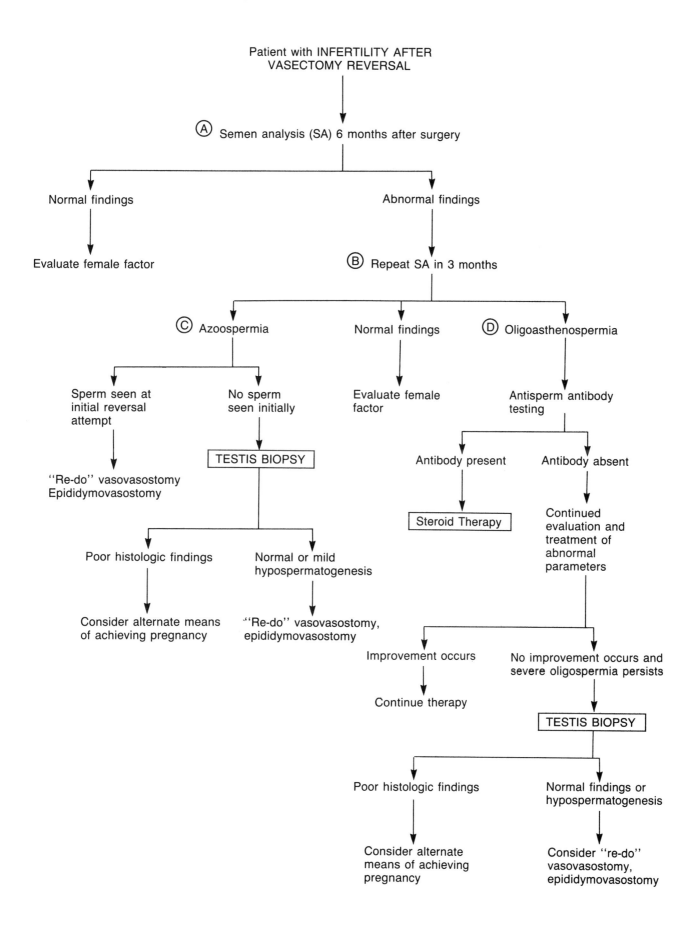

Patient with INFERTILITY AFTER VASECTOMY REVERSAL

(A) Semen analysis (SA) 6 months after surgery

Normal findings → Evaluate female factor

Abnormal findings → (B) Repeat SA in 3 months

(C) Azoospermia

- Sperm seen at initial reversal attempt → "Re-do" vasovasostomy Epididymovasostomy
- No sperm seen initially → TESTIS BIOPSY
  - Poor histologic findings → Consider alternate means of achieving pregnancy
  - Normal or mild hypospermatogenesis → "Re-do" vasovasostomy, epididymovasostomy

Normal findings → Evaluate female factor

(D) Oligoasthenospermia → Antisperm antibody testing

- Antibody present → Steroid Therapy
- Antibody absent → Continued evaluation and treatment of abnormal parameters
  - Improvement occurs → Continue therapy
  - No improvement occurs and severe oligospermia persists → TESTIS BIOPSY
    - Poor histologic findings → Consider alternate means of achieving pregnancy
    - Normal findings or hypospermatogenesis → Consider "re-do" vasovasostomy, epididymovasostomy

IN VITRO FERTILIZATION

Mary Lake Polan, M.D., Ph.D.

A. Initially women with damaged or blocked fallopian tubes and those without fallopian tubes were the primary candidates for in vitro fertilization (IVF). However, after several years of experience with the procedure, other indications for IVF have become common. Couples with poor postcoital test results because of inadequate mucus or antibody formation, men with severe oligospermia or asthenospermia, and women with endometriosis who have not conceived despite surgical therapy are now considered candidates for IVF. Finally, couples with many years of infertility of unknown etiology have successfully initiated pregnancies through IVF.

B. Couples are seen and examined by a physician member of the IVF team. Prior diagnostic work-ups are evaluated to insure that a complete infertility work-up has been performed. Semen analysis and sperm migration tests are carried out as well as a psychologic evaluation by a social worker. After an examination, which includes uterine sounding, the patient is presented to the in vitro fertilization team and accepted into the program.

C. In order to maximize the chances for pregnancy, multiple follicular development is induced so that multiple oocytes can be fertilized and transferred. Ovulation induction has been accomplished most commonly with clomiphene citrate, human menopausal gonadotropin (Pergonal), or a combination of the two drugs. In addition, pulsatile luteinizing hormone releasing factor and pure follicle stimulating hormone have been used in special situations to induce multiple follicular development for IVF.

D. In order to time ovulation so that human chorionic gonadotropin (hCG) may be given at the point of maximal follicular development, all cycles are monitored daily with ultrasound to assess follicular size and serum estradiol levels, beginning on day 8. When follicular maturity has been documented with ultrasound showing two follicles at least 1.5 cm in diameter and a serum estrogen level above 400 pg per milliliter, hCG (10,000 IU per milliliter) is given.

E. Follicles are harvested 36 hours after the administration of hCG just prior to spontaneous ovulation. Laparoscopy is performed and follicles are aspirated under direct vision. The use of percutaneous or transvaginal ultrasound-directed aspiration is becoming more common as technology improves.

F. Oocytes are fertilized approximately 8 hours after collection with 200,000 to 500,000 washed motile sperm. The medium surrounding the embryos is changed 16 hours later and fertilization and division are assessed. After another 24 hours of growth in the incubator, the embryos are again inspected just prior to transfer.

G. Forty-eight hours after oocyte aspiration, the fertilized embryos, usually at the four to eight cell stage, are transferred into the uterine fundus. A metal introducer is inserted into the cervix, and a special Teflon catheter with a side opening is passed through the introducer into the fundus. After the embryos are transferred, the patient remains supine for several hours.

H. Beta-human chorionic gonadotropin (β-hCG) titers and serum estradiol levels are monitored every 3 days during the luteal phase. β-hCG titers drop to near zero about 14 days after hCG administration; a subsequent rise in both the β-hCG titer and serum estradiol level indicates a pregnancy. A transient rise in the β-hCG titer followed by a menstrual period within several days is termed a chemical pregnancy. All pregnancies are assessed at 6 to 8 weeks by ultrasound to document an intrauterine pregnancy and the fetal heart beat. Once a successful pregnancy is established, the obstetric monitoring and mode of delivery depend upon the mother's history and the course of her pregnancy.

References

Johnston IWH, Lopata A, Speirs A, et al. In vitro fertilization: the challenge of the eighties. Fertil Steril 1981; 35:699-706.

Jones HW, Jones GS, Andrews MC, et al. The program for in vitro fertilization at Norfolk. Fertil Steril 1982; 38:14-21.

Laufer N, Tarlatzis B, Naftolin F. In vitro fertilization: state of the art. Reprod Endocrinol 1984; 2:197-219.

Liu JH, Durfee R, Muse K, Yen SCC. Induction of multiple ovulation by pulsatile administration of gonadotropin-releasing hormone. Fertil Steril 1983; 40:18-21.

Vargyas JM, Marrs RP, Kletzky OA, Mishell DR. Correlation of ultrasonic measurement of ovarian follicle size and serum estradiol levels in ovulatory patients following clomiphene citrate for *in vitro* fertilization. Am J Obstet Gynecol 1982; 144:569-573.

Patient undergoing IN VITRO FERTILIZATION

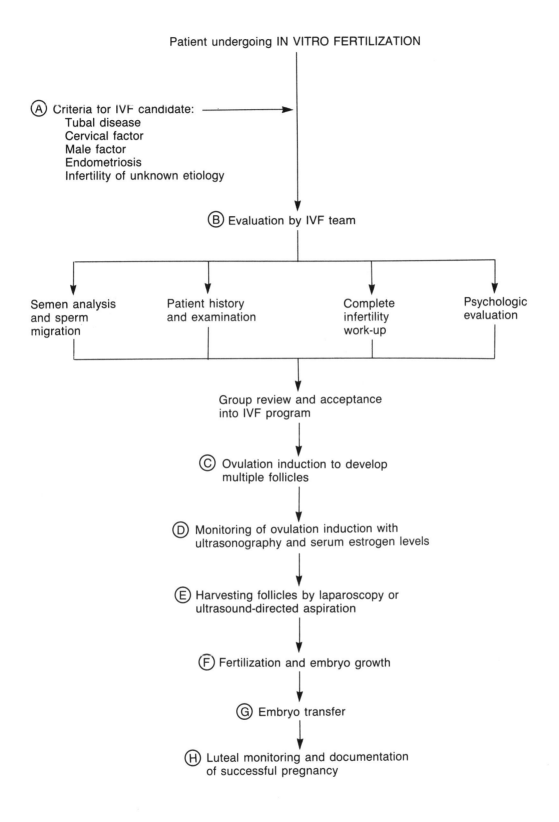

(A) Criteria for IVF candidate:
    Tubal disease
    Cervical factor
    Male factor
    Endometriosis
    Infertility of unknown etiology

(B) Evaluation by IVF team

Semen analysis and sperm migration

Patient history and examination

Complete infertility work-up

Psychologic evaluation

Group review and acceptance into IVF program

(C) Ovulation induction to develop multiple follicles

(D) Monitoring of ovulation induction with ultrasonography and serum estrogen levels

(E) Harvesting follicles by laparoscopy or ultrasound-directed aspiration

(F) Fertilization and embryo growth

(G) Embryo transfer

(H) Luteal monitoring and documentation of successful pregnancy

CRITERIA FOR IN VITRO FERTILIZATION CANDIDATES

Jeffrey B. Russell, M.D.
Mary Lake Polan, M.D., Ph.D.

A. In vitro fertilization (IVF) and embryo transfer (ET) were originally developed for patients with infertility due to irreparable tubal disease. The process of bypassing the mechanical barrier of severely damaged fallopian tubes offered a small but finite possibility of pregnancy for patients who would otherwise be unable to conceive. Since the incidence of success with IVF is about 20 to 25 percent, tubal surgery must remain the first line of therapy for patients with tubal disease; IVF is reserved for those without tubes or those in whom tubal repair has failed.

B. When there have been good results on semen analysis but persistent poor postcoital test (PCT) results without evidence of antibodies, infection, or ovulatory problems in a woman who fails to conceive after 6 months of intrauterine insemination with the husband's sperm, the option of in vitro fertilization should be offered.

C. IVF has also been offered as an alternative treatment for oligospermic males whose partners have normal findings on evaluation and for those who fail to conceive after empiric intrauterine artificial inseminations. IVF bypasses the reproductive tract and allows in vitro gamete contact.

D. Endometriosis continues to be a major problem associated with infertility. Once danazol or corrective surgery for endometriosis has been shown to be unsuccessful, IVF may be offered as therapy. As the number of conservative surgical procedures for endometriosis increases, the chances for successful pregnancy decrease. We usually allow the patient 18 months postoperatively to conceive prior to IVF.

E. Unknown etiology or unexplained infertility occurs in the second largest group of patients who may benefit from IVF. We empirically use 4 months of human menopausal gonadotropin (hMG) therapy with or without intrauterine inseminations prior to the IVF cycle in patients with unexplained infertility. The empiric use of hMG alone yields a 12 percent pregnancy incidence.

F. Over 2,000 infants have been delivered by in vitro fertilization and embryo transfer. IVF-ET is an accepted therapy for infertility but should not be considered until an exhaustive preliminary evaluation has been performed. The patient should be offered the therapy with an understanding of its incidence of success, fully realizing the limitations of IVF-ET.

References

DeCherney AH. Tubal disease: surgery and in vitro fertilization. In: Kase NG, Weingold AB, eds. Principles and practice of clinical gynecology. New York: John Wiley, 1983:461.

Mahadevan MM, Trounson AO, Leeton JF. The relationship of tubal blockage, infertility of unknown cause, suspected male infertility, and endometriosis to success of in vitro fertilization and embryo transfer. Fertil Steril 1983; 40:755–762.

Welner S, Polan ML, Graebe RA, Barnea ER, DeCherney AH. The use of empiric Pergonal therapy in patients with infertility of unknown origin. Presentation, 41st American Fertility Society Meeting, Chicago, October 1985 (abstract P45).

Criteria for IN VITRO FERTILIZATION

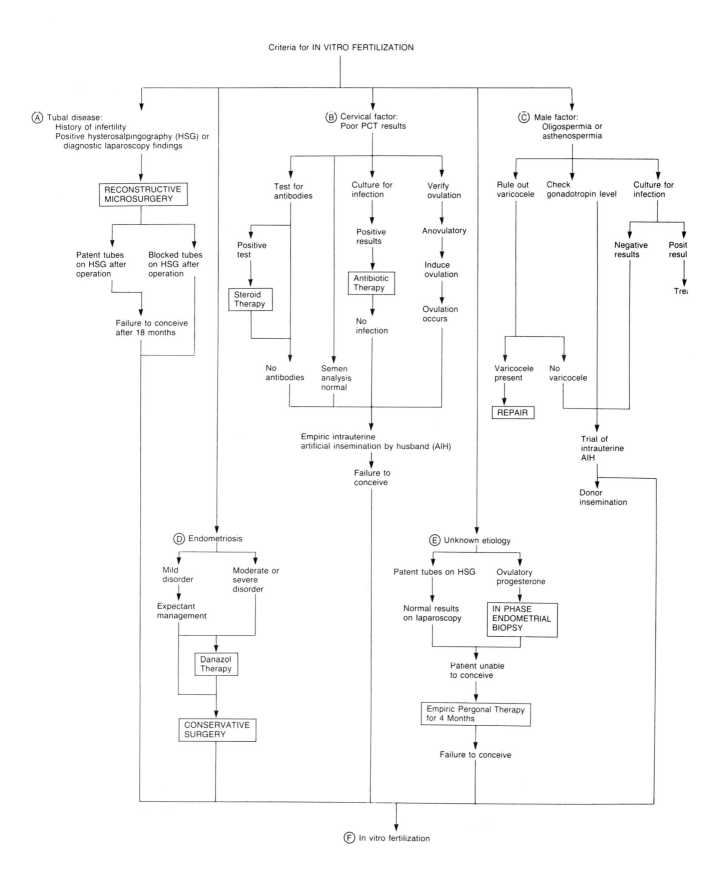

A Tubal disease:
  History of infertility
  Positive hysterosalpingography (HSG) or
  diagnostic laparoscopy findings

RECONSTRUCTIVE
MICROSURGERY

Patent tubes
on HSG after
operation

Blocked tubes
on HSG after
operation

Failure to conceive
after 18 months

B Cervical factor:
  Poor PCT results

Test for
antibodies

Culture for
infection

Verify
ovulation

Positive
test

Positive
results

Anovulatory

Steroid
Therapy

Antibiotic
Therapy

Induce
ovulation

No antibodies

Semen
analysis
normal

No
infection

Ovulation
occurs

Empiric intrauterine
artificial insemination by husband (AIH)

Failure to
conceive

C Male factor:
  Oligospermia or
  asthenospermia

Rule out
varicocele

Check
gonadotropin level

Culture for
infection

Negative
results

Posit
resul

Tre:

Varicocele
present

No
varicocele

REPAIR

Trial of
intrauterine
AIH

Donor
insemination

D Endometriosis

Mild
disorder

Moderate or
severe
disorder

Expectant
management

Danazol
Therapy

CONSERVATIVE
SURGERY

E Unknown etiology

Patent tubes on HSG

Ovulatory
progesterone

Normal results
on laparoscopy

IN PHASE
ENDOMETRIAL
BIOPSY

Patient unable
to conceive

Empiric Pergonal Therapy
for 4 Months

Failure to conceive

F In vitro fertilization

EVALUATION BY THE IN VITRO FERTILIZATION TEAM

Jeffrey B. Russell, M.D.
Mary Lake Polan, M.D., Ph.D.

A. A semen analysis and a migration test provide important preliminary information required prior to acceptance into the in vitro fertilization–embryo transfer (IVF-ET) program. At least 2 million motile sperm are needed for adequate fertilization. A migration test involves the washing of the sperm followed by swim-up of motile sperm for accurate assessment of sperm morphology and quality.

B. The initial evaluation of the couple includes a history and physical examination. The woman's first visit is usually scheduled at the time of her menses and a uterine sounding is performed. This allows the position and depth of the uterus to be evaluated and alleviates the need for additional examinations or uterine manipulation prior to the IVF cycle.

C. The psychologic assessment offers the couple an opportunity to discuss concerns or fears about their infertility problem or the demanding schedule of in vitro fertilization with a social worker. It also allows the social worker to evaluate the level of stress and the ability of the couple to cope with problems associated with their long history of infertility.

D. Presentations and a group discussion of the couple's work-up allow a thorough investigation of each aspect of the couple's infertility evaluation. If all appropriate avenues have been explored, and additional testing or therapy has been covered, the patient is accepted. We routinely administer human menopausal gonadotropins (hMG) for 4 months in patients with patent tubes as empiric therapy while awaiting the IVF cycle.

E. Information about ovarian accessibility aids in retrieving oocytes. If the ovaries have been previously described as being inaccessible, an exploratory laparotomy with ovarian suspension or ultrasonographic retrieval of the oocytes is considered.

References

Greenfeld D, Mazure C, Haseltine F, DeCherney AH. The role of the social worker in the in vitro fertilization program. In: Social work in health care. Vol. 10. New York: Haworth Press, 1984:71.

Mahadevan MM, Trounson AO. The influence of seminal characteristics on the success rate of human in vitro fertilization. Fertil Steril 1984; 42:400–405.

Seibel M, Taymor M. Emotional aspects of infertility. Fertil Steril 1982; 37:137-145.

Wikland M, Nilsson L, Hansson R, Hamberger L, Janson PO. Collection of human oocytes by the use of sonography. Fertil Steril 1983; 39:603–608.

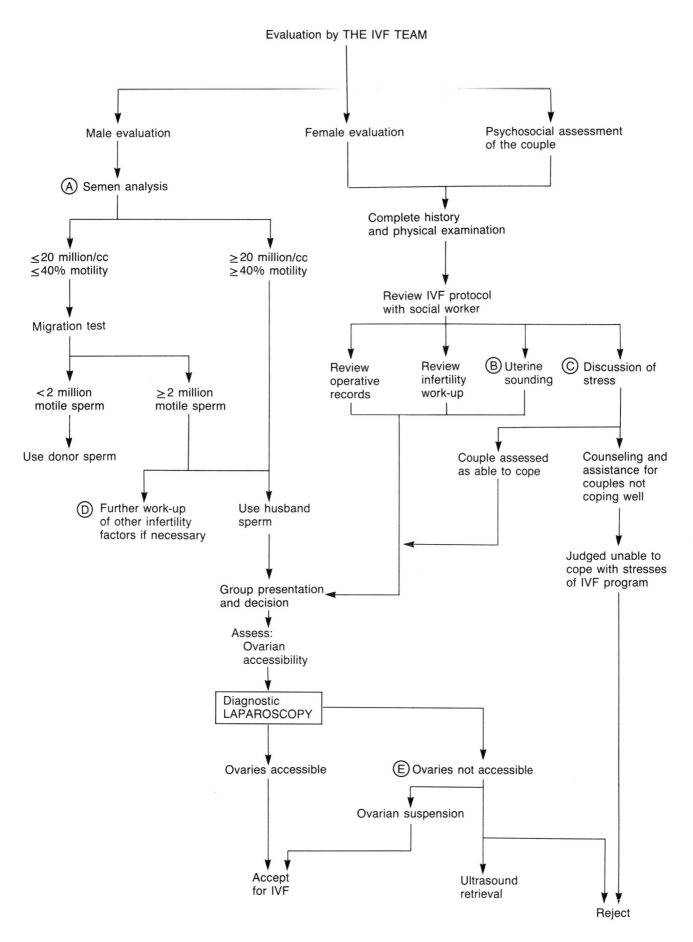

Evaluation by THE IVF TEAM

Male evaluation · Female evaluation · Psychosocial assessment of the couple

Ⓐ Semen analysis

≤20 million/cc
≤40% motility

≥20 million/cc
≥40% motility

Migration test

<2 million
motile sperm

≥2 million
motile sperm

Use donor sperm

Ⓓ Further work-up
of other infertility
factors if necessary

Use husband
sperm

Complete history
and physical examination

Review IVF protocol
with social worker

Review
operative
records

Review
infertility
work-up

Ⓑ Uterine
sounding

Ⓒ Discussion of
stress

Couple assessed
as able to cope

Counseling and
assistance for
couples not
coping well

Judged unable to
cope with stresses
of IVF program

Group presentation
and decision

Assess:
Ovarian
accessibility

Diagnostic
LAPAROSCOPY

Ovaries accessible

Ⓔ Ovaries not accessible

Ovarian suspension

Accept
for IVF

Ultrasound
retrieval

Reject

197

OVULATION INDUCTION PROTOCOLS

Jeffrey B. Russell, M.D.
Mary Lake Polan, M.D., Ph.D.

A. Ovulation induction (OI) is used to stimulate the development of multiple follicles in in vitro fertilization–embryo transfer (IVF-ET) patients and has been shown to increase the incidence of pregnancy. Multiple OI protocols using clomiphene citrate, human menopausal gonadotropins (hMG), luteinizing hormone releasing factor (LRF), pure follicle stimulating hormone (FSH), or a combination of each have been described.

B. The ovulation induction protocol for normal ovulatory women is similar to the protocols in anovulatory women. Once a protocol has been selected, a consistent dose is administered until days 6 to 8 of the cycle. The protocol is adjusted according to the follicular size and the estradiol (E_2) response.

C. Daily ultrasound testing and estradiol levels have been shown to be important parameters in assessing follicular development. Ultrasound and estradiol monitoring are initiated between days 6 to 8 of the cycle. We administer hMG in the evening after the estradiol level and the ultrasound data are available. An excellent correlation between the maturing oocyte and the follicular estradiol measurements has been reported.

D. The criteria for administering human chorionic gonadotropin (hCG) are contingent upon two follicles reaching a diameter of 1.5 cm (2.0 cm for clomiphene citrate) with an estradiol level above 400 pg per milliliter. Patients who were stimulated with FSH have been allowed to "coast" for 50 hours after the last FSH injection prior to hCG administration.

E. Laparoscopy is scheduled 34 to 38 hours after hCG is administered. Preoperative ultrasound evaluation is performed to confirm the number of follicles and to insure that the patient has not ovulated. Although spontaneous luteinizing hormone surges are rare in hMG treated patients, the possibility should always be entertained.

References

Jones GS, Acosta AA, Garcia JE, Bernardus RE, Rosenwaks Z. The effect of follicle stimulating hormone without additional luteinizing hormone on follicular stimulation and oocyte development in normal ovulatory women. Fertil Steril 1985; 43:696–702.

Laufer N, DeCherney AH, Haseltine FP, et al. The use of high dose human menopausal gonadotropins in in vitro fertilization program. Fertil Steril 1983; 40:734–741.

Vargyas JM, Marrs RD, Kletzky OA, Mishell DR Jr. Correlations of ultrasonic measurement of ovarian follicle size and serum estradiol levels in ovulatory patients following clomiphene citrate for in vitro fertilization. Am J Obstet Gynecol 1982; 144:569–573.

OVULATION INDUCTION TO DEVELOP MULTIPLE FOLLICLES

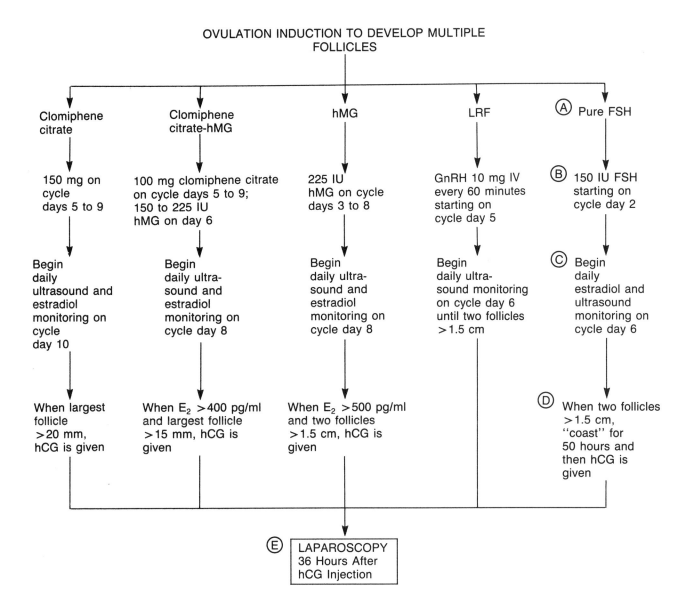

MONITORING OVULATION INDUCTION WITH SERUM ESTRADIOL AND ULTRASONOGRAPHY

Jeffrey B. Russell, M.D.
Mary Lake Polan, M.D., Ph.D.

A. Once the appropriate ovulation induction protocol has been selected for the patient, serial ultrasound monitoring and estradiol (E_2) level monitoring should begin between cycle days 6 to 8. Ultrasonography is performed with a real time sector scanner, and estradiol assays are performed using sensitive radioimmunoassay kits.

B. The ovulation induction protocols should continue until the estradiol level is higher than 400 pg per milliliter and two follicles have a diameter greater than 1.5 cm. Estradiol levels are an index of follicular development and maturation of the oocytes. An excellent correlation is shown with the size of the largest follicle and the time of the spontaneous luteinizing hormone (LH) surge in normal ovulatory cycles.

C. Once the criteria for follicular development have been fulfilled, human chorionic gonadotropin (hCG), 5,000 to 10,000 units, is given. Follicular scans and estradiol determinations are continued daily until laparoscopy.

D. If the estradiol levels decrease by 50 percent or more and the follicles decrease in size and number, or fluid is present in the cul de sac, the cycle is aborted. Ultrasonography is performed in all patients just prior to laparoscopy to make sure that they have not already ovulated and that at least two follicles are still present.

E. If the E_2 level continues to rise or plateaus in the face of continued follicular development, laparoscopy or ultrasound retrieval is performed 36 hours after hCG administration.

References

Buttery B, Trounson A, McMaster R, Wood C. Evaluation of diagnostic ultrasound as a parameter of follicular development in an in vitro fertilization program. Fertil Steril 1983; 39:458–463.

Hackeloer B, Fleming R, Robinson H, Adam A, Coutts J. Correlation of ultrasound and endocrinologic assessment of human follicular development. Am J Obstet Gynecol 1979; 135:122–128.

Vargyas JM, Marrs RP, Kletzky OA, Mishell DR Jr. Correlation of ultrasonic measurement of ovarian follicle size and serum estradiol levels in ovulatory patients following clomiphene citrate for in vitro fertilization. Am J Obstet Gynecol 1982; 144:569–573.

MONITORING OVULATION INDUCTION WITH SERUM ESTRADIOL AND ULTRASONOGRAPHY

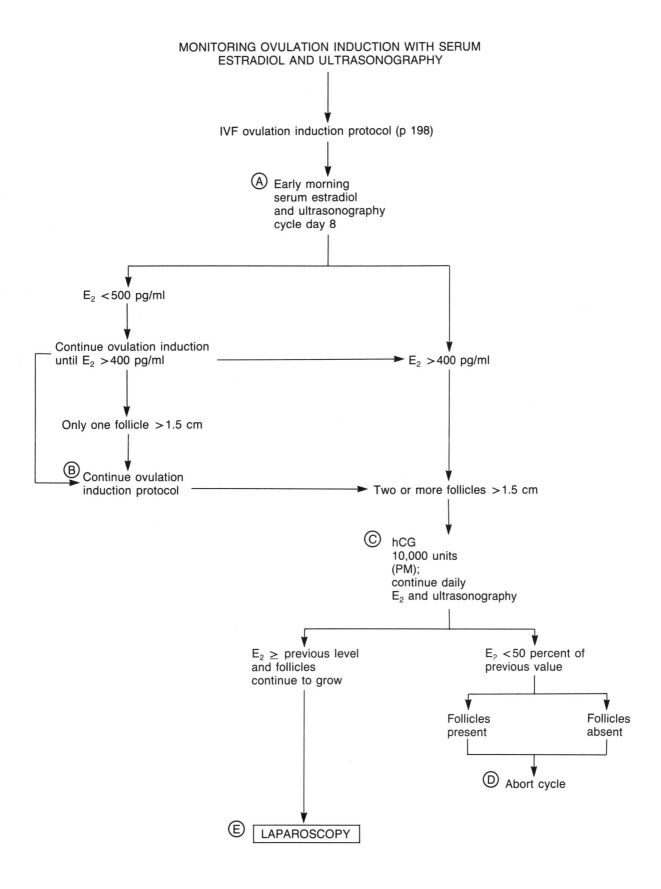

HARVESTING FOLLICLES BY LAPAROSCOPY AND ULTRASONOGRAPHY-DIRECTED ASPIRATION

Jeffrey B. Russell, M.D.
Mary Lake Polan, M.D., Ph.D.

A. Oocyte aspiration is performed 34 to 38 hours after the administration of human chorionic gonadatropin (hCG). Scanning is done prior to surgery to insure that follicular development has continued and that ovulation has not occurred. Endogenous luteinizing hormone (LH) surges may precipitate premature ovulation and luteinization of follicles, decreasing the success of oocyte retrieval. A rapid determination of the urine LH level may be helpful for assessment in the small number of patients with an endogenous elevation.

B. The triple puncture technique is commonly used for visualization and aspiration of follicles. The laparoscope is placed below the umbilicus, and a second puncture is made above the symphysis pubis. The aspiration needle is placed between the two punctures. We use a 14 gauge, 15.2 cm, modified liver biopsy needle to aspirate follicles.

C. Ultrasound aspiration is performed in patients with severe pelvic adhesions or previous laparoscopic failure as a primary procedure. Several European groups in a preliminary study have reported a 60 to 70 percent incidence of oocyte retrieval with ultrasound techniques. Laparoscopic retrieval or ultrasound aspiration has been reported with either local or general anesthesia (Fig. 1).

D. Ultrasound aspiration can be performed transabdominally through the vesicle window, transvaginally, or transurethrally. Follicular proximity of the ovary to the bladder is essential for use of the transvesical approach. The transvaginal approach allows access to ovaries that are adherent or immobilized by adhesions in the cul de sac.

E. Oocytes are aspirated with 100 mm water pressure from standard wall suction. The aspirated fluid within the collection trap follicle is flushed with Ham's F-10 medium. Heparin is added to the medium if the follicular fluid contains a moderate number of red blood cells. The traps in which the oocytes are transported to the laboratory are placed in a temperature controlled environment as quickly as possible.

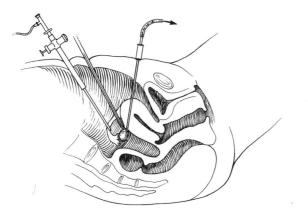

Figure 1 Laparoscopic retrieval of ovum. The ovary is stabilized by grasping forceps and the follicles are penetrated by the needle.

References

Renou P, Trounson AO, Wood C, Leeton JF. The collection of human oocytes for in vitro fertilization. I. An instrument for maximizing oocyte recovery rate. Fertil Steril 1981; 35:409–412.

Steptoe PC, Edwards RG. Laparoscopic recovery of preovulatory human oocytes after priming of ovaries with gonadotropins. Lancet 1970; 1:683–689.

Wikland M, Nilsson L, Hansson R, Hamberger L, Janson PO. Collection of human oocytes by the use of sonography. Fertil Stertil 1983; 39:603–608.

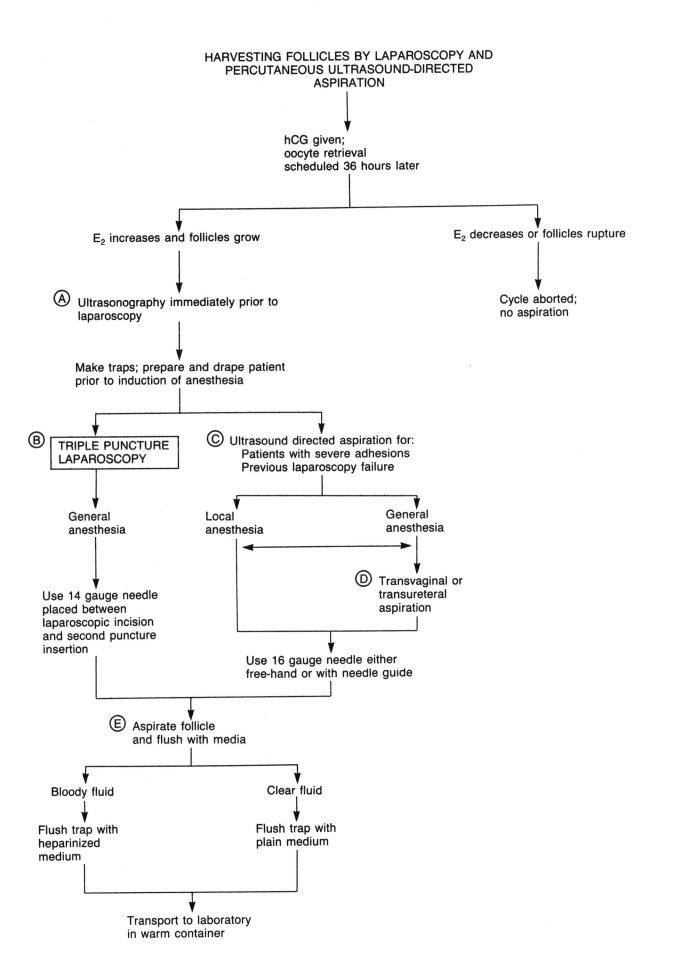

HARVESTING FOLLICLES BY LAPAROSCOPY AND
PERCUTANEOUS ULTRASOUND-DIRECTED
ASPIRATION

hCG given;
oocyte retrieval
scheduled 36 hours later

E₂ increases and follicles grow

E₂ decreases or follicles rupture

Ⓐ Ultrasonography immediately prior to
laparoscopy

Cycle aborted;
no aspiration

Make traps; prepare and drape patient
prior to induction of anesthesia

Ⓑ TRIPLE PUNCTURE
LAPAROSCOPY

Ⓒ Ultrasound directed aspiration for:
Patients with severe adhesions
Previous laparoscopy failure

General
anesthesia

Local
anesthesia

General
anesthesia

Ⓓ Transvaginal or
transureteral
aspiration

Use 14 gauge needle
placed between
laparoscopic incision
and second puncture
insertion

Use 16 gauge needle either
free-hand or with needle guide

Ⓔ Aspirate follicle
and flush with media

Bloody fluid

Clear fluid

Flush trap with
heparinized
medium

Flush trap with
plain medium

Transport to laboratory
in warm container

FERTILIZATION

Jeffrey B. Russell, M.D.
Mary Lake Polan, M.D., Ph.D.

A. Modified Delee suction traps with the aspirated follicular contents are transported to the laboratory in a temperature controlled container. The follicular fluid with Ham's F-10 medium added is divided into 7.5 ml Petri dishes on a 37° C heating plate. The dishes are quickly scanned for oocyte-corona-cumulus complexes (OCCC) over a light box to detect a clear area containing a "white dot," which may be grossly identified as an oocyte.

B. The clear area is quickly scanned for the oocyte. The OCCC is aspirated with a pipet and placed in insemination medium consisting of Ham's F-10 medium with 10 percent patient serum. The OCCC is graded according to the maturity of the oocyte and the corona and cumulus dispersion.

C. Oocytes graded as intermediate and mature are inseminated 6 to 8 hours after laparoscopic retrieval. Immature oocytes are incubated for 24 hours prior to insemination. Reports have shown an increase in the fertilization incidence when immature oocytes are incubated and allowed to mature in vitro. Sperm is collected by masturbation and prepared using a double wash and swim-up technique. Approximately 500,000 sperm are placed with each oocyte in the Petri dish.

D. Fertilization is confirmed about 18 hours after insemination by the presence of two pronuclei. If two pronuclei are not visualized, the embryo may have progressed through syngamy, or fertilization may not have occurred. The embryo is checked for viability at 24 hours. All oocytes and embryos are re-evaluated prior to transfer for the presence of pronuclei or the stage of development and number of blastomeres.

References

Laufer N, DeCherney AH, Haseltine FP, et al. The use of high dose human menopausal gonadotropin in an in vitro fertilization program. Fertil Steril 1983; 40:734–741.

Quigley MM, Schmidt CL, Beauchamp PJ, et al. Enhanced follicular recruitment in an in vitro fertilization program: clomiphene alone versus a clomiphene/human menopausal gonadotropin combination. Fertil Steril 1984; 42:25–33.

Trounson AO, Mohr LR, Wood C, Leeton JF. Effect of developed insemination on in vitro fertilization, culture and transfer of human embryos. J Reprod Fertil 1982; 64:285–294.

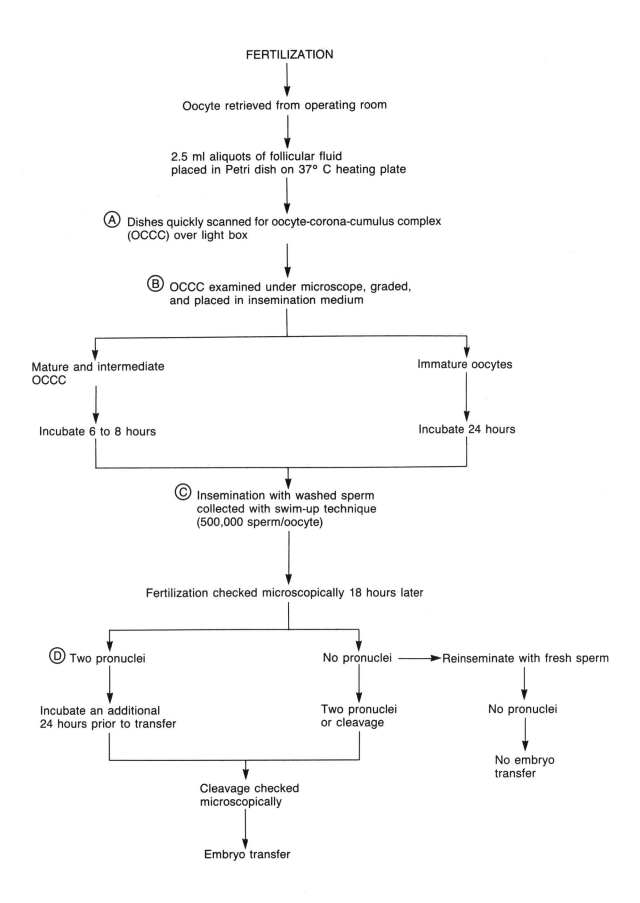

FERTILIZATION

Oocyte retrieved from operating room

2.5 ml aliquots of follicular fluid
placed in Petri dish on 37° C heating plate

(A) Dishes quickly scanned for oocyte-corona-cumulus complex
(OCCC) over light box

(B) OCCC examined under microscope, graded,
and placed in insemination medium

Mature and intermediate
OCCC

Immature oocytes

Incubate 6 to 8 hours

Incubate 24 hours

(C) Insemination with washed sperm
collected with swim-up technique
(500,000 sperm/oocyte)

Fertilization checked microscopically 18 hours later

(D) Two pronuclei

No pronuclei ⟶ Reinseminate with fresh sperm

Incubate an additional
24 hours prior to transfer

Two pronuclei
or cleavage

No pronuclei

No embryo
transfer

Cleavage checked
microscopically

Embryo transfer

EMBRYO TRANSFER

Jeffrey B. Russell, M.D.
Mary Lake Polan, M.D., Ph.D.

A. Embryo transfer is usually performed 48 hours after laparoscopy. The embryos are examined for fertilization, cleavage, or degeneration prior to transfer. All fertilized oocytes are moved to a transfer medium composed of Ham's F-10 medium with 90 percent patient serum. The Petri dish is placed on a 37° C heating plate under a hood and gassed with a nitrogen, oxygen, carbon dioxide mixture until the transfer is performed.

B. The patient is placed in the knee-chest position if the uterus is anteverted or the lithotomy position if it is retroverted. We employ a side opening catheter with a Teflon tip (Norfolk) design. The catheter is irrigated with transfer medium followed in sequence with 5 μl of medium, 10 μl of air, 10 μl of medium containing the embryos, 10 μl of air, and 5 μl of medium (Fig. 1A). A total of 20 μl of medium is used for the transfer.

C. The catheter is premeasured and marked according to the depth of the uterus measured during uterine sounding at the initial examination. The Teflon tip is advanced through the metal introducer, and both are placed just inside the external cervical os (Fig. 1B). The catheter is then advanced to the fundus. The embryos are slowly injected with the microliter syringe.

D. The catheter is kept in place for 60 seconds and withdrawn gently. It is grossly examined under a spotlight and quickly moved to the microscope to insure that all embryos have been expelled into the uterus. The transfer medium is aspirated and the catheter is flushed. Embryos that have not been successfully transferred are reloaded in a sterile catheter and the procedure is repeated.

E. The patient remains prone for at least 3 hours. Symptoms such as slight cramping or spotting are rare but may occur. We sometimes administer progesterone supplementation (50 mg intramuscularly daily). We request a 24-hour resting period, although the variety in posttransfer instructions for patients reflects the lack of knowledge concerning implantation.

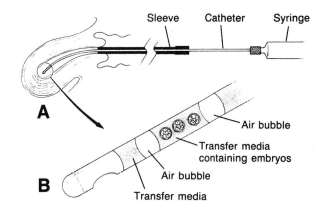

Figure 1 *A*, Tip of the catheter containing embryos suspended in medium between cushions of air and medium. *B*, The Teflon tip is advanced through the metal inducer and both are placed just inside the cervical os. The catheter is then advanced to the fundus and the embryos are slowly injected using the microliter syringe.

References

Jones HW, Acosta AA, Garcia JE, Sandow BA, Veeck L. On the transfer of conceptuses from oocytes fertilized in vitro. Fertil Steril 1982; 39:241–243.

Laufer N, DeCherney AH, Haseltine FP, et al. The use of high dose human menopausal gonadotropin in an in vitro fertilization program. Fertil Steril 1983; 40:734–741.

Leeton J, Trounson A, Jessup D, Wood C. The technique for human embryo transfer. Fertil Steril 1982; 38:156–161.

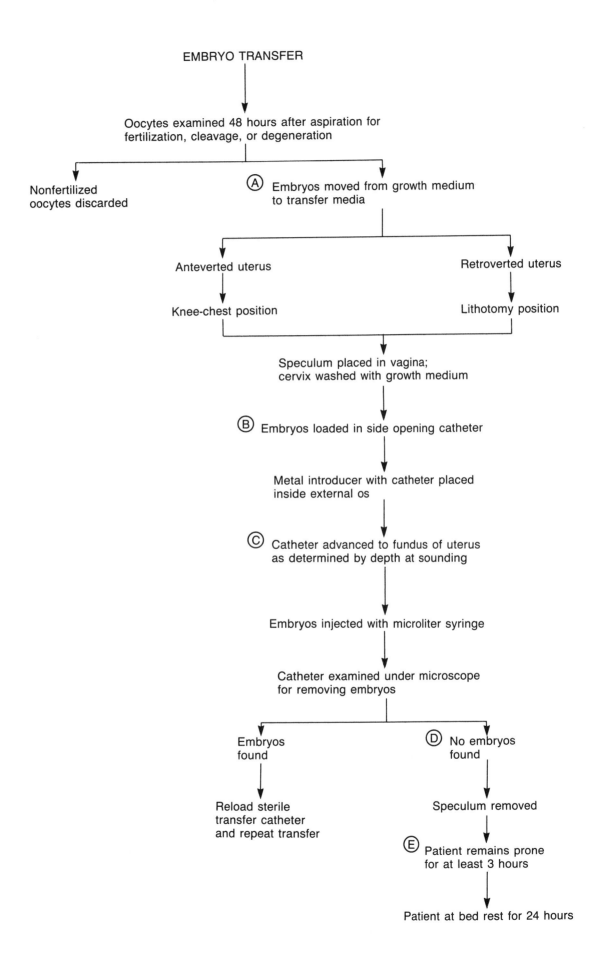

EMBRYO TRANSFER

Oocytes examined 48 hours after aspiration for
fertilization, cleavage, or degeneration

Nonfertilized
oocytes discarded

Ⓐ Embryos moved from growth medium
to transfer media

Anteverted uterus

Knee-chest position

Retroverted uterus

Lithotomy position

Speculum placed in vagina;
cervix washed with growth medium

Ⓑ Embryos loaded in side opening catheter

Metal introducer with catheter placed
inside external os

Ⓒ Catheter advanced to fundus of uterus
as determined by depth at sounding

Embryos injected with microliter syringe

Catheter examined under microscope
for removing embryos

Embryos
found

Reload sterile
transfer catheter
and repeat transfer

Ⓓ No embryos
found

Speculum removed

Ⓔ Patient remains prone
for at least 3 hours

Patient at bed rest for 24 hours

LUTEAL MONITORING AND DOCUMENTATION OF SUCCESSFUL PREGNANCY

Jeffrey B. Russell, M.D.
Mary Lake Polan, M.D., Ph.D.

A. Controversy exists over the use of progesterone supplementation during the luteal phase of an in vitro fertilization (IVF) cycle. Since ovulation inducing drugs are routinely used, the question of luteal phase inadequacy or dysynchrony with high levels of estradiol (E_2) is unanswered. One study revealed an advanced endometrium in stimulated IVF cycles at the time of the embryo transfer. Opinion regarding progesterone supplementation is divided, reflecting our lack of knowledge about the luteal phase and implantation.

B. Estradiol and human chorionic gonadotropin (hCG) levels rise at about the time of embryo transfer and then gradually decline. The estradiol pattern is similar to the normal physiologic curve. The hCG level rises after the initial injection and then slowly decreases over the next 10 days. Early trophoblastic activity of the embryo is detectable about 12 days after embryo transfer. This is followed by a gradual rise in the estradiol level.

C. Once the hCG titer rises and bleeding has not occurred, ultrasonography should be performed to visualize the fetal sac. Usually a fetal sac can be visualized at an hCG titer of 6,000 to 6,500 mIU per milliliter. If a fetal sac is initially not seen, the ultrasound examination is repeated 1 week later and correlated with the rise in hCG titer. The incidence of ectopic pregnancies has been as high as 10 percent in some series, and precautions should be taken when the hCG level is greater than 6,000 and an intrauterine sac is not visualized.

D. When an intrauterine sac is identified, a repeat ultrasound examination should be performed at about 8 to 9 weeks. A fetal heartbeat usually can be visualized on ultrasound examination when the hCG titer is greater than 50,000.

E. Near the end of the first trimester, when a fetal heartbeat has been confirmed, the patient should be treated as any other obstetric patient, although the incidence of cesarean section is high in successful IVF patients. Special care is not required unless other obstetric reasons require intervention.

References

Garcia JE, Acosta AA, Jones HW Jr. Advanced endometrial maturation after ovulation induction with hMG/hCG for in vitro fertilization. Fertil Steril 1983; 39:426(abstract).

Jones HW, Acosta AA, Andrews MC, et al. Three years of in vitro fertilization at Norfolk. Fertil Steril 1984; 42:826–834.

Steptoe PC, Edwards RG. Reimplantation of a human embryo with subsequent tubal pregnancy. Lancet 1976; 1:880–882.

LUTEAL MONITORING AND DOCUMENTATION
OF SUCCESSFUL PREGNANCY

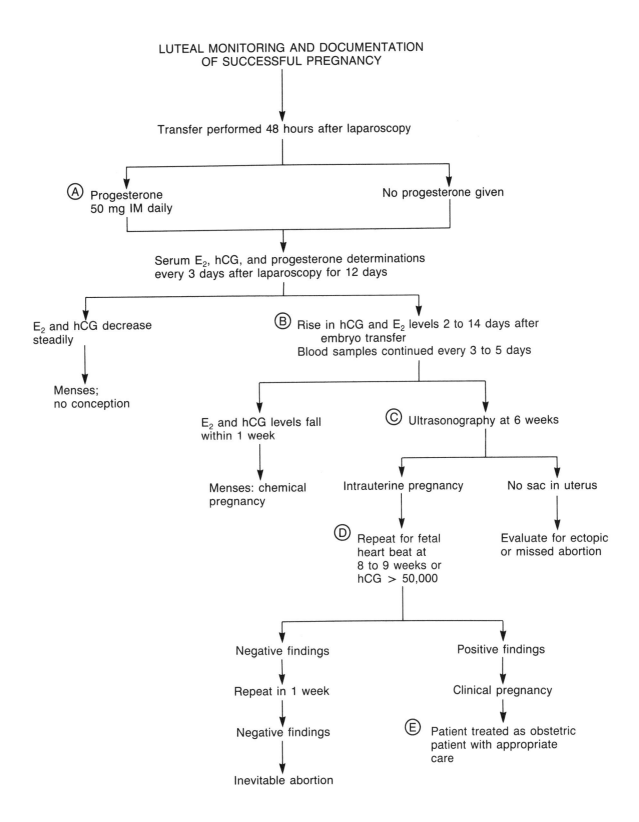

Transfer performed 48 hours after laparoscopy

(A) Progesterone 50 mg IM daily

No progesterone given

Serum E_2, hCG, and progesterone determinations every 3 days after laparoscopy for 12 days

E_2 and hCG decrease steadily

Menses; no conception

(B) Rise in hCG and E_2 levels 2 to 14 days after embryo transfer
Blood samples continued every 3 to 5 days

E_2 and hCG levels fall within 1 week

Menses: chemical pregnancy

(C) Ultrasonography at 6 weeks

Intrauterine pregnancy

No sac in uterus

(D) Repeat for fetal heart beat at 8 to 9 weeks or hCG > 50,000

Evaluate for ectopic or missed abortion

Negative findings

Repeat in 1 week

Negative findings

Inevitable abortion

Positive findings

Clinical pregnancy

(E) Patient treated as obstetric patient with appropriate care